Gender Differences in Metabolism

Practical and Nutritional Implications

MODERN NUTRITION

Edited by Ira Wolinsky and James F. Hickson, Jr.

Published Titles

Edited by Ira Wolinsky

Published Titles

Forthcoming Titles

Gender Differences in Metabolism

Practical and Nutritional Implications

edited by

Mark Tarnopolsky

CRC Press

Boca Raton   London   New York   Washington, D.C.

Library of Congress Cataloging-in-Publication Data

Catalog record is available from the Library of Congress.

Acknowledgments

I would like to thank my wife, Jackie and my children, Stephanie and Alanna, for their support and patience when I had none. This project could not have been completed without Joan Martin. Also, thanks to Scott and Daffodil.

Series Preface for Nutrition in Exercise and Sport

The CRC Series on Nutrition in Exercise and Sport, provides a setting for in-depth exploration of the many and varied aspects of nutrition and exercise, including sports. The topic of exercise and sports nutrition has been a focus of research among scientists since the 1960s, and the healthful benefits of good nutrition and exercise have been appreciated. As our knowledge expands, it will be necessary to remember that there must be a range of diets and exercise regimes that will support excellent physical condition and performance. There is not a single diet-exercise treatment that can be the common denominator, or the single formula for health, or panacea for performance.

This Series is dedicated to providing a stage upon which to explore these issues. Each volume provides a detailed and scholarly examination of some aspect of the topic, and, as such, will be of interest to professionals as well as educated laymen.

Contributors from any bona fide area of nutrition and physical activity, including sports and the controversial, are welcome.

We welcome to the Series a timely and authoritative monograph on *Gender Differences in Metabolism: Practical and Nutritional Implications* by the very knowledgeable Mark Tarnopolsky.

Ira Wolinsky, Ph.D.
University of Houston
Series Editor

Preface

In the mid-1980s I was reading some physiology literature and was taken by the fact that the majority of the participants were predominantly or exclusively males. I began to review some of the literature exploring potential gender differences in metabolism, for at the time my undergraduate physiology teaching had stressed that essentially there were no gender specific metabolic or muscle structural differences between males and females. In fact, the conclusion of several text books at the time was that there were no gender differences and no further consideration of a potential difference was discussed.

The first thing that was apparent, was the paucity of studies specifically designed to investigate gender differences in a metabolic response to exercise. It was clear that some studies with appropriate outcome measures had low subject numbers, and a few with higher subject numbers had outcome variables that were either non-specific or highly variable.

Perhaps some of the reason for the paucity of gender difference studies relates to the difficulty in matching the genders for training status. This issue will be discussed further in Chapter 1. In addition, to training status, the known menstrual cycle and hormonal differences between males and females poses further difficulties in research designs, and aspects of hormonal differences will be discussed by myself and Dr. Ron Cortright in Chapter 2. Following discussion of potential differences in the structure of skeletal muscle, the overall neuromuscular function will be discussed by Drs. Chorneyko and Bourgeois and Sale, respectively. This organization was purposeful in that structure per se may partially dictate function. The sympathetic nervous system operates through neurotransmitters and hormones and may, in part, influence metabolism, and interesting potential gender differences in sympathetic nerve activity are next discussed by Dr. Steve Ettinger.

Interesting potential gender differences in macronutrient utilization during exercise are discussed by Drs. Ruby, Phillips and myself in the ensuing three chapters. Overall, it appears that in response to sub-maximal endurance exercise females oxidize greater lipid, less carbohydrate and protein as compared to their male counterparts.

The ensuing two chapters deal with overall metabolic energy balance in growth in both animal (Dr. Cortright) and human (Dr. Westerterp) studies. I felt it important to include a section specifically on animal models, as certain controls and manipulations are possible to further explore mechanism(s). The contribution of animal research to potential gender differences in metabolism has been large, particularly from studies examining a role for estrogen per se to mediate many of the metabolic differences that are seen. Furthermore, influences of exercise and dietary intake on growth and maturation are more easily studied in this model. There is an overall impression that the female animal is more resistant to energy deprivation. Interesting anthropological speculation may indicate that this is a reflection of selective pressure in evolution. For example, it is of phylogenetic advantage for a female animal that can conserve energy through periods of starvation and still be fertile and reproduce such that their progeny eventually survives and perpetuates the species.

Another interesting potential gender difference is that of oxidative stress which is linked intimately with muscle damage. Animal models have been particularly helpful in showing evidence that oxidative stress (free radical generation) and muscle damage may be lesser for female animals vs. males. This data is somewhat more controversial in humans, and discussed extensively by Drs. Tiidus and Clarkson.

Throughout most of this book an attempt has been made to relate the basic science research to applied physiology, and where possible to make some practical suggestions. Along this lines, the final chapter examines the potential for an ergogenic aid (caffeine) to influence metabolism differentially in males and females. The reader should find this topic comprehensively covered by Dr. Graham and Ms. McLean.

The overall hope of the editor is that this book provides "food for thought" for researchers to consider potential gender differences in metabolism when designing research studies, and when implementing health care policy, and formulating nutritional and exercise guidelines. I think at this point there are far more questions than answers, and it is hoped that this book becomes a catalyst for well-controlled further research studies.

The Editor

Mark Tarnopolsky, MD, PhD, FRCP(C), Assistant Professor
Departments of Medicine (Neurology/Neurological Rehabilitation) and Kinesiology
McMaster University Medical Center
Hamilton, Ontario, Canada.

My clinical practice is dedicated entirely to patients with neuromuscular disease. Along this line, my research is focused around understanding of skeletal muscle metabolism. More specifically, I am interested in the metabolic differences between males and females at rest and during exercise, and in the study of protein metabolism and the effects of pharmacological, nutritional and exercise interventions in the promotion of protein synthesis. I am also involved in teaching of graduate students, medical students, and medical residents/fellows.

My wife, Jackie (Pediatric Pathologist), and I live near the hospital in Hamilton. I have two children, Stephanie (14) and Alanna (11), who form the main focus of my non-academic endeavours.

Contributors

Ronald N. Cortright, PhD
School of Medicine
Department of Biochemistry
Brody Medical Sciences Building
600 Moye Blvd.
Greenville, North Carolina 27858-4354
USA

Katherine Chorneyko, MD, FRCP(C)
Director, Electron Microscopy
Hamilton Health Sciences Corporation
McMaster University Medical Centre
1200 Main St. W.
Hamilton, ON
L8N 3Z5
CANADA

Jacqueline Bourgeois, MD, FRCP(C)
Department of Pathology
Hamilton Health Sciences Corporation
McMaster University Medical Centre
1200 Main St. W.
Hamilton, ON
L8N 3Z5
CANADA

Digby Sale, PhD
Department of Kinesiology
McMaster University
IWC-AB118
Hamilton, ON
L8S 4K1
CANADA

Steve Ettinger, MD, FACP
PennState Geisinger Health System
Department of Medicine, Section of
    Cardiology
The Milton S. Hershey Medical Centre
M.C. H047
PO Box 850
500 University Drive
Hershey, PA 17111
USA

Brent Ruby, PhD
The University of Montana
Director, Human Performance
    Laboratory
Department of Health and Human
    Performance
McGill Hall #121
Missoula, MT 59813
USA

Stuart M. Phillips
Dept. of Kinesiology — IWC
McMaster University
1280 Main St. West
Hamilton, ON
L8S 4K1
Ph: (905) 525-9140 x23574
Fax: (905) 523-6011
E-mail: phillis@mcmaster.ca

Klaas R. Westerterp, PhD
Department of Human Biology
Maastricht University
PO Box 616
6200 MD Maastricht
THE NETHERLANDS

Peter M. Tiidus, PhD
Associate Professor & Chair
Department of Kinesiology & Physical
    Education
2nd Floor
226-232 King St. N.
Waterloo, ON
N2L 3C5
CANADA

Priscilla M. Clarkson, PhD
University of Massachusetts
Department of Exercise Science
Totman Bldg.
Amherst, MA 01003
USA

Stephen P. Sayers, MSc
University of Massachusetts
Department of Exercise Science
Totman Bldg.
Amherst, MA 01003
USA

Terry E. Graham, PhD
University of Guelph
Department of Human Biology and
   Nutrition Science
Guelph, ON
N1G 2W1
CANADA

Cyndy McLean, MSc
University of Guelph
Department of Human Biology and
Nutrition Science
Guelph, ON
N1G 2W1
CANADA

Contents

CHAPTER 1

Introduction

Mark Tarnopolsky, M.D., Ph.D., F.R.C.P.(C)

CONTENTS

I. INTRODUCTION

Most of the research in the area of muscle metabolism, nutrition, and exercise physiology has been conducted using male participants. The resultant conclusions and recommendations, therefore, have an inherent gender bias. Even if one ignores the inequality of such an approach, the applicability of some conclusions to females lacks scientific validation. For example, it has been shown that the provision of a high carbohydrate (CHO) diet (~75% of energy from CHO or ~8g of CHO/kg) and a tapering of exercise training for four to five days prior to a sporting event (carbohydrate loading), resulted in an improvement in endurance exercise performance.[1] Close examination of the carbohydrate loading studies demonstrated that the study participants were predominantly or exclusively males.[1,2,3,4] Our group[5] showed that

Table 1.1 Body Composition from Four Studies in the Same Laboratory

		Weight (kg)	Height (cm)	Lean Mass (kg)	Body Fat %
Tarnopolsky, L. et al., 1991	6 ♂	70(2)	175(2)	57(2)	15(1)
	6 ♀	58(2)	168(2)	46(2)	22(1)
Phillips, S.M. et al., 1993	6 ♂	64(5)	173(5)	57(5)	11(2)
	6 ♀	58(5)	168(5)	47(2)	19(1)
Tarnopolsky, M.A. et al., 1995	7 ♂	75(3)	179(4)	64(4)	14(2)
	8 ♀	58(8)	166(5)	47(5)	18(4)
Tarnopolsky, M.A. et al., 1997	8 ♂	73(5)	N/A	65(5)	11(3)
	8 ♀	61(9)		47(4)	22(6)
Total Mean (±S.D.)	28 ♂	71(4)	176(3)	61(4)	13(1)
	27 ♀	59(1)	167(1)	47(0)	20(2)

Note: All between-group comparisons were significantly different ($p \leq 0.05$).

males increased muscle glycogen by ~45% with a corresponding increase in endurance performance time, whereas females did not increase muscle glycogen nor time to exhaustion in response to a CHO-loading protocol (four-day increase in CHO to 75% of energy intake). This result will be discussed in more detail in Chapter 6, but it serves to illustrate that conclusions based solely upon results obtained in males may not be directly applicable to females.

My interest in the area of gender differences in metabolism arose from observations of the paucity of gender-specific research. I also had a curiosity as to why females are generally smaller than males and have greater amounts of adipose tissue (Table 1.1), and whether this influenced, or was a consequence of, gender differences in metabolism.

I became intrigued with the possibility that these phenotypic differences may have some basis in evolutionary selective pressures conferring a phylogenetic advantage upon each of the respective genders and what role this may have in exercise metabolism. Hoyenga and Hoyenga[6] presented a theoretical review that provided support for the hypothesis that the propensity of females to have a higher body fat was linked to a sexual dimorphism arising from evolutionary pressures for energy conservation in times of starvation. Put another way, a female who, perhaps out of a random genetic polymorphism, is able to withstand a period of starvation and still remain fertile, would be most likely to have these genetic traits passed on to subsequent generations. Although of adaptive benefit during starvation, metabolic energy conservation during times of food abundance would lead to a propensity towards obesity. An enhanced energy conservation in females may, in part, explain the observation of reduced energy intake in female athletes that we (Table 1.2) and others[7,8] have demonstrated. This area remains controversial[9] and will be discussed in more detail in Chapters 9 and 10.

Over thousands of years, energy conservation and body fat distribution traits may become sex linked (i.e., sex chromosome) or sex-limited (i.e., sex hormones).[6] It is interesting to note that among Emperor penguins, where the males are the sole egg incubators (and fast for up to 120 days), the males have the higher percent body fat.[10] I shall leave the debate about societal roles, childbearing, and gender roles

Table 1.2   Habitual Energy and Macronutrient Intake from Four Studies in the Same
Laboratory

		Energy (kcal/d)	Energy (kcal/kgLBM)	%FAT	%PRO	%CHO
Tarnopolsky, L. et al., 1991	6 ♂	3475(214)	61	30	15	55
	6 ♀	2308(178)	50	30	15	55
Phillips, S.M. et al., 1993	6 ♂	3233(216)	57	31	15	53
	6 ♀	1809(133)	38	32	13	56
Tarnopolsky, M.A. et al., 1995	7 ♂	3372(323)	53	24	15	59
	8 ♀	1866(318)	40	27	12	59
Tarnopolsky, M.A. et al., 1997	8 ♂	3218(328)	50	31	17	52
	8 ♀	2059(363)	44	26	14	60
Total Mean (±S.D.)	28 ♂	3325(106)	55(4)	29(3)	16(1)	55(3)
	27 ♀	2010(195)	43(5)	29(2)	14(1)	58(2)

during evolution to these experts (i.e., anthropologists, sociologists, etc.). If these hypotheses hold some truth, then there may be a sexual dimorphism in the response of the genders to other physiological stimuli such as exercise.

Only in recent exercise physiology textbooks has there been even a comment about the potential for gender differences in the metabolic response to exercise.[11] I became interested in this area in the late 1980s for some of the reasons mentioned previously and started into a series of investigations designed to look for potential gender differences in the metabolic response to the quantitative physiological stress of exercise.[5,12,13,14] All of our studies were conducted after careful matching of the genders, rigorous dietary controls, and control for phase of menstrual cycle. All were performed at an exercise intensity of between 65 and 75% VO_{2max}. A summary of four of our studies demonstrated a significantly higher fat and a lower protein and carbohydrate oxidation during sub-maximal endurance exercise for females as compared to males (Table 1.3). Similar findings are evident in a brief summary of respiratory exchange ratio (RER) data from some of the better-known studies in this area (Table 1.4).

The main reason for this book is to provide a catalyst for future research in this interesting area and to encourage researchers to consider that there are sex differences in metabolism that need to be controlled for in research designs. It is important to note that there are some individuals who feel that any talk of comparison between the genders bears a negative connotation. It is my contention that quite the opposite is true, namely, ignorance of potential gender differences in metabolism breeds prejudice, exclusion, and a perpetuation of the gender bias in the literature. One of the goals of this book was to present the scientific data for and against gender differences in metabolism in an unbiased manner. It is also important to note that there was some debate as to the terminology of "sex" vs. "gender." According to Webster's Dictionary, "sex" is listed as the first definition under "gender" and under "sex" one finds the definition, "either of two divisions of organisms distinguished respectively as male or female."[15] After extensive review of the scientific literature there appears to be no general semantic consensus; therefore, I have allowed the chapter authors their choice of terminology. Given a slight preponderance of the

Table 1.3 Energy and Substrate Utilization from Four Studies in the Same Laboratory

		kcal/hr	kcal/kg/hr	kcal/kgLBM/hr	FAT(%)	PRO(%)	CHO(%)
Tarnopolsky, L. et al., 1991	6 ♂	797	11.9	14	10	9	81
	6 ♀	620	10.1	13.5	41	0	61
Phillips, S.M. et al., 1993	6 ♂	729	11.4	12.7	49	3	47
	6 ♀	590	10.2	12.5	61	2	35
Tarnopolsky, M.A. et al., 1995	7 ♂	1019	13.6	15.9	8	6	83
	8 ♀	666	11.6	14.2	24	1	72
Tarnopolsky, M.A. et al., 1997	8 ♂	806	11.1	12.5	23	2	75
	8 ♀	616	10.1	13.0	29	3	68
Total Mean (±S.D.)	28 ♂	838(126)**	12(1)*	13.7(1.6) +	22(19)**	5(3)**	72(17)**
	27 ♀	623(32)	10.5(0.7)	13.3(0.7)	39(16)	2(1)	59(17)

Note: **, $p \leq 0.001$; *, $p \leq 0.05$; +, NS.

Table 1.4 Respiratory Exchange Ratios from Several Gender Comparative Studies

Study	Subjects	Exercise	RER Males	RER Females
Phillips, S.M. et al., 1993	6 ♂ 6 ♀	90 min. treadmill run @ 65% VO_2 peak	0.86	0.83 p ≤0.001
Tarnopolsky, L. et al., 1991	6 ♂ 6 ♀	97 min. ♀ & 93 min ♂ treadmill run @ 63% VO_2 peak	0.94	0.87 p ≤0.0001
Tarnopolsky, M.A. et al., 1995	7 ♂ 8 ♀	90 min. cycle ergometry @ 65% VO_2 peak	0.92	0.89 p ≤0.05
Tarnopolsky, M.A. et al., 1997	8 ♂ 8 ♀	60 min. cycle ergometry @ 72% VO_2 peak	0.99	0.93 p ≤0.001
Blatchford, F.K. et al., 1985	6 ♂ 6 ♀	90 min. treadmill walk @ 35% VO_2 max.	0.85	0.81 p ≤0.05
Froberg, K. et al., 1984	6 ♂ 6 ♀	53.8 min. ♀ & 36.8 min. ♂ cycle ergometry @ 80% VO_2 max.	0.97	0.93 p ≤0.01
Costill, D. et al., 1979	13 ♂ 12 ♀	60 min. treadmill run @ 70% VO_2 max.	0.84	0.83 NS

Note: ♀ = females; ♂ = males; NS = non-significant.

term "gender" in the literature, I have chosen this term to be part of the title (although, a social science colleague of mine has told me that the term "sex" is technically more correct).

This book is meant to provide a review of the literature in the area of gender/sex differences in the metabolic response(s) to exercise. Another goal is to provide the reader with some ideas for future research directions and also some idea of the tools available for investigating each topic. The reader will be aware that there are significant differences in the length of the chapters, which is a result of large differences in the available literature on the topic. For example, in the area of carbohydrate metabolism (Chapter 6), much of the focus is on a comparison of the potential for gender differences. Much less work is available in the area of gender differences in sympathetic nerve activity (Chapter 5); thus, more of the chapter is dedicated to educating the reader about techniques for further investigating this interesting area. The book is roughly organized into the following sections: general issues in gender-based research; hormonal differences; muscle structure, function, and sympathetic ennervation; substrate metabolism; energy metabolism; muscle damage; potential for gender differences in the ergogenic response to caffeine; conclusions and future directions. The book follows a logical progression of structure to functional applicability.

By design, I have focused upon the aforementioned topics as there has been very little work and attention given to these issues. I have specifically chosen not to include the issues of the Female Athlete Triad (Disordered Eating, Amenorrhea, and Osteoporosis), because there is a significant body of literature already in existence in this area. This is not meant in any way to downplay the extreme importance of these issues. The reader is referred to articles in this area.[16,17]

II. STUDY DESIGN ISSUES

A. Matching the Genders for Comparative Studies

One of the most important and most difficult issues to deal with in comparing the metabolic response of males and females is that of equality of comparison between the groups. It is inherently obvious why most researchers try to control for age, weight, height, and exercise training status in between-group comparative research studies. It is therefore surprising that fewer studies have taken care to control for gender. As outlined in this section, one reason may be the lack of consensus as to the optimal criteria for such comparisons. For the most part, this section will deal with the issues surrounding gender comparative studies of exercise metabolism.

Habitual exercise training results in significant physiological adaptations in humans. These adaptations to the training stimulus can be even larger than potential gender differences in metabolism. For example, the increase in intra-muscular triglycerides as a result of endurance training[18] is greater than the difference between the genders (Chapter 8). Thus, gender-based muscle metabolic studies need to address the issue of cross-sectional between-group comparative training status. For endurance sports, one commonly accepted indicator of aerobic power is the maximal oxygen uptake (VO_{2max}), while for strength and resistance sports it is the one repetition maximum (1RM) or number of repetitions at a percentage of the 1RM (%1RM).

As seen in Table 1.1, a summary of four gender difference studies in our laboratory, showed that comparably trained females have lower body and lean mass weights and a higher percent body fat (%BF) as compared to males. Thus, comparison between genders based upon absolute VO_{2max} would lead to the selection of females who were heavier than the males. Even when expressed relative to body weight (relative VO_{2max}), comparably trained females will have a lower VO_{2max} as compared to males, or the females may be excessively lean. For example, in a gender comparison study reported in 1979, the males and females were matched based upon training history (running from 80 to 115 km/wk) and VO_{2max} (mL/kg/min).[19] It is unlikely, and not stated in the paper, whether the females were eumenorrheic, and it is clear from this paper that the males were significantly older than the females (35 vs. 23 years old, respectively).[19]

Sparling has promoted a gender-matching scheme based upon careful assessment of habitual activity in the year antecedent to the testing.[20] Cureton presented convincing arguments for comparing the genders based upon training history for trained individuals, and as VO_{2max} expressed relative to lean mass in untrained individuals.[21]

It is my feeling that the only way to compare between genders in human studies is to match the groups based upon assessment of both training history and aerobic capacity expressed relative to lean mass (mL/O_2/kg LBM). Furthermore, in studies using exclusively trained athletes, it is important to test at intensities of 75% of VO_{2max} or below for potential differences in lactate threshold (LT) not to alter the results. Using this selection criteria, we find that the LT is about 80% for well-trained males and females (males = 79.4 ± 1.4%; females 80.1 ± 2.7%).[13]

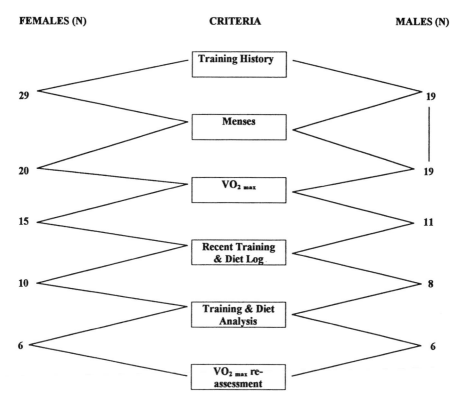

FEMALES (N)   **CRITERIA**   **MALES (N)**

Figure 1.1 Selection criteria used in a gender comparative study. (From Tarnopolsky, L. J., MacDougall, J. D., Atkinson, S. A., Tarnopolsky, M. A., and Sutton, J. R., *J. Appl. Physiol.*, 68, 302, 1990.)

Our matching approach takes into account both the genetic (genetically determined "window of VO_2 potential") and environmental (state of training) factors contributing to VO_{2max}, and expresses them relative to the mass of metabolically active tissues. There are several reasons why some studies have not gone to the aforementioned rigor in gender comparison studies; however, I feel that the labor intensity required is a major deterrent. As an example, in a study that our group conducted in the late 1980s, we screened a total of 28 female and 19 male participants to arrive at a final 6 females to match with the 6 males[12] (Figure 1.1). In our study in 1993,[13] we screened 26 females and 19 males before being able to match them according to our strict criteria. In our 1995 study,[5] it took nearly one year to recruit the females to match the males.

For gender comparison studies of strength and power, it is the author's view that training status is the most important factor to equate and that total volume or number of repetitions be determined relative to the 1RM for each individual. It is likely that for absolute strength, there will be equivalence in leg but not arm strength between the genders even when comparing for lean mass (Chapter 4). Distinctions also need to be made in weight dependent and independent activities between the genders.

B. Models to Study Potential Gender Differences

1. Human Models

Probably the most frequently used model to examine for potential gender differences in metabolism is to use the cross-sectional, between-group, comparative design in which males and females are matched according to the previously mentioned criteria. Both males and females are then exposed to some intervention, (i.e., running on a treadmill, cycling, etc.), and have various outcomes measured (i.e., muscle glycogen, oxygen consumption, etc.). In addition to the problems with matching between the genders, this approach requires that many other factors be strictly controlled (Table 1.5). This approach is probably the only way to truly compare between males and females because it takes into account both the phylogenetic and ontogenic (developmental) aspects of being male or female. An example of ontogenic gender dimorphism that may affect metabolism comes from the observation that females and males both deposit the majority of their energy as protein at age four to five years, whereas only males have a second peak at between 13 to 15 years.[22] Because these developmental differences are present, it is important to control for sexual maturity in gender comparison studies.

It is likely that much of the metabolic and physical characteristic differences between males and females is due to the influence of the sex hormones (see Chapter 2). For this reason, another model may be used for gender comparison studies involving either the withdrawal, or provision of, sex hormones. Technically, these

**Table 1.5   Factors to Control in Between-Gender
Comparative Studies for Endurance Exercise**

1. Age
2. VO_{2max} (mL/kg LBM/min)
3. Timing of:
   - a) Menstrual Cycle
   - b) Testing (a.m. or p.m.)
   - c) Diet (fed vs. fasted) (Rest day prior to testing)
   - d) Exercise Status
4. Training Status:
   - a) Years of Training
   - b) Frequency (times/week)
   - c) Duration (hours/week)
5. Testing Intensity:
   - a) Well trained → $\leq 75\%$ VO_{2max}
   - b) Untrained → determine LT → exercise $\leq 70\%$ VO_{2max}
6. Diet:
   - a) Measure habitual intake
     - i) Checklist diet
     - ii) Pre-packaged diet
     - iii) Metabolic ward (Gold Standard)
7. Menstrual Status:
   - a) Follicular vs. luteal
   - b) Eumenorrhea, oligoamennorrhea vs. amenorrhea

approaches are not gender comparative, but rather examine the effect of addition or withdrawal of the sex hormones (which are felt to be largely responsible for many gender differences in metabolism). One approach would be to study males and females before sexual maturity (pre-pubertal); however, this is limited in terms of the invasiveness of the testing for metabolic studies. A similar model would be the study of pre- and post-menopausal females; however, age would be a confounding variable. Another possibility that has been used is to compare amenorrheic to eumenorrheic females.[23] A problem with this latter approach is that there are likely to be a number of other confounding variables that could account for the ammenorrhea (i.e., dietary intake, amount and/or intensity of exercise, other psychological stressors, endogenous hypothalamic set-point, etc.).

The provision of exogenous hormones provides an opportunity for longitudinal studies within a given subject group. The advantage of such an approach is that the randomized, cross-over study design controls for many intrinsic and extrinsic variables and inherently improves statistical power. One example is to provide hormone replacement to post-menopausal[24] or amennorheic[25] females. In our laboratory we have been interested in the metabolic effects of estrogen and have been exploring the potential for a model of estrogen administration to males. Our first few attempts consisted of the provision of 17-β-estradiol (E_2) by a transdermal patch (Estraderm®, Ciba-Geigy, Summit, NJ).

We have used a number of doses and durations, but were unable to get the testosterone into the female range and could only get the E_2 into the early-follicular range (Chapter 2). The only side effects were skin irritation from the patch (40%) and a slight propensity for headaches. A study by Ettinger and colleagues (Chapter 5), used a single dose of oral estrogen (Estrace®, Roberts Pharmaceutical, Mississauga, Ontario) to study the effects of E_2 upon muscle sympathetic nerve activity (MSNA). We have recently tried this oral preparation (Estrace®, Roberts Pharmaceutical, Mississauga, Ontario) for a longer duration and were pleased with the lack of side effects and the high E_2 concentrations that were obtained (luteal phase equivalent; Chapter 2).

One obvious problem with the provision of an exogenous hormone is that it does not mimic all of the factors that distinguish male from female. For example, the pulsatility and interactions with progesterone may be important to metabolism (see Chapter 2). Furthermore, it is possible that a long duration of exposure to a hormone is required to observe the phenotypic expression(s) relevant to metabolism. There are obvious ethical constraints on such an approach in males.

A final approach to the study of potential gender differences in metabolism is a long-term, longitudinal training study. One should start with relatively untrained males and females and expose them both to the same intensity, frequency, and duration of training. The advantage would be equivalence of the training stimulus and an increase in statistical power due to the repeated measures design.

This approach has been taken by G. M. E. Janssen and F. tenHoor from the University of Limburg, Netherlands. They performed a longitudinal study of untrained males (N = 60) and females (N = 18) who trained to complete a marathon after 20 months.[26] The reader is referred to a comprehensive journal supplement summarizing the design and results. Briefly, they found many of the gender difference findings that are described in this book, including:

1. Females had a greater percent body fat before and after training.
2. Post-exercise plasma urea was greater for males.
3. Females preserved lean body mass loss due to training better than males.
4. Plasma CK activity rise was lower for females following the marathon.
5. Hemoglobin, hematocrit, and ferritin were higher in males.

Although the study design was excellent, i.e., longitudinal, it was unfortunate that for the muscle metabolite and substrate measurements, there was a highly variable period between the completion of exercise and obtaining the tissue (range = 30 min → 7 h). Thus, important issues such as acute metabolite changes and glycogen depletion were unanswerable questions. Still, this remains an excellent study of gender specific responses to endurance exercise training.

2. Animal Models

As with humans, one can compare between the sexes in animal studies. A major advantage, is the fact that environmental and dietary controls can be rigorously enforced. Most of the gender comparative work in animals reported in this book was based upon studies in rats. Matching issues do arise because the female is always lighter than the male rat throughout the life cycle (Chapter 9). This however, should be considered a gender difference *per se,* which is perhaps related to gender differences in metabolism.

Several studies have provided exogenous hormones to male and oophorectomized female rats.[27,28,29] Removal of either the testicles or ovaries is termed gonadectomy, whereas removal of the ovaries in a female rat is termed ovariectomy or oophorectomy. In this book either term may be used and will be abbreviated as OVX.

In the future, I expect that researchers will be using transgenic (i.e., overexpression of estrogen receptor gene in a male rat), knockout (i.e., removal of estrogen receptor in female rat), and clonal (i.e., genetically identical animals exposed to differing hormonal stimuli during development) animal models.

III. IMPLICATIONS OF RESEARCH

A. Policy (Journals, Grants)

As one will see from this book, there is already substantive evidence upon which to recommend that there are certain gender differences that need to be considered in research design and interpretation of the results. Unless there are obvious reasons why a study was conducted with only males or females, the authors should be required to justify the model. It is critical in some studies to account for potential gender differences in metabolism in the statistical analysis. For example, as stated above, males and females respond differently to carbohydrate loading. Thus, a study with four males and four females may conclude that carbohydrate loading does not increase muscle glycogen concentration. The resultant statistical power calculations may be based upon $N = 8$, but, it is more accurate to base these upon $N = 4$ given the known differential outcomes.[5] Therefore, studies with both male and female participants that reported negative outcomes could have committed a Type II error (falsely concluding that there is no difference in outcome when in reality there is) if they did not consider the potential for a gender-specific response.

In addition to the scientific aspects of considering gender-specific responses in physiology experiments, it is important from a gender equality perspective that both males and females be given equal opportunity to volunteer as participants in research studies. Recently, the National Institute of Health has made it a policy that research grant recipients recruit equal numbers of males and females for studies. Although this is an excellent policy, I hope that the researchers consider that there may be a sexual dimorphism in the response to a given physiological stimulus, and that the granting agencies realize that recruitment numbers may have to be doubled in some instances, which would require more funding.

B. Human Performance

Given the larger muscle mass of the males as compared to the females, it is unlikely that females will outperform males in strength or power events. On the other side of the metabolic coin are the ultra-endurance sports where an enhanced lipid oxidation and glycogen sparing,[5,12,13,14] may favor the female athlete. Because most of the metabolic fuel for the completion of a marathon (42 km) comes from carbohydrate oxidation, it is likely that males will have a slight metabolic advantage up to this distance, but as the distance exceeds 42 km, females should have an increasing advantage over males.

Anecdotally, there are more female ultra-endurance swimmers, and others have commented on the relative ease with which females finish ultra-runs as compared to males. A scientific approach was taken to explore this question by Speechley and colleagues in 1996, where they found that equally trained males and females performed identically over a distance of 42 km, yet the females outperformed the males over 90 km.[30] They accurately claimed that this was not due to a greater maximal aerobic capacity, training history, or running economy; however, they erroneously claimed that it was not due to differences in lipid oxidation based upon plasma free fatty acid concentrations (see Chapter 8).[30] Another study from South Africa matched males and females for performance times at the 56 km distance and found that the females outperformed the males at the 90 km distance.[31] Regression analysis showed that the males outperformed the females at 5 to 42 km, and that there were no gender differences in performance until an intercept of 66 km, after which the females had an increasing advantage.[31] It is plausible that the differences were multi-factorial and included differences in muscle fiber type (Chapter 3), oxidative stress (Chapter 11), and muscle damage (Chapter 12), as well as to differences in metabolic substrate (Chapters 6, 7, and 8).

It is important to note that gender difference research should not be used for exclusion nor segregation of groups nor to confer values or judgements of superiority upon one group or another. I have even seen an article in a magazine about "the Battle of the Sexes" to describe some of the aforementioned research. We must remember that ignorance and prejudice were instrumental in women's not being allowed to participate in an official marathon until 1972 and the Olympic Marathon until 1984!

I hope that this book provides the impetus for future researchers to consider that gender differences in metabolism do exist and there may be significant practical implications. The research in this area is quite embryonic and I hope that the answer to many of the current questions will be found in the next few years. Each chapter will provide some ideas for future research as well as information on some techniques that may be used in answering the questions.

REFERENCES

1. Sherman, W. M., Costill, D. L., Fink, W. J., et al., The effect of exercise-diet manipulation on muscle glycogen and its subsequent utilization during performance, *Int. J. Sports Med.,* 2, 114, 1981.
2. Bergstrom, J., and Hultman. E., A study of the glycogen metabolism during exercise in man, *Scand. J. Clin. Lab. Invest.,* 19, 218, 1967.
3. Hultman, E., Studies on muscle metabolism of glycogen and active phosphate in man with special reference to exercise and diet, *Scand. J. Clin. Lab. Invest.,* 19, 94, 1967.
4. Karlsson, J. and Saltin, B., Diet, muscle glycogen, and endurance performance, *J. Appl. Physiol.,* 31(2), 203, 1971.
5. Tarnopolsky, M. A., Atkinson, S. A., Phillips, S. M., and MacDougall, J. D., Carbohydrate loading and metabolism during exercise in men and women, *J. Appl. Physiol.,* 78(4), 1360, 1995.
6. Hoyenga, K. B. and Hoyenga, K. T., Gender and energy balance: sex differences in adaptations for feast and famine, *Physiol. Behav.,* 28(3), 545, 1982.
7. Marcus, R. C., Madvig, C. P., Minkoff, J., Goddard, M., Bayer, M., Martin, M., Gaudiani, L., Haskell, W., and Genant, H., Menstrual function and bone mass in elite women distance runners, *Ann. Inter. Med.,* 102, 158, 1985.
8. Drinkwater, B. L., Nilson, K., Chestnut, C. H. III, Bremner, W. J., Shainholtz, S., and Southworth, M. B., Bone mineral content of amenorrheic and eumenorrheic athletes, *N. Engl. J. Med.,* 311, 277, 1984.
9. Wilmore, J. H., Wambsgans, K. C., Brenner, M., Broeder, C. E., Paijmans, I., Volpe, J. A., and Wilmore, K. M., Is there energy conservation in amenorrheic compared with eumenorrheic distance runners? *J. Appl. Physiol.,* 72(1), 15, 1992.
10. Mrosovsky, N. and Sherry, D. F., Animal anorexias, *Science,* 297, 837, 1980.
11. Brooks, G. A., Fahey, T. D., and White, T. P. *Exercise Physiology: Human Bioenergetics and Its Applications.* Macmillan Publishing Co., New York, 1996.
12. Tarnopolsky, L. J., MacDougall, J. D., Atkinson, S. A., Tarnopolsky, M. A., and Sutton, J. R., Gender differences in substrate for endurance exercise, *J. Appl. Physiol.,* 68, 302, 1990.
13. Phillips, S. M., Atkinson, S. A., Tarnopolsky, M. A., and MacDougall, J. D., Gender differences in leucine kinetics and nitrogen balance in endurance athletes, *J. Appl. Physiol.,* 75(5), 2134, 1993.
14. Tarnopolsky, M. A., Bosman, M., MacDonald, J. R., Vandeputte, D., Martin, J., and Roy, B. D., Post-exercise protein-carbohydrate and carbohydrate supplements increase muscle glycogen in men and women. *J. Appl. Physiol.,* 83(6), 1877, 1997.
15. *Webster's Dictionary,* Thomas Allen and Son., Ltd., Toronto, Ont., 1981.

16. Nativ, A., The female athlete triad: managing an acute risk to long-term health, *Phys. Sportmed.,* 22(1), 60, 1994.

17. Smith, A. D., The female athlete triad: causes, diagnosis, and treatment, *Phys. Sportmed.,* 24(7), 67, 1996.

18. Hurley, B. F., Nemeth, P. M., Martin, W. H. III, Hagberg, J. M., Dalsky, G. P., and Holloszy, J. O., Muscle triglyceride utilization during exercise: effect of training, *J. Appl. Physiol.,* 60(2), 562, 1986.

19. Costill, D. L., Fink, W. J., Getchell, L. H., et al., Lipid metabolism in skeletal muscle of endurance-trained males and females. *J. Appl. Physiol.,* 47(4), 787, 1979.

20. Sparling, P. B., A Meta-Analysis of studies comparing maximal oxygen uptake in men and women. *Med. Sci. Ex. Sport,* 51(3), 542, 1980.

21. Cureton, K. J., Matching of male and female subjects using $VO_{2\,max}$, *Research Quarterly for Exercise and Sport,* 52(2), 264, 1981.

22. Dugdale, A. E. and Payne, P. R., Pattern of lean and fat desposition in adults, *Nature,* 266, 349, 1977.

23. Baer, J. T., Endocrine parameters in amenorrheic and eumenorrheic adolescent female runners, *Int. J. Sports Med.,* 14, 191, 1993.

24. Jensen, M. D., Martin, M. L., Cryer, P. E, and Roust, L. R., Effects of estrogen on free fatty acid metabolism in humans, *Am. J. Physiol.,* 266, E914, 1994.

25. Ruby, B. C., Robergs, R. A., Waters, D. L., Bruge, M., Mermier, C., and Stolarczyk, L., Effects of estradiol on substrate turnover during exercise in amenorrheic females, *Med. Sci. Sports Exerc.,* 29(9), 1160, 1997.

26. Janssen, G. M. E. and ten Hoor, F., Sport and health in a general perspective, *Int. J. Sports Med.,* S3(10), S118, 1989.

27. Kendrick, Z. V., Steffan, C. A., Ramsay, W. L., and Golberg, D. I., Effects of estradiol on tissue glycogen metabolism and lipid availability in exercised oophorectomized rats, *J. Appl. Physiol.,* 63(2),492, 1987.

28. Kendrick, Z. V., Steffen, C. A., Rumsey, W. L., and Goldberg, D. I., Effect of estradiol on tissue glycogen metabolism in exercised oophorectomized rats, *J. Appl. Physiol.,* 63(2), 492, 1987.

29. Hatta, H., Atomi, Y., Shinohara, S., Yamamoto, Y., and Yamada, S., The effects of ovarian hormones on glucose and fatty acid oxidation during exercise in female ovariectomized rats, *Horm. Metab. Res.,* 20, 609, 1988.

30. Speechly, D. P., Taylor, S. R., and Rogers, G. G., Differences in ultra-endurance exercise in performance-matched male and female runners, *Med. Sci. Sports Exerc.,* 28(3), 359, 1996.

31. Bam, J., Noakes, T. D., Juritz, J., and Dennis, S. C., Could women outrun men in ultramarathon races? *Med. Sci. Sports Exerc.,* 29(2), 244, 1997.

CHAPTER 2

Hormonal Differences Between Males and Females

Mark Tarnopolsky, M.D., Ph.D., F.R.C.P.(C) and
Ronald N. Cortright, Ph.D.

CONTENTS

I. INTRODUCTION

The phenotypic, and possibly many of the metabolic, differences between the genders are influenced by sex hormones. The predominant sex hormones discussed in this chapter will be the "male" hormone testosterone and the "female" hormones estrogen and progesterone. "Male" and "female" are generalizations, since testosterone is also present in females, and estrogen and progesterone are present in males. This chapter is not meant to be a comprehensive review of the endocrinology of the sex hormones, but rather to provide a brief overview of the physiology of these hormones, particularly as they relate to substrate metabolism and the physiology of growth. An overview of some of the models to manipulate the sex hormones will be discussed as they pertain to an understanding of gender differences in metabolism. We would also like to provide some human reference values that can be used to determine the sex hormone status of a group of individuals in a given study.

In addition to the study of gender differences in metabolism, an understanding of the effects of the sex hormones is important because of the prevalence of sex hormone supplementation in post-menopausal females.[1] Estrogen replacement therapy (ERT) has been shown to decrease cardiac associated mortality (Chapter 5). It is possible that this effect is mediated by an attenuation of oxidative damage (Chapter 11), or through a reduction sympathetic outflow (Chapter 5). ERT is also used in the prevention and treatment of osteoporosis.[2] Given the significant potential for morbidity and mortality reduction, and the fact that current dosing schemes do not increase the risk for endometrial carcinoma, it is likely that the prevalence of ERT will increase in the future.

In addition to the replacement therapy described above, synthetic steroids are commonly used by females as oral contraceptives (OCT). Many of these preparations try to mimic the normal female menstrual cycle in that they increase the concentration of estrogen and progestins progressively throughout a 21-day cycle, followed by withdrawal and subsequent menses. The most common synthetic estrogen is ethinyl estradiol (35 ug/d) and levonorgestrel or norethindrone (the latter in increasing concentrations). There have been several studies of the effects of oral contraceptives on female metabolism which will only briefly be summarized.

The endogenous concentrations of 17-β-estradiol, progesterone, luteinizing hormone (LH), and follicle stimulating hormone (FSH) are suppressed in OCT users.[3] In females with previous gestational diabetes, the provision of OCTs did not alter the response to an oral glucose tolerance test, nor was plasma cortisol, FFA, lipoproteins, nor cholesterol altered.[4] An exercise-induced increase in cortisol was slightly attenuated in OCT users, with minimal changes in growth hormone (GH) and insulin responses to exercise.[3] More important, however, was the finding of no significant difference between the OCT and non-OCT users in the substrate utilization during endurance exercise.[3] Another study found that GH was greater in OCT users during exercise and they also had a slightly lower exercise RER.[5] In this latter study, however, RER was lower at two time points and yet calculated total fat oxidation at those times was reportedly not different between the groups.[5] Given the comprehensiveness of the study by Bonen and colleagues,[3] it appears likely that current OCT preparations do not significantly alter substrate metabolism during exercise in healthy young females.

There is an extensive body of literature and whole volumes dedicated to understanding the psychology and physiology of taking large doses of exogenous androgenic-anabolic steroids.[6] There have even been investigations of the lipoprotein profiles of females taking exogenous androgenic-anabolic steroids during resistance exercise training.[7] We will not attempt to cover this literature to any large extent.

We hope that if there proves to be convincing ergogenic benefits derived from the administration of estrogen preparations (possibly in ultra-endurance sports[8]), that this does not become a doping agent to gain an ergogenic advantage. As some athletes will undoubtedly employ their use during competition, it is important for the International Olympic Committee and doping control agencies in each country to be cognizant of this potential.

Finally, the physiology of the sex hormones and the anabolic hormone insulin will be briefly discussed in the context of growth and substrate metabolism. Information gained from animal studies has been extremely important to our understanding of how these hormones orchestrate the growth process and subsequent control of body composition in humans as well other mammals. The interaction of sex steroids and insulin during periods of acute and chronic exercise and disease is discussed in detail in Chapter 9.

II. ANATOMY AND PHYSIOLOGY OF THE SEX HORMONES

A. Menstrual Cycle

The menstrual cycle refers to the cyclical changes in the concentrations of sex hormones seen for females. The duration of this cycle is usually 28 days and in divided roughly in half by ovulation (~ Day 14 is release of the ovum from the ovary). The period prior to ovulation is called the pre-ovulatory phase or the follicular phase and starts on day one of the menstrual blood flow (menses usually lasting about three to five days). The post-ovulatory phase is termed the luteal phase where the corpus luteum secretes progesterone to maintain the uterine lining for potential implantation with a fertilized ovum. The luteal phase ends with the onset of menses and the process starts again. The menstrual cycle usually starts between the ages of 11 to 14 (menarche) and terminates in the 40s (menopause). Estrogen secretion is under control of luteinizing hormone (LH) and follicle stimulating hormone (FSH), both of which are secreted from the anterior pituitary. Secretion of LH and FSH is regulated by gonadotropin releasing hormone (Gn-RH), released from the hypothalamus. A complex interaction of positive and negative feedback regulates the timing and amount of secretion of these hormones.

As will be seen below, there are large differences in the concentration of the sex hormones across the menstrual cycle. Therefore, within a given female, the phase of the menstrual cycle will significantly influence the hormonal mileau. Although the menstrual cycle adds a level of complexity to a research design, it also affords a fantastic opportunity to study the potential influence of the female sex hormones upon aspects of metabolism. Possible study designs include pre- vs. post-menarche, pre- vs. post-menopause, follicular vs. luteal phase, and hormonal replacement in menopausal females. The complex interactions of the hormones relevant to the menstrual cycle are illustrated in Figure 2.1.

The effect of the menstrual cycle upon metabolism will be considered individually in each of the chapters; however, it will become increasingly apparent that the menstrual cycle phase can significantly affect glycogen storage[9] (Chapter 6), caffeine

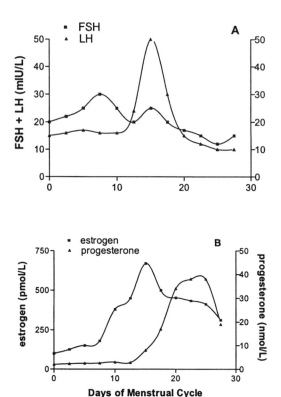

Figure 2.1 Sex hormone changes throughout the menstrual cycle. A. Pituitary hormones. FSH
= follicle stimulating hormone; LH = leuteinizing hormone. B. Ovarian hormones.
Estrogen (estradiol) and progesterone. Typical menstrual cycle length is about 28
days.

metabolism (Chapter 13), protein metabolism (Chapter 7), food selection,[10] and
interleukin concentrations (see below), to name only a few.

B. Estrogen

In addition to its role in regulating the ovarian cycle and in developing female
secondary sexual characteristics, estrogen has widespread effects on many physiological and metabolic processes. In females, most 17-β-estradiol is produced by the
ovaries, with lesser amounts from the adrenal cortex and from peripheral testosterone
aromatization. In males, the latter two pathways are responsible for estrogen production. Males have similar 17-β-estradiol to females in the early follicular phase
of the menstrual cycle (males = 6–44 pg/ml, 22–161 pmol/L; females = 10–50 pg/ml,
37–184 pmol/L). The female concentration increases progressively through the follicular phase of the menstrual cycle (Figure 2.1; Table 2.1).

In humans, estrogens are thought to cause deposition of increased quantities of
fat in the subcutaneous tissues. As a result, overall specific gravity of the female

body is considerably less that of the male.[11] Females also appear to selectively stimulate lipoprotein lipase (LPL) activity in the gluteofemoral adipocytes and thus promote fat storage in this area (Chapter 8). In the abdominal region, estrogen appears to stimulate lipolysis.[12,13] Estrogens are also believed to cause a slight increase in total body protein, which is evidenced by a slightly positive nitrogen balance when estrogens are administered.[11] This probably results from the growth-promoting effect of estrogen on the sexual organs, the bones, and other tissues. Estrogens also cause increased osteoblastic activity. Therefore, at puberty, growth rate becomes rapid for several years. However, estrogens cause the closure of the epiphyseal plate in the long bones, and thus act to terminate linear growth. This effect is much stronger in the female than is the similar effect of testosterone in the male. Therefore, linear growth in the female usually ceases several years earlier than in the male.

The role of estrogen in growth and body composition has been extensively studied in the rat. In the adult female rat, withdrawal of ovarian hormones by ovariectomy (OVX) induces hyperphagia and a rapid gain in body mass which lasts for approximately one month. Then hyperphagia subsides, and body mass is maintained at 20 to 25% above sham-operated controls.[14] In addition, running wheel activity is permanently suppressed by OVX. These effects of OVX can be reversed with estrogen replacement.[15] Following replacement, a transient hypoph-agia is accompanied by a sharp decrease in body mass gain. Food intake gradually returns to prehormone levels, and body mass is maintained below the level of the OVX controls as long as estrogen is administered. OVX produces a significant increase in carcass fat. Conversely, total carcass lipid is lowered following estrogen administration.

Estradiol also acts directly in the brain to alter regulatory behaviors. Implants of estradiol in the vicinity of the ventromedial hypothalamus decrease food intake, whereas implants in the medial preoptic area stimulate running wheel activity. These effects are achieved in the absence of direct effects on peripheral tissues.[20] Alterna-tively, an estrogen-induced change in fat concentrations in the blood has been proposed as a means by which the hypothalamus controls food intake[12] (i.e., the so-called lipostatic theory). Rat liver contains cytoplasmic estrogen receptors which have been shown to alter hepatic RNA and protein synthesis.[16] Through alterations in hepatic lipoprotein lipase activity, estrogens could influence liver lipid output and thus regulate feeding behavior.

Estradiol-induced alterations in insulin secretion have also been reported. Cos-trini and Kalkhoff[17] have shown that ovarian hormones can act on pancreatic islets to stimulate insulin production. It has also been demonstrated that estrogen increases liver glycogen content, decreases hepatic gluconeogenesis, and improves glucose tolerance.[18] These changes should act to increase both fat storage and body mass. However, this concept conflicts with the unequivocal finding that estrogen replacement in castrated rats decreases body mass and adiposity.[20] Furthermore, Dudley et al.[20] have shown that estradiol-induced changes in body mass are not dependent on changes in pancreatic insulin secretion. In support, Wade and Gray[14] suggested there appears to be a weak causal relationship between altered carbohy-drate metabolism and ovarian actions on food intake and body mass in rats. Therefore, it appears that ovarian hormones can affect eating behavior and body weight in the absence of changes in pancreatic insulin output. The contrasting effects of estrogens on carbohydrate (increased liver glycogen storage) and fat (decreased wholebody storage) metabolism merit further study.

As with humans, high-affinity, hormone-specific cytoplasmic[21] and nuclear[22] binding sites for estrogen have been demonstrated in rat adipose tissue. Consequently, estrogens have been shown to increase *in vitro* catecholamine-stimulated lipolysis in adipocytes[23] which could contribute to estradiol-induced decreases in adiposity. In addition, estradiol is able to decrease adipose tissue lipid uptake by decreasing lipoprotein lipase activity. In contrast, ovariectomy has been shown to increase white adipose tissue lipoprotein lipase activity, and this change can be prevented or reversed by treatment of physiological doses of estradiol.[19] Collectively, it appears that estradiol could reduce adiposity by lowering the rate of uptake and storage of circulating triglycerides in white adipose tissue via modulation of lipoprotein lipase. This may act to divert lipids to other metabolically active tissues like skeletal muscle for oxidation.[19]

In conclusion, the effects of estradiol on body mass and body composition may involve alterations in central and peripheral control of eating behavior and substrate (lipid) mobilization and metabolism. Further research is needed to understand better how estrogens interact with the neural and endocrine control of metabolism. In this regard, studies employing estrogen antagonists (e.g., Tamoxifen®) may aid in furthering our understanding of the processes of growth and differentiation.[25] Furthermore, given the current information on leptin's effects on eating behavior and peripheral metabolism, studies involving potential interactions between estrogen and leptin expression and regulation of secretion are extremely important (Chapter 9).

C. Progesterone

In humans, progesterone is secreted by the corpus luteum, the placenta, and the follicle. In women, the plasma level is approximately 0.9 ng/ml (3 nmol/L) during the follicular phase of the menstrual cycle (in men, the plasma level is ~ 0.3 ng/mL [1 nmol/L]). During the luteal phase, the corpus luteum produces large quantities of progesterone, and ovarian secretion increases ~30 fold. Progesterone is also an important intermediate in steroid biosynthesis in all tissues that secrete steroid hormones, and small amounts enter the circulation from the testes and the adrenals.[26] The principal target organs of progesterone are the uterus, the breasts, and the brain.

Progesterone is the most active naturally occurring antagonist of androgens. Progesterone antagonizes the effects of both testosterone and dihydro-testosterone by competing for the androgen-dependent tissues and thus prevents target tissues from responding to the normally low concentration of androgens in the female.[27]

In the rat, progesterone has definite effects on body mass and composition. Galletti and Klopper[28] showed that the increase in the daily mass gain of progesterone-treated rats (80 days old) was significantly greater (2.62 g/d) than controls (1.53g/d). The greater weight gain was due to fat accumulation because the protein and ash content was not significantly higher in the progesterone-treated rats. Additional analysis of the distribution of the various depots indicated that progesterone induced a proportional and uniform increase of body fat. In the same study, Galletti and Klopper[28] also showed that the hormonal changes accompanying puberty are necessary for progesterone to exert its biological effect(s) on fat deposition. Female rats (25 days old), treated with progesterone prior to commencement of the ovarian cycle, were compared to similarly aged controls. Under this condition, the mass gain (approximately 5 g/d) and components of body composition were the same for both groups. Collectively, these studies indicate that progesterone leads to fat deposition, but is dependent on an intact, mature reproductive system.

It has been hypothesized that progesterone, in the presence of estradiol, determines the amount of fat stored by altering lipoprotein lipase activity in the adipocyte. In gonadal-intact rats, progesterone treatment approximately doubles adipose tissue lipoprotein lipase activity and this increases fat storage.[29] Gray and Wade[30] have shown that rat adipose tissue contains specific, high affinity progestin receptors which are induced by estrogen treatment. *In vitro* cell culture work has confirmed that estradiol acts directly on adipocytes to induce progestin receptors.[19] In contrast, in OVX rats, progesterone neither affects lipoprotein lipase activity nor increases carcass fat content.[28] The highly significant correlation between regional differences in adipose tissue estrogen receptor content and induction of progestin receptors strongly suggest that it is the interaction of these two hormones that regulates tissue adiposity.[30]

In summary, estradiol and progesterone appear to affect tissue mass and composition, at least in part, by altering lipoprotein lipase activity in adipose tissue. Estradiol acts to lower adiposity by lowering lipoprotein lipase activity, while progesterone increases fat storage by increasing the activity of this enzyme. Other potential mechanisms which regulate body mass and tissue composition in the female include ovarian action on the hypothalamus, the pituitary, and the liver to alter feeding behavior and substrate availability.

D. Testosterone

Testosterone (androgens in general) is produced by the Leydig cells of the testes. Its secretion (normal rate ~4–9 mg/d [13.9–31.2 nmol/d]) is under control of luteinizing hormone (LH) which is dependent upon the stimulatory effects of the hypothalamic trophic factor, gonadotropin releasing hormone (Gn-RH). The majority of testosterone is produced by the testes while the adrenal cortex produces the remainder. These sources act to control blood concentrations (free plus bound: male ~525 ng/ml [~20 nmol/L], female ~30 ng/dL [~1.0 nmol/L]) by feedback inhibition of both LH and Gn-RH.[31] In general, androgens develop and maintain male secondary sex characteristics. They also exert important protein-anabolic, growth-promoting effects. They increase the synthesis and decrease the breakdown of protein, leading to increased growth rate. However, like estrogen, they cause the epiphyses of long bones to fuse and eventually stop growth.[27]

There is a burst of testosterone secretion in the male fetus before birth. In the neonate, there is another burst, but thereafter the Leydig cells become quiescent until puberty. Increased secretion of testosterone is the direct cause of puberty at which time sexual maturation and the adolescent growth spurt occurs. Testosterone produces these effects in part by increasing GH production and hence IGF-1.[32] Testosterone concentration decreases with fasting[33] and chronic malnutrition.[34] This may be related to the finding that the gonadotrophins and Leydig cells require a certain minimal glucose delivery to function normally.[35] This implies that testosterone concentration is dependent upon the energy balance of the body.

In the rat, the presence and timing of testosterone secretion is critical for the attainment of maximal body mass. It is not known whether androgens act directly on the brain to influence body weight and food intake, but testosterone (males$_{plasma}$ 2.3 ± 0.6 ng/ml, females 63.6 ± 13.7 pg/ml, mean ± SEM) does act on a variety of non-neural tissues to alter tissue mass and composition. In addition to its stimulatory effects on the male genitalia, testosterone has growth-promoting effects in several other tissues. Androgens stimulate the growth of kidney and liver, both of which contain androgen receptors.[36] Rat skeletal muscles also contain androgen receptors.[65] *In vitro* studies indicate that testosterone can directly alter biochemical processes in rat skeletal muscle.[38] In some reproductive tissues (prostate) testosterone must first be reduced by 5α-reductase to dihydrotestosterone which is then bound by the androgen receptor to stimulate tissue growth. Rat skeletal muscle and kidney have no 5α-reductase activity, and so testosterone is much more effective in stimulating mass gain as has been shown in orchidectomized rats.[39]

In the male rat, the effects of androgens on eating and body mass appear to vary with the type and dose of the hormone, but adiposity is suppressed by testosterone in a wide range of doses. High doses of testosterone, like estrogen, reduce body mass primarily by decreasing body fat.[40] It is possible, via its estrogenic metabolites, that testosterone is acting on adipose tissue in the male. Adipose tissue contains the enzymes which aromatize testosterone to estradiol.[41] This effect of testosterone occurs naturally in the intact animal. The increased secretion of testosterone associated with copulatory activity in the male can cause significant decreases in both body mass and carcass fat content.[42]

Orchidectomy decreases running wheel activity and increases fat content in male rats.[43] Both of these changes are reversed by testosterone replacement.[44] According to Wade and Gray[14] it is possible that testosterone is aromatized to estrogen in the brain to stimulate running activity, just as it may be aromatized before being bound to adipose tissue. Testosterone, via estrogenic metabolite(s) might simultaneously stimulate activity and divert triglyceride for oxidation in muscles of male rats.

In summary, it appears that testosterone alters body mass and composition in rats by:

1. Stimulating growth in genital tissues via 5α-reductase metabolite dihydro-testosterone
2. Its anabolic actions on kidney and skeletal muscle
3. Estrogenic metabolites of testosterone acting directly on adipose tissue to suppress adiposity. An overview of the basal sex hormone concentrations for males and females is presented in Table 2.1.

Table 2.1 Basal Sex Hormone Concentrations

Hormone	Male	Female (Follicular)	Female (Luteal)
Testosterone (ng/ml)	~525	~25	~35
Estrogen (pg/ml)	6–24	10–50	120–375
Progesterone (ng/ml)	<0.6	0.1–1.5	2.5–28

Note: To convert to SI units: testosterone (ng/ml → nmol/L) * 0.0347; estrogen (pg/ml → pmol/L) * 3.67; progesterone (ng/ml → nmol/L) * 3.16. Values derived from References 3, 9, 46, 50, 51, 53, and 54.

E. Response of Sex Hormones to Acute Exercise and Chronic Exercise Training

In response to mild endurance exercise (~40% VO_{2max}), plasma $[E_2]$ usually does not change.[3] In more intensive endurance exercise, the plasma $[E_2]$ increases during both the follicular[3,9,45] and luteal phase of the menstrual cycle.[9,3] Progesterone shows a similar pattern, with a proportionate increase that has been shown to be similar between the two menstrual cycle phases[3,45] or increased only in the luteal phase.[9] A potentiation of the acute exercise induced progesterone elevations is seen in the third trimester of pregnancy (when progesterone is about 15 times above non-parous concentrations).[3]

Both plasma FSH and LH generally do not show a significant acute change in response to either low or high intensity endurance exercise.[3,45] It has been suggested that the acute increase in plasma sex steroid concentration is due predominantly to an increased secretion as opposed to a reduced clearance, based upon the finding that when endogenous secretion is attenuated with oral contraceptives, there is no significant exercise-induced increase.[3] However, if LH and FSH concentrations do not increase, an increased estrogen and progesterone release must occur via receptor, post-receptor alterations or possibly through synergistic interactions between other hormones.

In response to chronic exercise training, the female may not show any alteration in menstrual cycle; however, there is a complex interplay between percent body fat, exercise intensity, psychological stress, biological predisposition, rapidity of weight loss, or rapidity of exercise stress imposition that may ultimately result in oligoamenorrhea (infrequent periods) or amenorrhea (absence of periods for 6 months).[45,47,48] Probably the first change is a shortening of the luteal phase duration, followed by anovulatory cycles and finally, cessation of menses. It is well established that this phenomenon is mediated at the level of the hypothalamus (decreased GnRH pulsatility).[49] From an endocrine standpoint, a female athlete with secondary amenorrhea has E_2 concentrations that are about 33%, and progesterone concentrations that are 10–20% of otherwise comparable eumenorrheic females[48,50,51] (Table 2.1). Furthermore, there is a loss of the cyclical changes in the amenorrheic female and this may have important long-term metabolic effects (it is possible that certain receptors may be regulated by prolonged stable concentrations of hormones, although this remains to be tested in the context of sex hormones and metabolic regulation). A cautionary note is that an athlete with primary or secondary amenorrhea should consult with her family doctor and appropriate referral should be arranged if deemed necessary. Potential repercussions may include premature osteopenia. Even in the late 20s and early 30s amenorrheic female athletes can already show low bone mineral content when compared to oligo- and eumenorrheic female athletes.[50]

Testosterone concentrations generally increase consequent to an acute bout of resistance exercise in males.[52,53,54] The increase in testosterone is not as reproducible for females as compared to males in response to resistance exercise.[54] Furthermore, the absolute testosterone concentration remains about 10- to 15-fold higher in males as compared to females even into the eighth decade of life.[54] In response to endurance exercise, an opposite effect is observed. Namely, in a longitudinal study of both males and females progressively training to finish a 15-, 25-, and 42-km race, it was observed that post-exercise plasma testosterone concentrations were about 50% lower than pre-exercise values.[55]

In response to chronic endurance training, there appears to be a significant gender differential response upon basal plasma testosterone concentrations, with males increasing and females remaining unchanged.[55] There does not appear to be any difference in testosterone concentration between amenorrheic and eumenorrheic female runners.[48] In chronic resistance exercise training there are increases in total plasma testosterone, FSH, LH, and testosterone:sex hormone-binding globulin concentrations.[54] One study examined the effects of nine weeks of heavy resistance exercise training upon plasma testosterone concentration in both males and females and found significant increase for males but not for females.[56] In summary, chronic endurance exercise training results in a lowering of testosterone concentrations for males and females. Conversely, resistance exercise training increases plasma testosterone concentration for males but not females.

III. POTENTIAL GENDER DIFFERENCES IN OTHER HORMONES

A. Growth Hormone

Growth hormone (GH) is secreted by the anterior pituitary gland in response to growth hormone releasing factor (GHRH) from the hypothalamus. Major stimuli leading to its release include; sleep, exercise, fasting, certain amino acids, and hypoglycemia.[58] In addition to its well-known effects on overall growth,[59] it also has lipolytic properties which could have potential interesting implications for gender differences in metabolism. There have been several studies in the elderly showing that GH supplementation can increase lean body mass,[60,61] nitrogen balance,[59] mixed muscle fractional synthetic rate,[59] and decrease adipose tissue mass by 14% (possibly via increased lipolysis[60]). Furthermore, these anabolic effects are present in females.[59]

Bunt and colleagues studied the effects of training status and acute exercise upon plasma growth hormone concentrations in both males and females.[62] In sedentary persons they found that resting [GH] was higher in females, yet the percent increase in response to exercise was greater for the males.[62] The higher resting [GH] was also seen in the female endurance-trained group, again with a greater percentage increase in males. Endurance training appeared to have a positive influence upon GH release for the absolute peak GH concentrations were higher in this group as compared to the sedentary group.[62] A nearly identical finding was reported by Friedmann and Kindermann in 1989,[63] where resting [GH] was higher for both endurance-trained and sedentary females as compared to males. This group also found that the exercise-induced peak percent increase in [GH] was greater for males (~900%) vs. females (~150%).[63] Tarnopolsky and colleagues showed similar results in well-trained endurance males and females with the females having a higher [GH] at rest and the males maintaining higher concentrations during endurance exercise at 65% VO_{2peak}.[64] We found that the female's [GH] returned to baseline by 60 minutes of exercise, while the male's remained significantly elevated.[64] Another study with exclusively female participants also showed that the post-exercise [GH] were no different from resting values.[9] A contradictory study found that 10 minutes of mild exercise resulted in a greater increase in [GH] for females as compared to males.[58] Furthermore, this latter group also showed that three and six days of estrogen treatment resulted in an accentuated GH response to exercise.[58] The contradictory results between the studies may be related to the duration of the exercise stimulus. For example, we found that [GH] were similar at 30 minutes of exercise for both genders. The females showed a progressive decline in [GH], whereas males showed a progressive increase in [GH] at later time points.[64] It is also important to control for phase of the menstrual cycle, for resting [GH] is about twice as high in the luteal compared to follicular phase in some,[9] but not all studies.[65]

Differences between the genders in GH response to endurance exercise appear to indicate a propensity for resting female concentrations to be higher than for males, whereas the percentage increase is greater for males. The GH response to acute exercise is potentiated in amenorrheic versus eumenorrheic female athletes,[65] suggesting that estrogen *per se* may be responsible for the blunted GH responsivity to acute exercise stress. The opioid antagonist, naloxone, attenuated GHRH induced GH release in females, yet there was no such effect in males.[66] This latter gender difference suggests that estrogen may blunt an opioid mediated GH release at the level of the hypothalamus.[66]

The biological significance of these differences to metabolism are far from clear. It is likely that GH is not a significant regulator of exercise-induced lipolysis for the [GH] and does not follow changes in RER in a consistent pattern. Additionally, the greater [GH] increase during endurance exercise in males is opposite to the observation of greater fat oxidation in females during sub-maximal endurance exercise (Chapters 1 and 8). For example, Tarnopolsky and colleagues found that females had a much lower RER as compared to males during endurance exercise and yet their [GH] fell to baseline concentrations by 60 minutes of exercise, while the males showed a slow progressive increase in [GH] with a higher RER (higher CHO oxidation).[64]

For male athletes during and following an acute resistance exercise bout,[52] there appears to be an increase in plasma [GH] that is similar in magnitude and timing to that seen for male endurance athletes (see above). Acute GH responses in females to resistance exercise have not, to our understanding, been reported. However, an excellent longitudinal study measured resting plasma [GH] in both males and females during a nine week resistance training period.[57] They found that the females had consistently higher basal [GH] as compared to the males and that there were no significant training effects.[57]

Overall, it appears that resting plasma [GH] is slightly greater in females, exercise is a stimulator of GH release, and that the responsivity of females to an acute exercise stress is attenuated compared to males. The implications of these changes to potential gender differences in metabolic substrate selection and muscle hypertrophy are not clear. If GH does play a role in gender specific responses to metabolic stressors, the relationship appears complex.

B. Cortisol

Cortisol is a steroid-based hormone that is secreted from the *zona fasiculata* and *reticularis* of the adrenal cortex in response to stimulation from adrenocorticotrophic hormone (ACTH), which itself is released from the anterior pituitary in response to cortisol-releasing hormone (CRH) from the hypothalamus. There are very strong diurnal variations in cortisol concentration with the highest concentrations seen between 0400h and 1200h and the lowest in the evening hours.[67] The diurnal variation is very important to consider in the design of research studies. Cortisol has important effects on gluconeogenesis, protein and lipid metabolism, and in the overall response to metabolic stress.

During endurance exercise, plasma cortisol concentrations generally show increases;[63,67,68] however, one study found that post-marathon cortisol concentrations were significantly elevated only for the male and not female runners.[55] The observed increase is mediated at the hypothalamic or pituitary level for ACTH also shows increases in response to exercise.[68] It has been suggested that opioid receptors do not play a role in the ACTH release during exercise from results of naloxone-blocking experiments.[68] However, in this study there were 12 male subjects and no females, which raises the possibility of a gender difference such as that described above for GHRH responsiveness to naloxone. Following resistance exercise there does not seem to be an acute elevation of cortisol concentrations in well-trained males.[53]

In response to chronic endurance training, basal plasma cortisol concentrations do not show changes.[55] Similarly, with resistance exercise training there does not appear to be an effect upon the basal cortisol concentration for females; in contrast, males show a progressive decline.[57]

In summary, plasma cortisol concentrations usually increase in response to an acute bout of endurance exercise and do not change in response to chronic endurance training. Concentrations may not be elevated after resistance exercise; however, chronic resistance exercise training may lower basal cortisol in males but not for females. The importance of the lowering of basal plasma concentrations in males is unclear; however, a resulting increase in the testosterone:cortisol ratio, may be physiologically relevant as an indicator of anabolic potential.[56] Future research could explore the potential for gender differences in glucocorticoid receptor activation[69] in addition to merely plasma cortisol concentrations.

C. Insulin

Insulin is an amino acid-based hormone that is secreted from the β-cells of the pancreas in response to elevated blood glucose concentrations and to a lesser extent by amino acids. Traditionally, insulin's role in metabolism has centered on its anabolic effects on body tissues by its positive action on lipogenesis in adipocytes and glucose disposal and resynthesis in skeletal muscle.[64] Less well understood is insulin's role in protein synthesis and amino acid transport.[71] We shall only highlight a few areas of interest including the most recent studies that aid in further defining insulin's role in protein synthesis as well as the interaction of exercise and gender on insulin regulation of metabolism. Further discussion of the effects of insulin upon carbohydrate metabolism is found in Chapter 6.

Recently, the role that insulin plays in protein anabolism is being redefined. For example, it has been suggested that insulin can affect the rate of protein synthesis in skeletal muscle under physiological conditions that alter protein mass (e.g., aging, disease, and exercise). It has been documented that age is associated with losses of muscle mass in both humans and animals. Accordingly, Fluckey et al.[72] examined whether insulin would elevate rates of protein synthesis in muscle following acute resistance exercise in elderly male, Fischer 344/BN FI rats, using the bilateral hindlimb perfusion technique. Rates of protein synthesis were assessed using a flooding dose protocol to measure incorporation of [3H] amino acids. It was found that rates of protein synthesis were higher following resistance exercise training in soleus muscle supplemented with physiological doses of insulin (6.5 ng · ml^{-1}). In addition, translational efficiency (rates of protein synthesis · unit of RNA^{-1} · h^{-1}) for gastrcocnemius muscle supplemented with insulin was also significantly greater.[72]

Some investigators have demonstrated insulin-regulated rates of protein synthesis in diabetic rodent models.[72,73,74] For example, Flaim et al.,[74] observed decrements in rates of protein synthesis in rat hindlimb resulting from reductions in insulin availability. The attenuated rates of protein synthesis occurred in muscles predominately composed of fast-twitch fibers and were quickly reversed by the administration of insulin. Insulin availability had little effect on rates of protein synthesis in slow-twitch muscle fibers. The mechanism(s) associated with insulin modulation of the rates of protein synthesis is not known but the hormone has potent actions at the level of peptide-chain initiation.[73]

Although these studies present strong evidence for the role of insulin in the regulation of protein synthesis in aged or diabetic muscles, it is not completely understood whether similar effects are evident in younger animals with normal (insulin responsive) muscle. Therefore Fluckey et al.[76] examined the effects of insulin on rates of protein synthesis in muscle following four days of resistance exercise in young, non-diabetic rats. Male rats were assessed for rates of protein synthesis using a bilateral hindlimb perfusion technique and a flooding dose protocol to measure incorporation of a [3H] amino acid. It was found that rates of protein synthesis in gastrocnemius and soleus were higher in the resistance exercised limb vs. the non-exercised limb only when supplemented with physiological doses of insulin (6.5 ng · ml^{-1}). In addition, rates of protein synthesis in the exercised limb without insulin were significantly lower vs. the non-exercised limb with or without insulin. Thus insulin appears to be a necessary component in elevated rates of protein synthesis under physiological conditions that perturb muscle protein mass.

Studies examining the potential role that gender may play on rates of protein synthesis have not been published. In fact, studies examining the interactions of gender and physiological perturbations of protein status on growth and body composition are not numerous. However, a gender dimorphism favoring females in terms of maintenance of muscle protein content in aged rats[78] and an attenuated muscle wasting following trauma[77] suggests that females may be better able to protect against loss of muscle mass. In support of this contention, two conditions that are known to affect protein metabolism, chronic endurance exercise and diabetes, will be described in Chapter 9.

In response to acute endurance exercise there is usually a progressive decrease in plasma insulin concentrations.[63,64,70] One study has found that females had an attenuation of the exercise induced decline during running exercise,[64] whereas other studies have found similar decreases for both genders in response to running[63] and cycling.[70] It has been demonstrated that females may have a greater receptor sensitivity to insulin as compared to males,[78] however, this appears to have a greater influence on its lipogenic effects.[79] In response to endurance exercise training, females show a greater increase in insulin sensitivity (+82%) as compared to males (+35%).[80]

In response to post-exercise glucose supplements (1 g/kg), the areas under the insulin/glucose curve (indicator of insulin sensitivity) are similar for males and females and the early (first four hours) rate of muscle glycogen re-synthesis is also similar between the genders.[70] We are not familiar with any gender comparative studies looking at the effects of glucose supplements given following resistance exercise. However, the resistance exercise induced a decrease in insulin concentration that was nearly identical to that seen in endurance exercise and the post-exercise area under the insulin and glucose curves was also similar between the two types of exercise.[81]

The only study that we are familiar with that measured plasma insulin concentrations in both trained and untrained males and females during endurance exercise found that neither gender nor training status affected the results.[63] Chronic endurance exercise training results in an enhanced ability to carbohydrate load, and it is well known that insulin sensitivity is increased following endurance training.[80] It is therefore critical to control for training status in gender comparative studies of insulin sensitivity. A comprehensive review of the adaptations of insulin sensitivity to exercise training is beyond the scope of this chapter.

We hope that future gender comparative studies of insulin effects in athletes consider some of the very exciting developments showing the difference in glucose transporter (GLUT 4) translocation between the insulin- (P-I-3 kinase) and contraction- (nitric oxide) stimulated glucose transport[82] mechanisms.

D. Catecholamines

The catecholamines are amino acid-based hormones that are released from the adrenal medulla and sympathetic nerve endings. Epinephrine and norepinephrine are the ones most often investigated; however, dopamine is also reported in some studies.[64,83] In general, these hormones stimulate lipolysis, glycogenolysis,[84] and may have anabolic effects[84,84] in human skeletal muscle. The potential for a gender difference in muscle and overall sympathetic activation will be discussed in more detail in Chapter 5, and as such we will highlight only a few points relevant to gender and exercise.

In both trained and untrained males and females, epinephrine and norepinephrine concentrations have been reported to increase progressively during exercise in a similar fashion.[63] Tarnopolsky and colleagues found that norepinephrine increased progressively for both males and females running 15.5 km, yet the epinephrine concentration was greater for the males in the later stages of exercise.[64] An interesting interaction was found for dopamine following exercise with a further increase for males and a decrease for females.[64] One other study measured the effects of isometric handgrip exercise upon plasma dopamine, norepinephrine, and epinephrine concentrations in both genders and found that the exercise induced increases for each catecholamine were attenuated for the females.[83]

In well-controlled longitudinal studies in males, it has been demonstrated that the exercise-induced catecholamine concentrations are attenuated.[86] It will be interesting to see whether similar observations are made in a recent longitudinal gender comparative study that we have completed in our laboratory in early 1998 (MacKenzie, S., unpublished, 1998).

Overall, the general impression of an attenuation in the catecholamine response to acute exercise for females emerges, which is consistent with the general findings reviewed in Chapter 5.

E. Miscellaneous Hormones

The thyroid hormones, triiodothyronine (T3) and thyroxine (T4), are amino acid-based hormones released from the thyroid gland in response to anterior pituitary derived thyroid stimulating hormone (TSH). Both T3 and T4 are critical to the overall regulation of metabolic rate and also affect protein turnover.[87,88] The major interest in the potential for a gender difference in the thyroid hormones came from investigations looking into the possibility for females to have enhanced energy conservation (See Chapters 9 and 10). One study found no difference in T3, T4, TSH, nor the inactive, reverse T3, between eumenorrheic and amenorrheic female runners.[48] Another study found that both free (unbound) T3 and free T4 were lower in amenorrheic runners as compared to eumenorrheic runners and sedentary controls.[51] Gender differences in thyroid hormones may also play a role in some of the gender differences in fiber characteristics outlined in Chapter 3. For example, T3 induced a translational or post-translational myosin heavy chain type IIA to type IIB conversion for female, but not male rats.[88]

Also relevant to gender differences in metabolism is the hormone leptin. This is covered in much detail in Chapter 9, however, there are some clear gender differences. Firstly, females have higher leptin concentrations even when matched for body fat percentage and total content.[80] Secondly, females show an attenuation of plasma leptin concentrations in response to endurance training whereas males show

Table 2.2 Summary of Hormonal Responses to Acute Exercise and Endurance Training

Hormone	Acute Exercise		Chronic Exercise	
	Males	Females	Males	Females
Estradiol	↑	↑	?	→, ↓
Progesterone	?	↑	?	→, ↓
Testosterone	↑	→	↑	↓
Insulin	↓↓	↓	increased sensitivity	
GH	↑	↑*	→	→
Cortisol	↑	↑	→(↓)	→
Epinephrine	↑↑	↑	↓	?↓
Leptin	→	→	→	↓

Note: Arrows indicate usual directional change. * = basal concentrations are higher in females and the responsitivity to exercise is greater in males.

no change.[80] The short-term (nine days) administration of 17-β-estradiol to males resulted in an increase in plasma leptin and there was a significant positive correlation between leptin and estrogen with no such relationship for plasma testosterone in spite of significant testosterone reductions (Carter, S. and Tarnopolsky, M. A., unpublished disertations, 1998). Leptin vs. estrogen, P <0.05; r = 0.54; leptin vs. testosterone, P > 0.05; r = 0.17, 1998.

The potential for there to be a significant effect of gender upon leptin metabolism is very high and we expect that many studies will be forthcoming in the next few years that will clarify the relationship between gender, leptin, fat metabolism, uncoupling proteins (Chapter 9), and energy metabolism.

Although traditionally considered autocrine or paracrine factors, the interleukins (IL) have an undeniable role in the inflammatory response and immunology and also have endocrine functions. There are very large gender differences in plasma IL-1 secretion with female basal mononuclear cell secretion rates an order of magnitude greater than for the males.[89] Furthermore, the IL-1 stimulation index,[89] and the IL-1 secreted agonist/antagonist ratios,[89] were greater for females in the luteal phase of the menstrual cycle. It will be very instructive to explore the potential relationships between these large gender differences in an important cytokine and the observations of lesser exercise induced muscle damage (Chapter 12) and oxidative stress (Chapter 11).

An overview of some of the gender differences in the hormonal responses to acute and chronic exercise training is summarized in Table 2.2.

REFERENCES

1. Jensen, J., Riis, B. J., Strøm, V., Nilas, M. D., and Christiansen, C., Long-term effects of percutaneous estrogens and oral progesterone on serum lipoproteins in postmenopausal women, *Am. J. Obstet. Gynecol.*, 156, 66, 1987.

2. Ettinger, B., Genant, H. K., and Cann, C. E., Postmenopausal bone loss is prevented by treatment with low-dosage estrogen with calcium, *Annals of Internal Med.,* 106, 40, 1987.

3. Bonen, A., Haynes, F. W., and Graham, T. E., Substrate and hormonal responses to exercise in women using oral contraceptives, *J. Appl. Physiol.,* 70(5), 1917, 1991.

4. Skouby, S. O., Kühl, C., Mølsted-Pedersen, L., Petersen, K., and Christensen, M. S., Triphasic oral contraception: metabolic effects in normal women and those with previous gestational diabetes, *Am. J. Obstet. Gynecol.,* 153, 495, 1985.

5. Bemben, D. A., Boileau, R. A., Bahr, J. M., Nelson, R. A., and Misner, J. E., Effects of oral contraceptives on hormonal and metabolic responses during exercise. *Med. Sci. Sports Exerc.,* 24(4), 434, 1992.

6. Kleiner, S. M., Performance-enhancing aids in sport: health consequences and nutritional alternatives, *Journal of the American College of Nutrition,* 10(2), 163, 1991.

7. Moffatt, R. J., Wallace, M. B., and Sady, S. P., Effects of anabolic steroids on lipoprotein profiles of female weight lifters, *The Physician and Sports Medicine,* 18(9), 106, 1990.

8. Speechly, D. P., Taylor, S. R., and Rogers, G. G., Differences in ultra-endurance exercise in performance-matched male and female runners, *Med. Sci. Sports Exerc.,* 28(3), 359, 1996.

9. Nicklas, B. J., Hackney, A. C., and Sharp, R. L., The menstrual cycle and exercise: performance, muscle glycogen, and substrate responses, *Int. J. Sports Med.,* 10, 264, 1989.

10. Fong, A. K. H. and Kretsch, M. J., Changes in dietary intake, urinary nitrogen, and urinary volume across the menstrual cycle, *Am. J. Clin. Nutr.,* 57, 43, 1993.

11. Guyton, A. C., Female reproduction before pregnancy and the female hormones, *Textbook of Medical Physiology (8th ed.),* W.B. Saunders, Philadelphia, 1991, 905.

12. Mahan, L. K. and Arlin, M., Weight management in *Food, Nutrition, and Diet Therapy,* Mahan, L. K. and Arlin, M., Eds., W.B. Saunders, Philadelphia, 1992, 319.

13. Rebuff-Scrive, M. L., Crona, N., Lonnroth, P., Abrahasson, L., Smith, U., and Bjorntorp, P., Fay cell meyabolism in different regions in women, *J. Clin. Invest.,* 75, 1973, 1985.

14. Wade, G. N. and Gray, J. M., Gonadal effects of food intake and adiposity: a metabolic hypothesis, *Physiol. Behav.,* 22, 583, 1979.

15. Gavin, M. L., Gray, J. M., and Johnson, P. R., Estrogen-induced effects on food intake and body weight in ovarietomized, partially lipoectomized rats, *Physiol Behav.,* 32(1), 55, 1984.

16. Eisenfeld, A. J., Aten, R., Weinberger, M., Haselbacher, G., Halpern, K., and Ktakoff, L., Estrogen receptor in the mammalian liver, *Science,* 191, 862, 1976.

17. Costrini, N. V. and Kalkhoff, R. K., Relative effects of preganancy, estradiol, and progesterone on plasma insulin and pancreatic islet insulin secretion, *J. Clin. Invest.,* 50, 992, 1971.

18. Matute, M. L. and Kalkhoff, R. K., Sex steroid influence on hepatic gluconeogenesis and liver glycogen formation, *Endocrinology,* 92, 762, 1973.

19. Wade, G. N., Gray, J. M., and Bartness, T. J., Gonadal influences on adiposity, *Int. J. Obes.,* 9(1), 83, 1985.

20. Dudley, S. D., Gentry, T., Silverman, B. S., and Wade, G. N., Estradiol and insulin: independent effects of eating and body weight in rats, *Physiol. Behav.,* 22(1), 63, 1979.

21. Wade, G. N. and Gray, J. M., Cytoplasmic 17β-[3H]-estradiol binding in rat adipose tissues, *Endocrinology,* 103, 1695, 1978.

22. Gray, J. M., Dudley, S. D., and Wade, G. N., In vivo nuclear uptake of 17β-[³H] estradiol in rat adipose tissues, *Am. J. Physiol.,* 240, E43, 1981.

23. Hansen, F. M., Fahmy, and Neilson, J. H., The influence of sexual hormones on lipogenesis and lipolysis in rat fat cell, *Acta Endocrinol.,* 46, 279, 1964.

25. Etgen, A. M., Differential effects of two estrogen antagonists on the development of masculine and feminine sexual behaviour in hamsters, *Physiol. & Behav.,* 15, 299, 1981.

26. Ganong, W. F., The gonads: development and function of the reproductive system, *Review of Medical Physiology (16th ed.),* Lange Medical Publications, Los Altos, 1993, 400.

27. Rhoades, R. and Pflanzer, R., The Pituitary Gland, in *Human Physiology,* Rhoades, R. and Pflanzer, R., Eds., Saunders College Publishing, Philadelphia, 1989, 403.

28. Galletti, F. and Klopper, A., The effect of progesterone on the quantity and distribution of body fat in the female rat, *Acta Endocrinol.,* 46, 379, 1964.

29. Kim, H. J. and Kalkoff, R. K., Sex steroid influence on triglyceride metabolism, *J. Clin. Invest.,* 56, 888, 1975.

30. Gray, J. M. and Wade, G. N., Cytoplasmic progestins binding in rat adipose tissues, *Endocrinology,* 104, 1377, 1979.

31. Griffen, J. E. and Wilson, J. D., Disorders of the testes and male reproductive tract, J. D. Wilson and D. W. Foster (Eds.), *Williams Textbook of Endocrinology (7th ed.),* W.B. Saunders, Philadelphia, 1985, 239.

32. Blizzard, R. M., Martha, P. M., Kerrigan, J. R., Marus, N., and Rogol, A. D., Changes in growth hormone (GH) secretion and in growth during puberty. *J. Endocrinol. Invest.,* 12(Suppl. 3), 65, 1989.

33. Klibanski, A., Beitins, I. Z., Badger, T., Little, R., and McArthur, J. W., Reproductive function during fasting in men, *J. Clin. Endocrinol.,* 53(2), 258.

34. Smith, S. R., Chetri, M. K., Johanson, J., Radfar, N., and Migeon, C. J., The pituitary-gonadal axis in men with protein-calorie malnutrition, *J. Clin. Endocrinol. Metab.,* 41, 60, 1975.

35. Rodjmark, S., Influence of short-term fasting on the pituitary-testicular axis in normal men, *Hormone Research,* 25, 140, 1967.

36. Gustafsson, J. A., Pousette, A., Stenberg, A., and Wrange, O., High-affinity binding of 4-androstene-3,17-dione in rat liver, *Biochemistry,* 14, 3942, 1975.

37. Dube, J. Y., Lesage, R., and Tremblay, R. R., Androgen and estrogen binding in rat skeletal and perineal muscles, *Can. J. Biochem.,* 54, 50, 1976.

38. Powers, M. L. and Florini, J. R., A direct effect of testosterone on muscle cells in tissue culture, *Endocrinology,* 97, 1043, 1975.

39. Gentry, R. T. and Wade, G. N., Androgenic control of food intake and body weight in male rats, *J. Comp. Physiol. Psychol.,* 90, 18, 1976.

40. Hervey, G. R. and Hutchinson, I., The effects of testosterone on body weight and composition in the rat, *J. Endocrinol.,* 577, 24–25, 1973.

41. Nimrod, A. and Ryan, K. J., Aromatization of androgens by human abdominal and breast tissue, *J. Clin. Endocrinol. Metab.,* 40, 367, 1975.

42. Drori, D. and Folman, Y., Effects of cohabitation on the reproductive system, kidneys, and body composition, *J. Reprod. Fert.,* 8, 351, 1964.

43. Hoskins, R. G., Studies in vigor: II. The effect of castration on voluntary activity. *Am. J. Physiol.,* 72, 324, 1925.

44. Roy, E. J. and Wade, G. N., Role of food intake in estradiol-induced body weight changes in female rats, *Horm. & Behav.,* 8, 265, 1977.

45. Baker, E. R., Menstrual dysfunction and hormonal status in athletic women: a review, *Fertility and Sterility,* 36(6), 1981.

46. Bonen, A., Campagna, P., Gilchrist, L., Young, D. C., and Beresford, P., Substrate and endocrine responses during exercise at selected stages of pregnancy, *J. Appl. Physiol.,* 73(1), 134, 1992.

47. Sinning, W. E. and Little, K. D., Body composition and menstrual function in athletes, *Sports Medicine,* 4, 34, 1987.

48. Wilmore, J. H., Wambsgans, K. C., Brenner, M., Broeder, C. E., Paijmans, I., Volpe, J. A., and Wilmore, K. M., Is there energy conservation in amenorrheic compared with eumenorrheic distance runners? *J. Appl. Physiol.,* 72(1), 15, 1992.

49. Rogol, A.D., Weltman, A., Weltman, J. Y., Seip, R. L., Snead, D. B., Levine, S., Haskvitz, E. M., Thompson, D. L., Schurrer, R., Dowling, E., Walberg-Rankin, J., Evans, W. S., and Velhuis, J. D., Durability of the reproductive axis in eumenorrheic women during one year of endurance training, *J. Appl. Physiol.,* 72(4), 1571, 1992.

50. Snead, D. B., Weltman, A., Weltman, J. Y., Evans, W. S., Veldhuis, J. D., Varma, M. M., Teates, D., Dowling, E. A., and Rogol, A. D., Reproductive hormones and bone mineral density in women runners, *J. Appl. Physiol.,* 72(6), 2149, 1992.

51. Baer, J. T., Endocrine parameters in amenorrheic and eumenorrheic adolescent female runners, *Int. J. Sports Med.,* 14, 191, 1993.

52. Kraemer, W., Marchitelli, J., Gordon, L., Harman, S. E., Dziados, E. J. E., Mello, R., Frykman, P., McCurry, D., and Fleck, S. J., Hormonal and growth factor responses to heavy resistance exercise protocols, *J. Appl. Physiol.,* 69(4), 1442, 1990.

53. Volek, J. S., Kraemar, W. J., Bush, J. A., Incledon, T., and Boetes, M., Testosterone and cortisol in relationship to dietary nutrients and resistance exercise, *J. Appl. Physiol.,* 82(1), 49, 1997.

54. Häkkinen, K. and Pakarinen, A., Acute hormonal responses to heavy resistance exercise in men and women at different ages, *Int. J. Sports Med.,* 16(8), 507, 1995.

55. Keizer, H., Janssen, G. M. E., Menheere, P., and Kranenburg, G., Changes in basal plasma testosterone, cortisol, and dehydroepiandrosterone sulfate in previously untrained males and females preparing for a marathon, *Int. J. Sports Med.,* 10, S139, 1989.

56. Häkkinen, K., Pakarinen, A., Alen, M., Kauhanen, H., and Komi, P. V., Neuromuscular and hormonal adaptations in athletes to strength training in two years, *J. Appl. Physiol.,* 65(6), 2406, 1988.

57. Staron, R. S., Karapondo, D. L., Kraemer, W. J., Fry, A. C., Gordon, S. E., Falkel, J. E., Hagerman, F. C., and Hikida, R. S., Skeletal muscle adaptations during early phase of heavy-resistance training in men and women, *J. Appl. Physiol.,* 76, 1247, 1994.

58. Chakmakjian, Z. H. and Bethune, J. E., Study of human growth hormone response to insulin, vasopressin, exercise, and estrogen administration, *J. Lab. Clin. Med.,* 72(3), 1968.

59. Butterfield, G. E., Thompson, J., Rennie, M. J., Marcus, R., Hintz, R. L., and Hoffman, A. R., Effect of rhGH and rhIGF-I treatment on protein utilization in elderly women, *Am. J. Physiol.* 272 (*Endocrinol. Metab.* 35), E94, 1997.

60. Rudman, D., Feller, A. G., Nagraj, H. S., Gergans, G. A., Lalitha, P. Y., Goldberg, A. F., Schlenker, R. A., Cohn, L., Rudman, I. W., and Mattson, D. E., Effects of human growth hormone in men over 60 years old, *The New England Journal of Medicine,* 323(1), 1, 1990.

61. Cuneo, R. C., Salomon, F., Wiles, C. M., Hesp, R., and Sönksen, P. H., Growth hormone treatment growth hormone-deficient adults. I. Effects of muscle mass and strength, *J. Appl. Physiol.,* 70(2), 688, 1991.

62. Bunt, J. C., Boileau, R. A., Bahr, J. M., and Nelson, R. A., Sex and training differences in human growth hormone levels during prolonged exercise, *J. Appl. Physiol.*, 61(5), 1796, 1986.

63. Friedmann, B. and Kindermann, W., Energy metabolism and regulatory hormones in women and men during endurance exercise, *Eur. J. Appl. Physiol.*, 59, 1, 1989.

64. Tarnopolsky, L. J., MacDougall, J. D., Atkinson, S. A., Tarnopolsky, M. A., and Sutton, J. R., Gender differences in substrate for endurance exercise, *J. Appl. Physiol.*, 68, 302, 1990.

65. Kanaley, J. A., Boileau, R. A., Bahr, J. A., Misner, J. E., and Nelson, R. A., Substrate oxidation and GH responses to exercise are independent of menstrual phase and status, *Med. Sci. Sports Exerc.*, 24(8), 873, 1992.

66. Barbarino, A., De Marinis, L., Mancini, A., D'Amico, C., Passeri, M., Zuppi, P., Sambo, P., and Tofani, A., Sex-related naloxone influence on growth hormone-releasing hormone-induced growth hormone secretion in normal subjects, *Metabolism*, 36(2), 105, 1987.

67. Sutton, J. R. and Casey, J. H., The adrenocortical response to competitive athletics in veteran athletes, *J. Clin. Endocrinol. Metab.*, 40, 135, 1975.

68. Staessen, J., Fiocchi, R., Bouillon, R., Fagard, R., Lunen, P., Moerman, E., De Schaepdryver, A., and Amery, A., The nature of opioid involvement in the hemodynamic respiratory and humoral responses to exercise, *Circulation*, 72(5), 982, 1985.

69. Czerwinski, S. M. and Hickson, R. C., Glucocorticoid receptor activation during exercise in muscle, *J. Appl. Physiol.*, 68(4), 1615, 1990.

70. Tarnopolsky, M. A., Bosman, M., MacDonald, J. R., Vandeputte, D., Martin, J., and Roy, B. D., Postexercise protein-carbohydrate and carbohydrate supplements increase muscle glycogen in men and women. *J. Appl. Physiol.*, 83(6), 1877, 1997.

71. Biolo, G., Fleming, R. Y. D., and Wolfe, R. R., Physiological hyperinsulinemia stimulates protein synthesis and enhances transport of selected amino acids in human skeletal muscle, *J. Clin. Invest.*, 95, 811, 1995.

72. Fluckey, J. D., Vary, T. C., Jefferson, L. S., and Farrell, P. A., Augmented insulin action on rates of protein synthesis after resistance exercise in rats, *Am. J. Physiol.*, 270 (*Endocrinol. Metab.*, 33), E313-E319, 1996).

73. Karinch, A. M., Kimball, S. R., Vary, T. C., and Jefferson, L. S., Regulation of eukaryotic initiation factor-2B activity in muscle of diabetic rats, *Am. J. Physiol.*, 264 (*Endocrinol. Metab.*, 27), E101-E108, 1993.

74. Flaim, K. E., Copenhaver, M. E., and Jefferson, L. S., Effects of diabetes on protein synthesis in fast- and slow-twitch rat skeletal muscle, *Am. J. Physiol.*, 289 (*Endocrinol. Metab.*, 2): E88-E95, 1980.

75. Flaim, K. E., Kochel, P. J., Kira, Y., Kobayashi, K., Fossel, E. T., Jefferson, L. S., and Morgan, H. E., Insulin effects on protein synthesis are independent of glucose and energy metabolism, *Am. J. Physiol.*, 245 (*Cell Physiol.*, 14): C133-C143, 1983.

76. Fluckey, J. D., Vary, T. C., Jefferson, L. S., Evans, W. J., and Farrell, P. A., Insulin stimulation of protein synthesis in rat skeletal muscle following resistance exercise is maintained with advancing age, *J. Gerontol.*, 51A(5), B323-B330, 1996.

77. Yang, Q. and Birkhahn, R. H., Metabolic rate and nitrogen balance after skeletal trauma in female and male rats. *Nutrition*, 95(5): 433-438, 1993.

78. Nuutila, P., Knuuti, M. J., Mäki, M., Laine, H., Ruotsalainen, U., Teräs, M., Haaparanta, M., Solin, O., and Yki-Järvinen, H., Gender and insulin sensitivity in the heart and in skeletal muscles, *Diabetes*, 44, 31, 1995.

79. Rebuffe-Scrive, M., Enk, L., Crona, N., Lönnroth, P., Abrahamsson, L., Smith, U., and Bjomtorp, P., Fat cell metabolism in different regions in women, *J. Clin. Invest.,* 75, 1973, 1985.

80. Hickey, M., Houmard, J. A., Considine, R. V., Tyndall, G. L., Midgette, J. B., Gavigan, K. E., Weidner, M. L., McCammon, M. R., Israel, R. G., and Caro, J. E., Gender-dependent effects of exercise training on serum leptin levels in humans, *Am. J. Physiol.,* 272 (*Endocrinol. Metab.,* 35), E562, 1997.

81. Roy, B. D., Tarnopolsky, M. A., MacDougall, J. D., Fowles, J., and Yarasheski, K. E., Effect of glucose supplement timing on protein metabolism after resistance exercise, *J. Appl. Physiol.,* 82(6), 1882, 1997.

82. Roberts, C. K., Barnard, R. J., Scheck, S. H., and Balon, T. W., Exercise-stimulated glucose transport is skeletal muscle in nitric oxide dependent, *Am. J. Physiol.,* 273 (*Endocrinol. Metab.,* 36), E220, 1997.

83. Sanchez, J., Pequignot, J. M., Peyrin, L., and Monod, J., Sex differences in the sympatho-adrenal response to isometric exercise, *Eur. J. Appl. Physiol.,* 45, 147, 1980.

84. Fryberg, D. A., Gelfand, R. A., Jahn, L. A., Oliveras, D., Sherwin, R. S., Sacca, L., and Barrett, E. J., Effects of epinephrine on human muscle glucose and protein metabolism, *Am. J. Physiol.,* 268 (*Endocrinol. Metab.,* 31), E55, 1995.

85. del Prato, S., DeFronzo, R. A., Castellino, P., Wahren, J., and Alvestrand, A., Regulation of amino acid metabolism by epinephrine, *Am. J. Physiol.,* 258 (*Endocrinol. Metab.,* 21), E878, 1990.

86. Phillips, S. M., Green, H. J., Tarnopolsky, M. A., Heigenhauser, G. J. R., Hill, R. E., and Grant, S. M., Effects of training duration on substrate turnover and oxidation during exercise., *J. Appl. Physiol.,* 81(5), 2182, 1996.

87. Jepson, M. M., Bates, P. C., and Millward, D. J., The role of insulin and thyroid hormones in the regulation of muscle growth and protein turnover in response to dietary protein in the rat, *British Journal of Nutrition,* 59, 397, 1988.

88. Larsson, L. and Yu, F., Gender-related differences in the regulatory influence of thyroid hormone on the expression of myosin isoforms in young and old rats, *Acta. Physiol. Scand.,* 159, 81, 1997.

89. Lynch, E. A., Dinarello, C. A., and Cannon, J. G., Gender differences in IL-1β, and IL-1 receptor antagonist secretion from mononuclear cells and urinary excretion, *The Journal of Immunology,* 153, 300, 1994.

90. Cannon, J. G. and Dinarello, C. A., Increased plasma interleukin-1 activity in women after ovulation, *Science,* 227, 1247, 1985.

CHAPTER 3

Gender Differences in Skeletal Muscle Histology and Ultrastructure

Katherine Chorneyko, M.D., F.R.C.P.(C) and
Jacqueline Bourgeois, M.D., F.R.C.P.(C)

CONTENTS

I. INTRODUCTION

Skeletal muscle is approximately 40 to 50% of total mammalian body weight. Muscle cells or fibers are structurally designed to convert chemical energy into mechanical work and they can undergo a variety of structural adaptations in response to different stresses and stimuli. Skeletal muscle fibers essentially consist of a highly ordered array of proteins, which interact in order to shorten the muscle fiber as necessary. The structure of muscle fibers and their constituent proteins are intimately related to their function. Based on histochemical ATPase staining three main fiber groups are readily identified. Type I fibers contract slowly and are resistant to fatigue. They are predominantly responsible for sustained activity and characteristically contain higher levels of intra-mitochondrial oxidative enzymes (succinyl dehydrogenase, NADH-TR). Correspondingly, they have a high lipid and mitochondrial content with a relatively low glycogen content. Type IIb fibers are capable of powerful actions: they contract quickly but have a low resistance to fatigue. They tend to be larger in size than Type I fibers (at least in males) but they have relatively lower lipid and mitochondrial content as well as lower oxidative enzyme levels. They have a higher glycogen content than Type I fibers and are considered glycolytic. Type IIa fibers are essentially a hybrid with both oxidative and glycolytic characteristics. They contain abundant glycogen and mitochondria but less lipid than Type I fibers. They are intermediate between Type I and Type IIb fibers with respect to their speed of contraction and resistance to fatigue.

The study of skeletal muscle structure at the light or electron microscopic level can give us insights about function. For example, fibers which have increased mitochondrial content, may have increased their oxidative and aerobic activity. In fact, a linear correlation has been found between mitochondrial volume and the maximal rate of oxygen consumption.[1] Therefore, the study of morphologic relationships and changes in these relationships under a variety of conditions can give us information regarding the function of skeletal muscle under these conditions.

II. THE MUSCLE BIOPSY FOR LIGHT AND ELECTRON MICROSCOPY

In order to study muscle optimally, proper acquisition of samples is essential. The muscle biopsy is obtained by first anaesthetizing the skin and subcutaneous tissue with local anaesthetic (lidocaine). A small incision is made in the skin and fascia over the muscle to be sampled. The Bergström needle with sliding trochar is commonly used.[2] The needle is introduced into the muscle and a small piece is clipped off using the cutting edge of the trochar. Approximately 20 to 30 mg of fresh muscle tissue can be obtained from a single pass in a healthy individual. Once obtained, the tissue can be allocated for biochemical studies, electron microscopy (EM), and light microscopy (LM). The tissue for light microscopy is oriented, using a dissecting microscope, in order to obtain a good cross section. It is then rapidly frozen in isopentane and liquid nitrogen and stored at −70°C in order to preserve enzyme activity and minimize freezing artifact. The frozen tissue is cut in a cryostat with sections varying from 7–10 μm in thickness. The routine hematoxylin and eosin (H&E) stain can give information regarding fiber size, capillary network, and the presence or absence of inflammation (Figure 3.1a); however, other histochemical stains, in particular enzyme reactions, are more informative for most studies of muscle, especially in pathological states. The most commonly used stains in physiologic studies are the ATPase stains. Fiber types can be determined by performing the stains at various pHs. Adenosine triphosphatase is a hydrolase enzyme and catalyzes the reaction:[3]

$$ATP + water \rightarrow ADP + orthophosphate$$

Table 3.1   Muscle Biopsy Histochemical Stains and Electron Microscopy

Determination	Light Microscopy	Semi-Thins (Toluidine Blue Stained)	Electron Microscopy
Fiber Morphology	Good with Hematoxylin and Eosin	Good	For fine structural details only
Glycogen	PAS*	Possible with PAS stain	Yes, directly seen
Lipid	Oil red O Sudan Black	Yes, directly seen	Yes, directly seen
Fiber Type and Distribution	ATPase pH 4.3, 4.6, and 10.0	Limited information	Fiber type only
Mitochondria	Modified Gormori Trichrome	Limited information	Good
Enzymes Distribution and Activity	NADH-TR*, SDH*, MADA*, COX*, Acid phosphatase, Alkaline phosphatase	No	No
Cytoskeletal	IHC* for Desmin, Vimentin Myosin, Actin	No	Possibly with IEM*
Damage	IHC* for Ubiquitin, HSP*, NOS*	Yes	Possibly with IEM*

Note: PAS = periodic acid schiff, IEM = immunoelectron microscopy, MADA = Myoadenylate deaminase, ATPase = Adenosine triphosphatase, COX = Cytochrome oxidase, NADH-TR = Nicotinamide adenine dinucleotide-tetrazolium reductase, SDH = Succinate dehydrogenase, HSP = Heat Shock Protein, IHC = Immunohistochemistry.

The released phosphate then can bind to calcium in solution and precipitates calcium phosphate formation. The Type I fibers are dark when performed at pH 4.3, and light at pH 4.6 and 10. The Type II a, b fibers are dark at pH 10.0 (Figure 3.1 c, d). To differentiate the two, the stain is performed at pH 4.6. The Type I fibers are light, Type IIb fibers are dark, and the Type IIa fibers are intermediate. The use of this stain not only helps identify the fiber type but provides information regarding their percent distribution and cross sectional area. The histochemical stains most commonly used for physiological studies are summarized in Table 3.1. Most sections are obtained serially to compare and contrast the differences in fibers with different stains (Figures 3.1 and 3.2).

More recently, immunohistochemistry has become an important adjunct in the study of muscle pathology (Figure 3.3). The principle of immunohistochemistry (IHC) is based on the availability of specific antibodies to cellular antigens. A muscle tissue section is initially incubated with a primary antibody (monoclonal or polyclonal) against the antigen of interest. After incubation, the unbound antibody is washed away. Then, a second biotin-conjugated antibody against the primary antibody is incubated with the section. The unbound secondary antibody is then washed away. The final bound antibody is incubated with avidin-biotin peroxidase enzyme to produce a colorimetric reaction which can be visualized on the tissue section

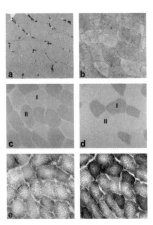

Figure 3.1 Serial cross-sections of skeletal muscle fibers from vastus lateralis (×250) of normal
untrained male. a) H & E; b) PAS; c) ATPase at pH 10.0; d) ATPase at pH 4.3; e)
NADH.TR; f) SDH.

(Figure 3.3a). This method of visualization is the most commonly used; however,
visualization can be obtained using other methods such as immunofluorescence.

Immunohistochemistry is routinely used in diagnostic pathology and the number
of antibodies available to various biologically important cellular proteins has become
enormous. The potential use of such technology in skeletal muscle research, specifically to investigate gender differences, is substantial. Some of the currently available
antibodies that may be potentially useful include different isoforms of myosin (fetal,
neonatal, slow, and fast), cytoskeletal proteins (desmin, dystrophin, and vimentin)
(Figure 3.4a), novel enzymes and proteins (nitric oxide synthetase, NOS; heat shock
protein, HSP; and ubiquitin), and inflammatory cells (leukocyte common antigen,
LCA; CD20, a B cell marker; and CD3, a T cell marker). These techniques could
be used to determine not only gender differences in structure but also to demonstrate
potential gender differences in tissue development, responses to injury and adaptations to stress.

For routine transmission electron microscopic studies, as soon as the biopsy
tissue is available, a small portion should be placed immediately in cold buffered
glutaraldehyde. Longitudinal portions of muscle measuring approximately 1–2 cm
in length by 1–2 mm^2 are ideal as tissue portions of this size will allow for adequate
penetration of fixative in one hour. After fixation in glutaraldehyde the tissue portions
can be trimmed to 1–2 mm^3 for either longitudinal or cross-sectional embedding.
Two percent glutaraldehyde buffered with 0.1% sodium cacodylate gives very good

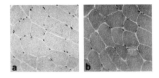

Figure 3.2 Serial cross-sections of skeletal muscle fibres from vastus lateralis (×250) of normal
untrained male. a) Oil reol O; b) Gomori trichome.

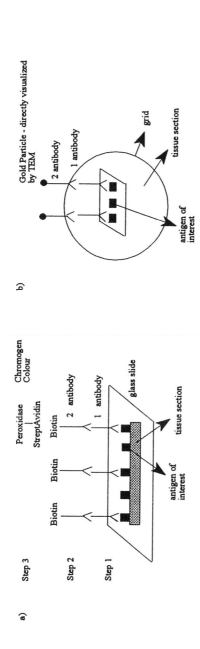

Figure 3.3 Schematic representation of immunolocalization methods: a) immunohistochemical method using streptavidin/biotin and peroxidase system; b) immunoelectron microscopic technique using gold particles which can be directly visualized under the transmission electron microscope.

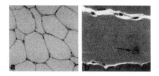

Figure 3.4 Serial cross-sections of skeletal muscle fibers from vastus lateralis. a) normal untrained male, dystrophin, (×400); b) normal acutely trained male with Z band streaming, Toluidine blue semi-thin section (×600).

ultrastructural preservation. The tissue is then post fixed in 1% osmium tetroxide, dehydrated in graded alcohols and embedded in a plastic resin, e.g., Spurr's or Epon. Semi-thin sections (approximately 0.5 um in thickness) are cut using a glass knife and stained with Toluidine blue for light microscopic evaluation (Figure 3.4b). With resin embedded, material shrinkage is minimal compared to paraffin embedded or frozen cryostat sections so that many fine details can be resolved even at the light microscopic level. In addition, Toluidine blue-stained sections allow lipid droplets and mast cell granules to be easily visualized. An area of interest can be chosen from the semi-thin sections. The tissue is trimmed to this area and a thin section (approximately 50 to 60 nm in thickness) is cut using a diamond knife. The thin sections are placed on a copper grid and stained with uranyl acetate and lead citrate for transmission electron microscopic examination.

For EM evaluation, muscle fibers can be embedded longitudinally or in cross section depending on the type of features being assessed. Longitudinal sections allow the sarcomere to be well visualized for the assessment of Z and M bandwidth. T-tubules are best assessed longitudinally. The capillary network in skeletal muscle is, for the most part, longitudinally orientated; therefore, morphometric data in regard to capillaries is best assessed in cross sections. Fiber typing, however, cannot be done on cross sections.[4]

Many variations and modifications to the routine EM procedure can be done depending on the questions being addressed. For example, glycogen can be high-lighted by addition of potassium ferrous cyanide to the fixation process or post fixation by treatment of thin sections with periodic acid-thiosemicarbazide-silver proteinate.[5,6] For immunoelectron microscopic studies, the issue must be handled differently in order to preserve antigenicity. Glutaraldehyde may be used; however, some antigens may be destroyed and frozen material may be necessary. In addition, plastic resins such as Spurr's or Epon destroy antigens necessitating the use of other embedding resins such as methacrylate or LR white. The basic principle of immu-noelectron microscopy is outlined in Figure 3.3b. An antibody is allowed to interact with an antigen on a thin section. A secondary antibody against the primary antibody of interest is tagged with a gold particle, and it is this gold particle which is visualized by transmission electron microscopy. It is a very elegant way to localize antigens to various cell compartments or organelles; however, it requires considerable time and patience as a number of modifications or variations of the technique might be necessary since antibodies may react differently and antigens are variably expressed and preserved.

In general, light microscopy using histochemical stains has the advantage of a greater sampling area compared to electron microscopy. However subcellular details and changes in organelles can only be assessed at the electron microscopic level. Therefore each technique is of value depending on the nature of the issues being addressed.

III. HISTOLOGIC GENDER DIFFERENCES

An individual muscle cell is also termed a muscle fiber. It can measure up to 10 cm in length and contains multiple nuclei. Individual cells are arranged in a bundle and held together by a fine collagenous support network (endomysium) to form fascicles. A more extensive collagenous network called perimysium further supports groups of fascicles. Most muscles are made of many fascicles, in which each group is surrounded by a dense collagenous sheath called the epimysium. Other structures essential to muscle function include nerves, blood vessels, and lymphatics.

During embryogenesis primitive myoblasts proliferate. At one point they fuse to form multinucleated cells called myotubes. Once fused, the contractile apparatus is produced. At birth much of the muscle mosaic development is completed and is similar to that seen in adults. A few major changes, however, occur after birth and before adulthood. The distribution of Type IIc cells (satellite, undifferentiated) decrease from approximately 20% in neonates to 1–2% in adults.[7] In addition, many of the Type IIa fibers convert to IIb during early childhood.[7]

Most morphologic studies of skeletal muscle in relation to function and gender differences have centered on fiber type, size, and fiber type distribution in men among different muscle groups. Johnson et al.[8] in a series of autopsies carried out one of the earliest, most extensive studies looking at muscle fiber distribution in men. They examined several muscle groups and found that postural muscle groups such as the *soleus* and *anterior tibialis* had a significantly higher number of Type I fibers (87% and 73%, respectively). The *rectus femoris* had a predominance of Type II fibers (70%) as did the brachial triceps (60 to 80%). The more commonly biopsied muscle groups showed less dramatic differences; for example, in the *vastus lateralis,* Type I fibers were 38% and in the *biceps brachii,* Type I were 42%. The authors expected to see such structural differences since they reflect the different functions these muscle groups perform. Postural muscle groups could be expected to have more Type I fibers for the sustained activity required to maintain an upright position.

Morphologic changes are known to occur with different modes of exercise. For example, in endurance sports, there is little change in fiber size but there appears to be an increase in Type I and IIa fibers over Type IIb fibers.[1,4,9] In contrast, resistance training has been shown to cause an increase in fiber size but few changes in fiber distribution.[10] Similar changes have been seen in women;[11,12] however, systematic investigations into gender differences have only been undertaken in a few studies. Some of the more commonly evaluated parameters in these studies have included distribution of fiber types (I/II ratio, %), and muscle fiber cross sectional area (CSA).

A. Differences in Fiber Distribution and Area in Untrained Individuals

Studies examining gender differences in muscle structure have been limited. Most studies have small numbers, biopsy different muscle groups, or compare both untrained and trained individuals together.

A study by Brooke and Engel[13] was one of the earliest to compare men and women. They examined 37 men and 66 women. The subjects were from three groups: Fifty-six were from asymptomatic relatives of neuromuscular patients, 29 were neuromuscular patients without symptoms, and 18 had organic disorders. They compared both the *biceps brachii* and *vastus lateralis* in men and women. They found that the percent of Type I/II fibers in the *biceps brachii* and *vastus lateralis* was higher in women (% ratio 0.9% in females and % ratio 0.6% in males in both muscle groups). The overall size of the Type II fibers was larger in men in both the *biceps brachii* and *vastus lateralis*. They also found that Type II fibers were larger than Type I in men in both muscle groups while the reverse was seen in women (particularly *biceps brachii*).

Later, Costill et al.[10] examined a group of untrained individuals (11 men and 10 women) and athletes (23 men and 17 women). They biopsied the *gastrocnemius*. In untrained individuals, they found that men had a higher ratio of Type I fibers (% ratio 1.15%) compared to women (% ratio 0.98%). The overall area of Type I fiber was greater than Type II fibers in men, while the opposite was seen in women. These results are the opposite to those previously noted by Brooke & Engel,[13] however, this can be partially attributed to the different muscle biopsied (*gastrocnemius*). That the overall cross sectional area of all fibers was smaller in women than men supports the previous study.

In 1978, Komi and Karlsson[14] examined gender differences in twin groups. Biopsies from the *vastus lateralis* of 20 men and 11 women were examined. Here the men tended to have a higher percent of Type I fibers (55.9%) than women (49.1%) but also had a wider range in fiber size.

Simoneau et al.[15] biopsied the *vastus lateralis* in 418 individuals. There were 270 sedentary and 148 active individuals. Men and women were equally distributed between groups. Unfortunately both the active and sedentary subjects were examined together as one gender group. Even so, their results were similar in the *vastus lateralis* to those previously seen by Brooke and Engel[13] but are in contrast to those seen by Komi and Karlsson.[14] The men had larger fibers than women. The women had a slightly higher number of Type I fibers than men. They also examined the glycolytic potential via measurement of glycolytic enzyme activities, and as expected, the activities were slightly lower in females than males. This may be due to the overall larger cross-sectional area of Type II fibers in men.

Finally, Miller et al.[16] examined eight women and eight men. They also had a mix of active, resistance trained, and sedentary individuals. The *biceps brachii* and *vastus lateralis* were biopsied. The men had a higher proportion of Type II fibers in the *vastus lateralis* as compared to women. In the *biceps brachii,* men had a larger area of Type I fibers than women, and in the *vastus lateralis,* men had a larger area of Type II fibers.

A few conclusions can be drawn from these studies even though the results in some instances are conflicting. In general, women have smaller muscle fibers than men. Gender differences seem to be more pronounced in the *biceps brachii* than in the *vastus lateralis*. It also appears that women may have a tendency to have more Type I fibers than Type II fibers especially in the *biceps brachii* although not all the studies support this observation.

B. Differences in Fiber Distribution and Area in Endurance and Resistance Training

It has been established that different types of training can alter fiber type distribution and size. A few studies have examined the effects of endurance exercise exclusively in women. Nygaard,[17] examined 54 women: 25 were sedentary, 20 were active, and 9 were endurance athletes. In the *vastus lateralis* of the runners and the deltoid of the swimmers, the Type I fibers were 60% of the total fiber distribution. Also, the Type I fibers of the *vastus lateralis* were larger than Type II fibers. This is in contrast to men who have a tendency to have larger Type II fibers than Type I fibers.[13]

Costill et al.[10] did look at the differences between men and women athletes. In this study, the only large group with both genders was that of the middle-distance runners (seven males and seven females). No women were in the long distance runner group. They found that the middle distance female runners had a higher percent of Type I fibers compared to men (60.6% vs. 51.9% respectively) but had a similar CSA (6099 vs. 6069 μm^2 respectively in the *gastrocnemius*). They suggested that the men had a greater individual fiber diameter which explains why the overall CSA is similar in both men and women. On average, both trained males and females had larger fibers (I and II) compared to sedentary individuals.

A more recent study by Howald et al.[18] took 10 untrained individuals (five males and five females) and trained them for six weeks. One person from each group continued for 24 weeks. They found that training increased the percent of Type I fibers (12%) and the volume of mitochondria per fiber. They did not comment on the difference in the increase of Type I fiber and decline of Type IIb fibers between genders.

Kuipers et al.[19] examined 21 men and eight women. In this study, the subjects underwent endurance training for a total of 18–20 months. After the first six month interval, a set of biopsies were taken from the *vastus lateralis*. They took the first biopsy five days before a 15 km race, 0.5 to 6 hours post race then 8 to 9 days post race. In the first set (five days pre-race [15 km]), men had 43% Type I fibers, and women had 49% Type I fibers. They did not find a significant difference between men and women with respect to diameter or fiber distribution in the subsequent biopsies. They did find subtle degenerative changes at the later stages of endurance training. Unfortunately, no biopsies were taken before the training program was initiated.

From these studies, endurance training tends to favor Type I fiber changes as compared to Type IIb in both men and women. This may be partially due to genetic selection as well as adaptation and it is still controversial whether these changes are due to hypertrophy or hyperplasia. Men probably still maintain slightly larger fibers in the *vastus lateralis* even after long periods of endurance training, although this is not directly supported by Kuipers et al.[19] The results of Simoneau et al.[15] and Miller et al.,[16] with both active and untrained individuals, suggest that this may be the case. This is another area which is still controversial. A pre- and post-long term endurance training study would clarify whether there are gender-specific differences in muscle fiber adaptations. Of course, the difficulty in identifying differences in these well-trained groups may be related to the menstrual cycle disruption which occurs at this level of activity (Chapter 2).

In terms of resistance training, the most direct gender study is by Alway et al.[20] They examined the biopsies from eight men and five female elite bodybuilders. The biopsies were obtained from the *biceps brachii*. They found that both Type I and II fibers were larger in men than women. The higher number of Type II fibers in men was thought to be because women have a lower lean body mass (LBM) and muscle CSA. Women had less variability in Type II fiber size. It may be that women have genetically smaller fibers and that at this upper limit of hypertrophy, they have obtained their diameter limit. In contrast, men may genetically have a larger potential CSA limit. Therefore they do not attain their upper CSA limit as readily and thus have more variability between fibers.

Bell and Jacobs[21] compared nine bodybuilders (five men and four women) to 10 untrained individuals (four men and six women). Biopsies from the *vastus lateralis* indicated that the male and female bodybuilders had larger Type IIa fibers than the controls. The males had greater CSA of all fibers than the females. They also found that the Type II fibers in the male bodybuilders were larger than those of the female bodybuilders, and that the ratio of Type II/I CSA was significantly increased in men but not in women bodybuilders. They concluded, as did Alway et al.,[20] that men selectively hypertrophy Type II fibers while women tend to hypertrophy both II and I, but to a lesser degree than men.

Staron et al.[11] examined the early phase effects of resistance training in men and women. In this study, 13 men and eight women commenced an eight week weight training program. These subjects where directly compared to sex-matched controls based upon biopsies obtained from the *vastus lateralis*. They found a decrease in Type IIb fibers after two weeks in trained women and four weeks in trained men. They found no other significant differences.

Sale et al.[22] looked at 13 untrained men and eight trained women, and compared them to eleven male bodybuilders. Again, in the untrained individuals, as seen previously by Brooke and Engel,[13] and Costill et al.,[10] men had greater fiber cross-sectional areas than women. In the bodybuilders (only men), they found a decrease in Type I fibers and increase in Type II fibers. They also noted an increase in variability in Type II size.

In summary, it appears that the long-term changes seen in body builders are gender dependent. Men clearly are able to hypertrophy both fiber types more readily than women. They are able to increase the CSA of the Type II fibers more dramatically while women tend to hypertrophy both fibers more equally. Alway et al.[20] and Bell and Jacobs[21] both note this difference. Men may also tend to have a greater percent of Type II fibers. This was noted by Alway et al.[20] but not by Bell and Jacobs.[20] These two studies looked only at established bodybuilders. Staron et al.[11] examined the changes in the early phases of resistance training and found little difference. The results suggest that the changes seen in both women and men are in part due to long-term adaptations.

The findings in these gender studies have been summarized in Tables 3.2, 3.3, and 3.4.

C. Capillary Supply

Muscle is well vascularized to ensure appropriate oxygenation during different activity requirements. Men and women have similar capillary concentrations per square unit of muscle. The vascularity is highly adaptable and changes to accommodate increases in oxygen demands in both men and women.[23,24] In a study by Bell and Jacobs,[21] they found that the number of capillaries/fiber was increased in body builders as compared to controls. They also found that the number of capillaries/fiber in men were similar to that seen in women. There was no gender difference seen in the number of capillaries/mm^2.

IV. ULTRASTRUCTURAL GENDER DIFFERENCES

A. Normal Muscle Ultrastructure

Human skeletal muscle is one of the most ordered and elegantly structured human organs. As previously mentioned, one skeletal muscle is composed of a bundle of muscle fibers in a connective tissue framework. These muscle fibers are 10 cm or more in length and vary in diameter from 10–100 um. Compared to light microscopy, which allows the assessment of fiber diameters, types, enzyme activity, and other parameters, ultrastructural examination allows one to focus on the fine structural components that make up the individual muscle.[25]

Individual muscle fibers are surrounded by a basal lamina which is extracellular material composed of amorphous Type IV collagen as well as other proteins such as fibronectin and laminin.[26] The basal lamina, which is approximately 20–30 nm thick, is separated from the muscle plasma membrane by an electron lucent area about 10–15 nm wide. This area represents the unstained portion of the glycocalyx of the muscle plasma membrane. The muscle plasma membrane (or plasmalemma) is also referred to as the sarcolemma and it is connected to the tubules of the transverse tubular (t-tubules) system. The intrinsic proteolipids and proteins of the sarcolemma are related to the sarcoplasm by a number of proteins felt to have a structural role. One such protein is desmin, a component of the 10 nm intermediate filaments which form a network around the myofibrils and link the edges of contiguous Z disks.

The major component of the muscle fiber are the myofibrils, which are composed of repeating segments of identical structures — the sarcomeres. An individual sarcomere consists of a dark central band (A band) flanked on either side by two paler bands (I band) which vary in length with the state of shortening of the myofiber. The Z lines or disks demarcate the longitudinal boundaries of individual sarcomeres. The dark central A band contains a dark narrow transverse line in its midpoint, the M band. The M band is flanked on either side by a paler band called the H zone,

Table 3.2 Gender Differences "Sedentary/Normal"

Study	Design	Muscle	Gender	Fiber Area (μm²)		Ratio % I/II	Conclusions
				I	II		
Brooke & Engel, 1969	37 ♂ 66 ♀ Asymptomatic patients Organic disorders	Biceps bracchii Vastus lateralis	♂ ♀ ♂ ♀	3247 2534 2781 2715	4151* 1757 3298 1956	0.6 (♂) 0.9 (♀)	1. ♂ had larger type II fiber 2. ♀ had larger type I fibers than type II 3. ↑ variation in ♂ II size 4. I/II greater in ♀ (0.9) than ♂ (0.6)
Costill et al., 1976	11 ♂ untrained 10 ♀ untrained	Gastrocnemius	♂ ♀	5699 3875	4965 4193	1.11 1.04	♂ have larger fibers
Komi and Karlsson, 1978	20 ♂ twins 11 ♀	Vastus lateralis	♂ ♀			1.27*** 0.96	No significant difference
Simoneau et al., 1989	418 biopsies 270 sedentary 148 active	Vastus lateralis	♂ ♀	4591 4044	4694**** 3412	0.85*** 1.04	1. ♀ had slight ↑ in the # of I fibers 2. ♀ slightly smaller fiber area 3. ♀ slightly lower glycolytic potential
Miller et al., 1993	8 ♂ 3 sedentary 5 active 8 ♀ 3 sedentary 5 active	Biceps brachii Vastus lateralis	♂ ♀ ♂ ♀	4597 3482 6142 4040	8207 4306 7700 4531	0.75*** 0.77 0.62 1.00	1. ♂ fibers larger than ♀ 2. ♂ type I fibers larger than ♀ (biceps) 3. ♂ type II fibers larger than ♀ (vastus) 4. No gender difference in fiber area ratio

Note: *Estimated from diameter; *** estimated from % Fiber type; **** calculated avg. of IIa and IIb; CSA = cross sectional area.

Table 3.3 Gender Differences in "Endurance Training"

Study	Design	Muscle	Gender	Fiber Area (μm²)		Ratio	Conclusions
				I	II	% I/II	
Costill et al., 1976	7 ♂ athletes 7 ♀ middle distance	*Gastrocnemius*	♂ ♀	6099 6069	7117 5642	1.08*** 1.54	1. ♀ have smaller type I & II fiber than ♂ 2. Athletes have larger fiber area than non-athletes (see Table 3.2)
Howald et al., 1985	5 ♂ 6 weeks of 5 ♀ cycling 5 x/wk. 1/grp. continued to 24 weeks	*Vastus lateralis*	Pre ♂ ♀ 6 wks ♂ ♀ 24 wks ♂ ♀			1.1** 0.9 1.5 1.9 1.5 1.0	1. Training cause a 12% ↑ in type I fibers & a 24% ↓ in Type IIb 2. ↑ in volume of mitochondria 3. ↑ in volume density of intracellular lipid
Kuipers et al., 1989	21 ♂ 18–20 mos. 8 ♀ endurance training Biopsies @ 5 mo (15 km) 6 mo (25 km) 7 mo (42 km)	*Vastus lateralis*	15 km ♂ ♀ 25 km ♂ ♀ 42 km ♂ ♀	2922* 3167 3147 3068 3107 3029	3088 2980 2971 3088 3463 2818	0.75*** 0.96	1. No shift in fiber type was seen 2. No change in diameter 3. Mild degenerative changes seen with ↑ training.

Note: * Estimated from diameter; ** estimated from average derived from graphed material; *** estimated from known % fiber type.

Table 3.4　Gender Differences in "Resistance Training"

Study	Design	Muscle	Gender	Fiber Area (µm²) I	II	Ratio % I/II	Conclusions
Sale et al., 1987	13 ♂ untrained	Biceps bracchii	♂	5500	7000**	0.63***	1. ♂ greater fiber area than ♀
	8 ♀ untrained		♀	4000	4500	0.63	2. ↑ variability in type II size in BB
	11 ♂ bodybuilders (BB)		♂	7000	12000	0.72	
Alway et al., 1989	8 ♂ elite	Biceps bracchii	♂	7259	11398	0.67***	1. ♂ have greater CSA in both I & II
	5 ♀ bodybuilders		♀	4760	5010	1.0	2. ♂ had greater II/I ↑ than ♀
Bell and Jacobs, 1990	5 ♂ bodybuilders	Vastus lateralis	♂	6696	8219	0.64***	1. ♂ & ♀ had larger type IIa fibers than controls
	4 ♀		♀	5989	6385	0.72	2. ♂ BB had larger CSA of fibers than ♀ BB
	4 ♂ controls		♂	4856	6512	0.41	3. BB had an increase of capillaries/fiber than controls
	6 ♀		♀	4861	5010	1.04	4. ♂ & ♀ had same # capillaries/fiber
Staron et al., 1994	13 ♂ early phase resistance training (8 wks.)	Vastus lateralis	Pre ♂	5000	6200**	0.69	1. Decrease IIb fiber number in both ♀ & ♂.
	8 ♀		♀	3800	3300	0.63	2. Early phase changes minimal between genders.
	12 ♀/♂ controls		Post ♂	6000	7500	0.67	
			♀	4000	4300	0.80	

Note:　** Estimated from average derived from graphed material; *** estimated from known % fiber type.

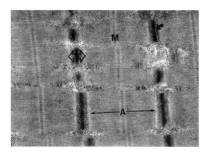

Figure 3.5 Electron micrograph showing the sarcomeres in a longitudinally cut skeletal muscle fiber (uranyl acetate and lead citrate, ×28,000, A band = thin arrows, I band = large open arrows, M band = M, Z disk = curved solid arrow, t-tubules = small double arrows).

which like the I band also varies in width with sarcomere length since it represents the portion of A filaments "unoccupied" by I filaments (Figure 3.5).

A detailed description of the proteins comprising the sarcomere is beyond the scope of this chapter, although some general comments can be made. The A (anisotropic) band of the sarcomere consists of a regular array of thick filaments 15–18 nm in diameter composed predominantly of myosin. Each filament is linked to its neighbor at its midpoint by a stable cross band, the M line. The I band is composed of thin myofilaments approximately 7 nm in diameter. The principal component of these myofilaments is the globular protein actin but they also contain troponin and tropomyosin. The I filaments of two halves of one I band find a common attachment in the dense matrix of the Z line.

The cytoplasm of the muscle fiber is also referred to as the sarcoplasm. It contains mitochondria, the membranes of the t-tubules and sarcoplasmic reticulum, free ribosomes, small cisternae of rough endoplasmic reticulum (RER), lipid droplets, microtubules, and intermediate filaments (8–12 um in diameter). Lipid droplets usually sit between myofibrils, adjacent to the mitochondria (Figure 3.6). They are more prominent in the Type I fibers. Intermediate filaments, which are not well visualized by routine electron microscopic techniques, are preferentially located in the Z disk region.[27] In the subplasmalemmal area, caveolae, coated vesicles, and rarely the outer end of the t-tubules may be seen. In the perinuclear region, ribosomes, Golgi membranes, and lipofuscin granules (heterogeneous, variably electron dense structures complexed with lipid) tend to be more prominent.

The t-tubules are extensions of the plasmalemma. They penetrate into the sarcoplasm between the myofibrils to form an interconnecting framework. Their connection to the plasmalemma however is rarely seen. The t-tubular system functions as an extension of the surface membrane.

The sarcoplasmic reticulum is the main internal membrane system of the muscle cell. It is considered to be from the RER, although ribosomes are not seen on its surface in mature muscle fibers. These membranes surround each myofibril and their terminal cisternae are closely related to the t-tubules.

Mitochondria are oblong-shaped, double membrane-bound organelles with a mean diameter of about 0.5–1.0 μm; however, their size and shape is quite variable.

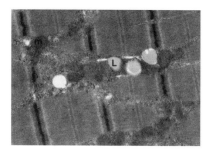

Figure 3.6   Electron micrograph showing the relationship of lipid droplets to the sarcomeres and mitochondria. (uranyl acetate and lead citrate, ×28,000, mitochondria = m, lipid = L).

They are found between the myofibrils and in a subsarcolemmal location. They are found in greater numbers in Type I fibers.

Although there is a great deal of variability in the ultrastructural features between individual muscle fibers, there is enough consistency between different fiber types to assign them with some degree of certainty to their respective fiber groups by using a constellation of ultrastructural features. Type I, slow twitch oxidative fibers, have relatively wide Z disks (between 85 to 105 nm), numerous mitochondria predominantly transverse in orientation, inconspicuous sarcoplasmic reticulum, very little glycogen, and small but consistent numbers of intermyofibrillar lipid droplets. Type IIb, fast twitch glycolytic fibers, have narrow Z bands (35 to 55 nm), few mitochondria also transversely orientated, well-developed sarcoplasmic reticulum and t-tubules, conspicuous amounts of intermyofibrillar glycogen, but essentially no intermyofibrillar lipid. The Type IIa, fast twitch, oxidative/glycolytic fibers, have intermediate Z band widths (45 to 85 nm), abundant mitochondria predominantly in longitudinal orientation and some in subplasmalemmal aggregates, sarcoplasmic reticulum, and t-tubules (approximately as developed or slightly more developed than Type I fibers), moderate amounts of intermyofibrillar glycogen and occasional intermyofibrillar lipid droplets (Figure 3.7).

B. Ultrastructural Differences in Untrained Individuals

There has been very little investigation into the fine structural differences in skeletal muscle between males and females. The studies which are available were done many years ago and they are limited by the small numbers of subjects studied as well as by the variable muscle sites biopsied.

Hoppler et al.[28] studied the volume density of myofibrils, sarcoplasm, intracellular lipid, peripheral and central mitochondria in the *vastus lateralis* muscle in nine untrained men and three untrained women. The mean age of the males was 28, and the females, 25. Their mean weight was 69 and 55 kg, respectively. They found a higher volume density of central mitochondria, a higher ratio of central mitochondria to volume of myofibrils, a higher surface of central mitochondria, and mitochondrial cristae in males compared to females. No significant difference in volume density of lipid was found between males and females.

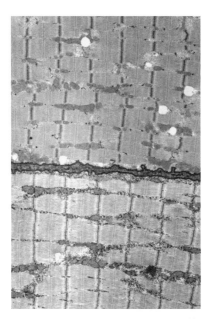

Figure 3.7 Electron micrograph illustrating a Type I (top) and Type II (bottom) fiber (potassium ferricyanide, uranyl acetate and lead citrate, ×11,500).

Jerusalem et al.[29] studied the ultrastructural features of muscle in 10 control subjects. Four were children (all female, ages one month to 12.6 years) and six were adults (two females, four males, ages 28 to 55 years). No consistent muscle site was studied: four triceps, three *vastus lateralis,* one *deltoid,* one *tibialis anterior,* and one *flexor carpi radialis* were examined. Mean mitochondrial size was significantly greater for children than for adults although there was no significant difference between adult males and females. Despite the small numbers, the difference is interesting in light of the fact that all of the children were female. No differences were found between the lipid droplet fraction of the fiber volume between children and adults and the data for adult females vs. adult males is not provided. There was no difference between children and adults in sarcotubular surface density.

In general, both studies are limited by the small numbers of subjects studied and the latter study by the heterogeneous group of subjects and biopsy samples. In addition, since these studies have been performed, more consistent data has accumulated in regards to the ultrastructural differences between different fiber types. It would be of interest to see if differences between males and females are present in different fiber types since we know that different fiber types are involved in different work and metabolic capacities.

It has been noted that muscle damage in the form of Z band streaming can be found in normal individuals (Figure 3.8). In a study looking at Z band streaming, some differences were found between males and females.[30] In this study, they found that the incidence of focal Z band streaming (defined as lesions occupying one to two adjacent myofibrils of one to two contiguous sarcomeres) was 62% while the incidence of extensive Z band streaming (defined as lesions occupying three or more

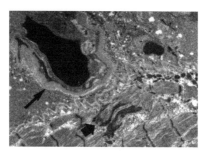

Figure 3.8 Electron micrograph showing Z band streaming in close proximity to a capillary (uranyl acetate and lead citrate, ×10,000, capillary = long arrow, Z band streaming = short arrow).

adjacent myofibrils and three or more contiguous sarcomeres) was 32%. Interestingly, there was a significant difference in focal Z band streaming between females and males (incidence 12/12 in females, 9/22 in males, p <0.005) but no difference between males and females with respect to extensive Z band streaming (incidence 5/12 in females, 6/22 in males, p = 0.10).

At the ultrastructural level, very little information is available about male and female skeletal muscle differences in untrained individuals at different ages. There is some data implying differences in mitochondrial volume densities between males and females but good data is not available as to gender differences in the different fiber types. There is also some data implying that male and female muscles differ in baseline amounts of muscle damage[30] (Chapter 12), and thus there probably are other baseline differences yet to be documented.

C. Gender Differences with Exercise Training

A number of studies have looked at light microscopic changes in response to exercise and some of these have looked at gender differences, but there are few studies looking at fine structural changes in response to exercise. In addition, those which are available have not systematically addressed gender differences.

In one small early study,[31] three male long distance runners and two world class power lifters were examined in comparison to nine active but untrained male controls. The muscle fibers from the long distance runners had an increased volume percent of mitochondria and lipid in both slow and fast twitch muscle fibers compared to the controls, while the world class power lifters had a lower mitochondrial volume percent in fast twitch fibers and decreased lipid stores in all fibers compared to controls. No females were studied.

Very little has been documented about ultrastructural changes in muscle at low exercise intensities although endurance training of moderate intensity and longer duration does evoke ultrastructural changes in muscle.[32] Twelve men on a six month home-based jogging program showed significant increase in VO_{2max} and submaximal power output. In their *vastus lateralis* muscles, the total mitochondrial volume density increased by 20% and the subsarcolemmal mitochondria volume increased preferentially compared to central mitochondrial volume. This training protocol had no effect on capillary to fiber ratio, fiber cross-sectional area or volume of intracellular lipid droplets.[32] Other studies have shown that with moderate long-term exercise, glycogen is preferentially lost from Type I fibers (mostly from subsarcolemmal and other sarcoplasmic locations); however, the glycogen loss is not complete and glycogen granules can still be found in the I band region.[4]

Endurance exercise training is known to produce alterations that allow the skeletal muscle to produce large mechanical power outputs over longer periods of time without becoming fatigued or damaged.[4] The muscle of endurance-trained individuals has been shown to have a higher volume density of mitochondria[33] with a preferential proliferation of subsarcolemmal mitochondria.[1,34] Type IIa fibers usually show a larger relative increase in mitochondrial volume density than Type I or Type IIb fibers.[18,33] The sarcoplasmic space tends to increase with endurance exercise programs and that increase may be due to an increase in glycogen content.[4] Endurance exercise causes increases in the volume density of intracellular lipid deposits which are often found in direct contact with mitochondria.[35] Changes in Z band width have not been documented after endurance exercise.[4]

The structural adaptations to strength training mainly involve the synthesis of new myofibrils. In addition, a higher incidence of structural abnormalities such as central nuclei and atrophic muscle fibers have been reported.[36] The volume density of mitochondria decreases with strength training.[36]

Despite the documented changes in ultrastructure with exercise, very little information is available in regards to structural differences between males and females. One study which looked at histologic and ultrastructural features of 21 males and 8 females after long distance training and running, primarily concentrated on muscle damage overall and gender differences were not specifically addressed.[19] Howald et al.[18] tested 10 sedentary women and men in a high-intensity endurance exercise training program. They found an increased volume density of intracellular lipid in Type II fibers of the *vastus lateralis* with training; however, there were significant differences between the volume density of lipid between males and females even before the exercise intervention. Significant differences in the increase of lipid volume density after the exercise training also occurred between males and females: in Type I fibers, males had an over fourfold increase in lipid volume density compared to females. These findings suggested that with high intensity endurance exercise muscle adaptations with respect to lipid metabolism are different between males and females.

V . FUTURE DIRECTIONS

Considering the limited data currently available regarding structural gender differences in skeletal muscle, it is safe to say that there are a wide variety of studies yet to be completed. Light microscopy utilizing enzyme plus other histochemical methods and electron microscopy are standard well-established techniques. Structural differences identified by these methods could reflect functional differences. For example, could the changes in lipid content between male and female muscle be reflected in different fatty acid oxidation potentials? Conversely, are the differences in glycolytic enzymes between male and female muscle reflected in differences in glycogen distribution seen at the ultrastructural or light microscopic level? In future studies, the use of histochemical stains for glycogen and lipid may help to characterize these changes. Glycogen and lipid can be directly visualized by electron microscopy and relationships of these compounds to fine structural compartments may give further insights into functional variations. In addition, future investigations of gender differences could potentially take advantage of new developments in antibodies to novel antigens by utilizing immunohistochemical and immunoelectron microscopic techniques. Molecular biologic methods which examine DNA and RNA may also have a role to play in future investigations.

Even before the application of immunohistochemical, immunoelectron microscopic, or molecular biologic techniques however, several issues need to be addressed. The influence of genetic selection to adaptation is yet to be fully investigated. Most of the studies to date have been limited by their small and cross sectional design. Ideally, to answer the question of whether or not there is genetic selection in endurance and resistance trained individuals, the range of fiber distribution in sedentary or untrained individuals needs to be established. There needs to be standardization within this group of individuals since variability of fiber distribution could be influenced by activities of daily living. For example, a woman who has young children will no doubt do a great deal of lifting and carrying, and will likely have a different cross-sectional area and fiber distribution compared to a woman without young children, although both are considered within the group of sedentary or untrained individuals. If a subgroup can be defined within the spectrum of sedentary individuals that has a relatively consistent fiber type phenotype, then an exercise protocol within the context of a longitudinal study can be implemented and fiber type switching can either be confirmed or refuted.

Hormone levels inherently and physiologically fluctuate throughout our lives. In addition, estrogens are known to have antioxidant and membrane-stabilizing properties (Chapter 2). Since exercise-induced muscle damage is felt to be related to oxygen free radical production,[37] a possible protective effect of estrogen on muscle damage is an intriguing hypothesis requiring further study (Chapter 11). However, hormonal influences on skeletal muscle differences could be also investigated by looking at skeletal muscle differences in children before and after puberty, as well as in females before and after menopause. Correlation with hormone levels in these groups may offer further insights into relationships between skeletal muscle changes and hormones.

A great deal of work can be done in all of these areas. Studies of this nature will have far-reaching implications for exercise and diet programs, not only in athletes but in the wide variety of fitness programs advocated for health reasons.

ACKNOWLEDGMENTS

We would like to acknowledge the technical staff in the EM department with special thanks to Rick for his work on the histological micrographs. We would like to also thank Dr. J. Provias for providing the sections of muscle for photography, and Marie Colbert, Joan Martin, and Sarah Fick for their assistance in preparing the manuscript.

REFERENCES

1. Hoppeler, H., Howald, H., Conley, K., Lindstedt, S. L., Claassen, H., Vock, P., and Weibel, E. R., Endurance training in humans: aerobic capacity and structure of skeletal muscle, *J. Appl. Physiol.,* 59 (2), 320, 1985.

2. Bergström, J., Muscle electrolytes in a man determined by neutron activation analysis on needle biopsy specimen: A study in normal subjects, kidney patients, and patients with chronic diarrhoea, *Scand. J. Clin. Lab. Invest.,* 14 (suppl. 68), 1, 1962.

3. Dubovicz, V., *Muscle Biopsy: A Practical Approach.* 2nd ed., Bailliere Tindall, London, 1985, 26.

4. Hoppeler, H., Exercise induced ultrastructural changes in skeletal muscle, *Int. J. Sports Med.,* 7, 187, 1986.

5. Thiery, J. P., Mise en evidence des polysaccharoides sur coupes fines en microscopie electronique, *J. Microsc.,* 6, 987, 1967.

6. Thornell, L. E., An ultrahistochemical study on glycogen in cow Purkinje fibers, *J. Mol. Cell Cardiol.,* 6, 439, 1974.

7. Colling-Saltin, A.-S., Enzyme histochemistry on skeletal muscle of the human foetus, *J. Neurol. Sci.,* 39, 169, 1978.

8. Johnson, M. A., Polgar, J., Weightman, D., and Appleton, D., Data on the distribution of fibre types in thirty-six human muscles. An autopsy study, *J. of the Neurological Sciences,* 18, 111, 1973.

9. Anderson, P. and Henriksson, J., Training induced changes in the subgroups of human type II skeletal muscle fibres, *Acta Physiol. Scand.,* 99, 123, 1977.

10. Costill, D. L., Daniels, J., Evans, W., Fink, W., Krahenbuhl, G., and Saltin, B., Skeletal muscle enzymes and fiber composition in male and female track athletes, *Journal of Applied Physiology,* 40 (2), 149, 1976.

11. Staron, R. S., Karapondo, D. L., Draemer, W. J., Fry, A. C., Gordon, S. E., Falkel, J. E., Hagerman, F. C., and Hikikda, R. S., Skeletal muscle adaptations during early phase of heavy-resistance training in men and women, *J. Appl. Physiol.,* 76(3), 1247, 1994.

12. Prince. F. P., Hikida, R. S., and Hagerman, F. C., Muscle fiber types in women athletes and non-athletes, *Pflügers Arch.,* 371, 161, 1977.

13. Brooke, M. H. and Engel, W. K., The histographic analysis of human muscle biopsies with regard to fiber types. 1. Adult male and female, *Neurology,* 19, 221, 1969.

14. Komi, P. V. and Karlsson, J., Skeletal muscle fibre types, enzyme activities and physical performance in young males and females, *Acta Physiol. Scand.,* 103, 210, 1978.

15. Simoneau, J.-A. and Bouchard, C., Human variation in skeletal muscle fiber-type proportion and enzyme activities, *Am. J. Physiol.,* 257, E567, 1989.

16. Miller, A. E. J., MacDougall, J. D., Tarnopolsky, M. A., and Sale, D. G., Gender differences in strength and muscle fiber characteristics, *Eur. J. Appl. Physiol.,* 66, 254, 1993.

17. Nygaard, E., Skeletal muscle fibre characteristics in young women, *Acta Physiol. Scand.,* 112, 299, 1981.

18. Howald, H., Hoppeler, H., Claassen, H., Mathieu, O., and Straub, R., Influences of endurance training on the ultrastructural composition of the different muscle fiber types in humans, *Pflügers Archiv.,* 403, 369, 1985.

19. Kuipers, H., Janssen, G. M. E., Bosman, F., Frederik, P. M., and Geurten, P., Structural and ultrastructural changes in skeletal muscle associated with long-distance training and running, *Int. J. Sports Med.,* 10, S156, 1989.

20. Alway, S. E., Grumbt, W. H., Gonyea, W. J., and Stray-Gunderson, J., Contrasts in muscle and myofibers of elite male and female bodybuilders, *J. Appl. Physiol.,* 67 (1), 24, 1989.

21. Bell, D. G. and Jacobs, I., Muscle fibre area, fibre type and capillarization in male and female body builders, *Can. J. Spt. Sci.,* 15(2), 115, 1990.

22. Sale, D. G., MacDougall, J. D., Alway, S. E., and Sutton, J. R., Voluntary strength and muscle characteristics in untrained men and women and male bodybuilders, *J. Appl. Physiol.,* 62 (5), 1786, 1987.

23. Nygaard, E., Women and exercise — with special reference to muscle morphology and metabolism, *Biochemistry of Exercise,* Poortmans, J. and Niset, G., Eds., University Park, Baltimore, MD, IV-B, 161, 1981.

24. Hudlicka, O., The response of muscle to enhanced and reduced activity, *Baillière's Clinical Endocrinology and Metabolism,* 4 (3), 419, 1990.

25. Engel, A. G., Santa, T., Stonnington, H. H., Jerusalem, F., Tsujihata, M., Brownell, A. K. W., Sakakibara, H., Banker, B. Q., Sahashi, K., and Lambert, E. H., Morphometric study of skeletal muscle ultrastructure, *Muscle and Nerve* (Poster Session) May/June: 229, 1979.

26. Sanes, J. R., Laminin, fibronectin and collagen in synaptic and extrasynaptic portions of muscle fiber basement membrane. *J. Cell Biol.,* 9, 442, 1982.

27. Thornell, L. E., Edstrom, L., Henrikson, K. G., and Angquist, K. A., The distribution of intermediate filament protein (skeletin) in normal and diseased human skeletal muscle, *J. Neur. Sci.,* 41, 153, 1980.

28. Hoppeler, H., Lüthi, P., Claassen, H., Weibel, E. R., and Howald, H., The ultrastructure of the normal human skeletal muscle. A morphometric analysis on untrained men, women and well-trained orienteers, *Pflügers Arch.,* 344, 217, 1973.

29. Jerusalem, F., Engel, A. G., and Peterson, H. A., Human muscle fiber fine structure: Morphometric data on controls, *Neurology,* 25, 127, 1975.

30. Meltzer, H. Y., Kuncl, R. W., Click, J., and Yang, V., Incidence of Z band streaming and myofibrillar disruptions in skeletal muscle from healthy young people, *Neurology,* 26, 853, 1976.

31. Prince, F. P., Hikida, R. S., Hagerman, F. C., Staron, R. S., and Allen, W. H., A morphometric analysis of human muscle fibers with relation to fiber types and adaptations to exercise, *J. of the Neurological Sciences,* 49, 165, 1981.

32. Suter, E., Hoppler, H., Claassen, H., Billeter, R., Aebi, U., Horber, F., Jaeger, P., and Marti, B., Ultrastructural modification of human skeletal muscle tissue with 6-month moderate-intensity exercise training, *Int. J. Sports Med.,* 16, 160, 1995.

33. Bylund, A. C., Bjuro, T., Cederblad, G., Holm, J., Lundholm, K., Sjostrom, M., Angquist, K. A., and Schersten, T., Physical training in man. Skeletal muscle metabolism in relation to muscle morphology and running ability, *Eur. J. Appl. Physiol.,* 36, 151, 1977.

34. Rosler, K., Conley, K. E., Claassen, H., Howald, H., and Hoppeler, H., Transfer effects in endurance exercise: adaptations in trained and untrained muscle, *Eur. J. Appl. Physiol.,* 54, 355, 1985.

35. Holloszy, J. O. and Coyle, E. F., Adaptations of skeletal muscle to endurance exercise and their metabolic consequences, *J. Appl. Physiol.,* 56 (4), 831, 1984.
36. MacDougall, J. D., Sale, D. G., Elder, G. C., and Sutton, J. R., Muscle ultrastructural characteristics of elite powerlifters and bodybuilders, *Eur. J. Appl. Physiol.,* 48, 117, 1982.

CHAPTER 4

Neuromuscular Function

Digby G. Sale, Ph.D.

CONTENTS

1-8493-8194-0/98/$0.00+$.50

I. INTRODUCTION

This chapter focuses on differences between young women and men in voluntary muscle strength and endurance and evoked muscle contractile properties. Gender differences in voluntary strength have received the most study and, therefore, comprise a major portion of the chapter. For many years, muscle strength was measured almost exclusively with isometric dynamometers. In the 1970s, isokinetic dynamometers increasingly became available, allowing concentric contraction strength to be measured at various velocities. More recently, the introduction of dynamometers with an eccentric loading feature has produced a growing literature on eccentric strength. As a result of these developments in strength-testing methodology, gender differences in strength now can be studied in all contraction types and in a wide range of velocities. There also are studies that have addressed gender differences in a particular coupling of eccentric and concentric contractions, known as the stretch-shorten cycle.

Although the emphasis of the chapter is on voluntary strength and endurance performance, a section on evoked muscle contractile properties is included. Measurement of evoked contractile properties permits study of aspects of muscle function that either cannot or only with difficulty can be tested with voluntary contractions. There is also the advantage that muscle function (evoked contractile properties) can be interpreted without having to consider the variability associated with voluntary effort.

Finally, an attempt is made, throughout the chapter, to identify factors such as muscle size, fiber type distribution, and motor unit activation, which might be responsible for observed gender differences in muscle function.

II. STRENGTH

A. Absolute Strength

Absolute strength refers to strength expressed in the units of measurement (e.g., newtons of force) without reference to (or not relative to) factors such as body mass or muscle cross-sectional area (CSA). Averaged across all muscle groups, women have ~60% of the absolute strength of men.[1] Women have 60 to 80% of men's leg strength,[2-13] but only 50 to 60% of men's upper limb strength.[5-7,14-17] The differences

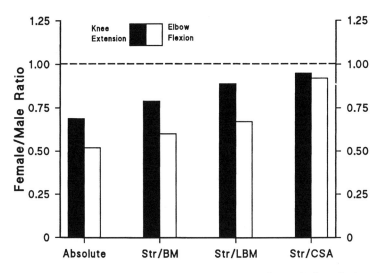

Figure 4.1 The ratio of female to male isometric knee extension and elbow flexion strength expressed absolutely and relative to body mass (Str/BM), lean body mass (Str/LBM), and muscle cross-sectional area (Str/CSA). * Significant difference between women and men, P < 0.05. Based on Miller et al.[10]

in absolute strength correspond to differences in muscle size;[5] thus, women have 50 to 60% of upper arm and 65 to 70% of thigh muscle CSA.[9,10,17-23] Men's larger muscles are due to larger muscle fibers[10,17,23-26] and possibly a larger number of fibers.[17,25] The greater gender difference in upper vs. lower limb muscle size corresponds to similar differences in skeletal size. Women have 65 to 75% of the humerus and 85% of the femur CSA of men.[10,17,20]

B. Relative Strength

1. Strength/Body Mass Ratio

In comparison to absolute strength, the gender difference is smaller when strength is expressed relative to body mass because on average men have a greater body mass.[9,10,27,28] This is evident in Figure 4.1, which shows a greater F/M ratio (i.e., ratio of female to male values) for the strength/body mass ratio than absolute strength. The F/M ratio for strength expressed in relation to lean body mass (fat-free mass) is greater still because women have a higher percentage of body fat.[9,10,29,30] Figure 4.1 also illustrates the greater F/M ratios for lower than upper body strength, regardless of how strength is expressed.

2. Specific Tension

Strength also may be expressed relative to muscle CSA, referred to as specific force or specific tension. In animal studies, specific tension is calculated using maximal isometric tetanic force. In humans, specific tension is determined more often from maximal voluntary contractions, which have the limitation that the values obtained could be affected by the ability to activate the muscles, as well as intrinsic contractile strength. Like animal studies, human specific tension measurements traditionally have been based on isometric contractions, but concentric contractions at a variety of velocities also have been used. As illustrated in Figure 4.1, the general finding has been little or no gender difference in specific tension in isometric and low velocity concentric contractions.[3,9,10,17,20,31-33] It should be noted, however, that some studies have reported a greater specific tension in men in knee extensors and flexors,[20,34] and in some of the studies showing no significant gender difference, men had larger (~10%) mean values.[9,10,32]

A difference in specific tension derived from voluntary contractions might be related to a difference in the ability to fully activate the muscles; however, the extent of motor unit activation is similar in women and men, at least for isometric contractions.[10,35,36] A lower specific tension in women might be expected on the basis of their greater relative amount of intramuscular fat[20,37,38] and connective tissue.[10,17] In isometric tests, the measured force and therefore the specific tension is affected by joint angle. In elbow flexion, for example, the optimal joint angle is greater in men than women.[39] However, in studies of elbow flexion using either a gender-neutral joint angle[10] or an angle favoring the women,[32] there was no significant difference in specific tension. Finally, women might be expected to have a lower specific tension because of their smaller type II to type I muscle fiber area ratio[10,17,40] because a lower II/I area ratio or percent type II fiber area has been associated with a lower specific tension.[10,41] Nevertheless, even if a small gender difference in specific tension favoring men is allowed, it is still muscle size rather than muscle quality (specific tension) that is mainly responsible for men's greater absolute strength.

3. *Relation of Absolute and Relative Strength to Performance*

In terms of performance, expressing strength measurements absolutely is most relevant when related to tasks such as lifting weights or moving objects. On the other hand, when performance consists of lifting or otherwise moving one's own body mass, strength relative to body mass is the most relevant expression of strength. Men, with their greater muscle mass and lower percentage of body fat, have the advantage over women in tasks requiring either absolute strength or a high strength/body mass ratio. As noted previously, the advantage is greater for activities involving the upper limbs. Although strength normalized to fat-free body mass or muscle CSA is useful in the study of muscle function, it is absolute strength and the strength/body mass ratio that are relevant to performance in sport or occupational settings.

C. Rate of Force Development

Isometric rate of force development (RFD), expressed absolutely (e.g., N/s), is consistently greater in men than women[42-45] (Figure 4.2A). Men's greater absolute RFD mainly reflects their greater absolute strength. In contrast, the time taken to attain various percentages of peak force (i.e., relative RFD) has been found to be

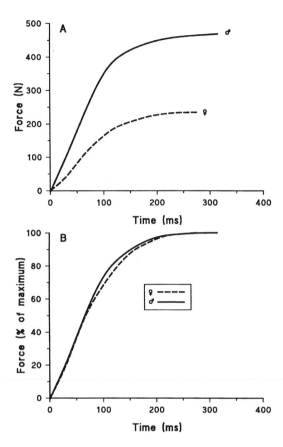

Figure 4.2 Force-time curves of isometric elbow flexion shown in absolute force units (A) and normalized to peak force (B). Men showed greater absolute rate of force development than women (A), but there was no gender difference in the time to attain various percentages of peak force (B). Other studies have shown different results (see text). Based on Bell and Jacobs.[43]

similar in women and men[43,44] (Figure 4.2B), shorter in women,[46] and shorter in men.[42,45] One study has compared RFD normalized to peak force (PF): (RFD/PF × 100); normalized RFD was similar in women and men, despite men having greater absolute RFD and shorter times to peak force.[42] The reason(s) for the discrepancies in relative RFD is unknown. On the basis of their greater type II to I fiber area ratio,[10,17,23,26,40,47-52] percent type II fiber area, and perhaps percent type II fibers,[10,40,52] and the positive correlation between RFD and percent type II fibers,[53,54] one might expect a greater relative RFD in men. Surprisingly, a study that found men to have greater relative RFD also found them to have a smaller percent type II fibers.[45]

D. Force-Velocity Relation

Muscles can generate force while shortening (concentric), being forcibly lengthened (eccentric), or at a fixed length (isometric). In concentric contractions, force

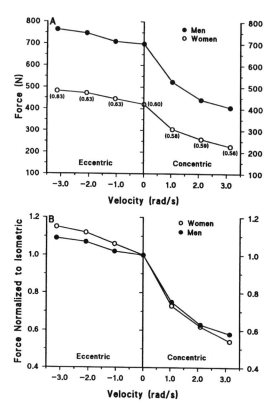

Figure 4.3 Knee extensor force-velocity relations in young women and men. A. Absolute strength. The numbers in parentheses with the women's values indicate the female/male (F/M) ratios. The ratios suggest that women do relatively better, compared to men, on the eccentric portion of the force-velocity relation. B. Concentric and eccentric values are normalized to the isometric value. In agreement with the F/M ratios in A, women do relatively best in high velocity eccentric, and worst in high velocity concentric strength. Based on Hortobágyi et al.[29]

decreases as velocity increases; in eccentric actions, force increases (and then plateaus) as velocity increases (Figure 4.3). Most of the research comparing strength in women and men has focused on isometric or relatively low velocity concentric strength tests. Fewer studies have included eccentric tests and a wide range of velocities.

1. ECC/CON Force Ratio

For a given rate of muscle length change (velocity), more force can be produced in eccentric (ECC) than concentric (CON) contractions; that is the ECC/CON force ratio is greater than 1.0. Figure 4.3 shows an example of the knee extension force-velocity relation in women and men. It is clear (Figure 4.3A) that the men had greater absolute strength in the three contraction types and at all veloctics. It is not

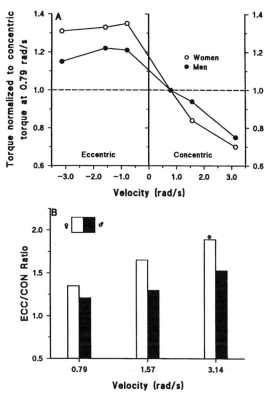

Figure 4.4 Knee extensor force-velocity relations in young women and men. A. Force (torque) is shown normalized to the concentric value at the lowest velocity tested. Compared to men, women show relatively greater normalized eccentric but smaller concentric force. B. Ratios of eccentric to concentric force (ECC/CON ratio) at the three velocities tested. Corresponding to the data shown in A, women had greater ECC/CON ratios than men, and the gender difference was greater at higher velocities. * Significant difference between women and men, P < 0.05. Based on Seger and Thorstensson.[28]

clear from this panel whether the shape of the relation differs between women, although the F/M ratios given under the women's values suggest that the women's performance is relatively better in eccentric than concentric contractions. This is better seen in Figure 4.3B, in which the force-velocity relations have been normalized to the isometric values. Women's eccentric values increase more above the isometric value, whereas their highest velocity concentric value decreases more below the isometric value. A second example is in Figure 4.4A, which shows the force-velocity relation normalized to the lowest velocity concentric value. Again it is evident that women do relatively better than men in eccentric contractions and relatively worse in concentric contractions at higher velocities. In Figure 4.4B, the eccentric and concentric forces are depicted as eccentric/concentric (ECC/CON) force ratios, which are greater in the women, particularly at higher velocities. Higher ECC/CON ratios have been observed in women for both upper and lower limb muscles.[27,28,55,56]

2. Mechanisms of Greater ECC/CON Ratios in Women

As shown in Figures 4.3 and 4.4, women's greater ECC/CON ratios appear to be the result of both enhanced eccentric force and diminished concentric force at higher velocities. The ECC/CON ratio is greater for electrically evoked than voluntary contractions,[57] and is increased by superimposing electrical stimulation on voluntary contractions.[58] In addition, motor unit activation, as assessed by electromyography (EMG), may be less in maximal eccentric than concentric contractions.[28,59-61] These lines of evidence indicate that neural inhibitory mechanisms sometimes may limit force production in maximal effort eccentric contractions. Thus, it might be suspected that the greater ECC/CON ratios in women may be attributed partly to less inhibition in eccentric contractions. However, higher knee extensor ECC/CON force ratios have been observed in women without a correspondingly greater ECC/CON EMG ratio.[28] In contrast, a recent study of elbow flexion showed a greater ECC/CON EMG ratio in women, but only a trend toward a greater ECC/CON force ratio.[62] More research is needed to determine whether there is a neural component to the greater ECC/CON ratio in women.

Enhanced eccentric force might reflect muscle fiber type distribution. If slow (type I) fibers have a slower myosin cross-bridge detachment rate, cross-bridges would be stretched more during forced lengthening, offering more braking force against stretch. There also might be a higher proportion of attached cross-bridges in a more slowly contracting muscle, as happens in fatigue.[63] Together, these effects would amplify eccentric relative to isometric force. The literature on a possible gender difference in fiber type distribution has not been consistent. The study[40] with the largest sample size (~400 subjects) found a significantly greater percentage of type I fibers in women, but the difference was small (51 ± 13 vs. $46 \pm 15\%$). Although some other studies with smaller samples have shown a similar difference,[10,52] others have failed to show a significant difference.[4,23,26,64-67] A more consistent finding has been a smaller type II/type I area ratio in women.[10,17,23,26,40,47-52] Women's similar or slightly greater percentage of type I fibers, combined with a greater type I/type II fiber area ratio, would give women a greater percent type I fiber area; that is, a greater proportion of the total muscle cross-sectional area occupied by type I fibers. This might give women an advantage in eccentric actions. It is possible that the relatively preserved eccentric strength in the elderly[29,68,69] may also be related partly to their greater type I/type II area ratio.[29,47,48,70-73]

A greater percent type I fiber area also might explain partly the relatively greater decline in force at high concentric velocities that has sometimes been observed in women.[4,8,28,30,55,56,74] It also has been shown that the gender difference (men > women) in specific tension is greater at high than low concentric velocities[33] (Figure 4.5). It should be noted, however, that at least one study has shown the opposite pattern; that is, a greater relative decline in high velocity concentric force in men.[42]

Measurements of maximal unresisted muscle shortening velocity (V_{max}) also have been made, but results have not been consistent. One study showed men having a greater V_{max} in elbow flexion;[14] in contrast, another study found no gender difference in knee extension, although men generated greater torque in producing V_{max}.[64]

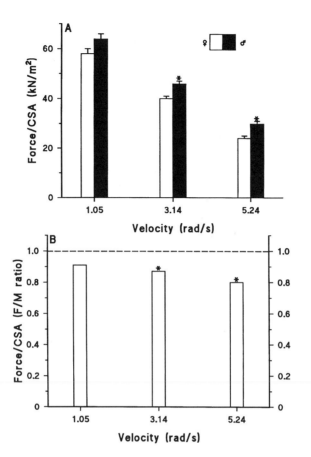

Figure 4.5 Knee extensor force per unit muscle cross-sectional area (Force/CSA) at three velocities of concentric contraction. A. Men had greater force/CSA (specific tension) than women. B. The data in A are expressed as F/M ratios, showing that the F/M ratio decreases at higher velocities. * Significant difference between women and men, P < 0.05. Based on Kanehisa et al.[88]

E. Stretch-Shorten Cycle

The force of a maximal concentric contraction is increased if it is immediately preceded by an eccentric contraction. This coupling of eccentric and concentric contraction is called the stretch-shorten cycle (SSC).[53] SSC potentiation has been observed in jumping,[53] on a sledge apparatus,[75] and in single joint actions on isokinetic dynamometers.[76] SSC potentiation of concentric force is attributed largely to a combination of the high force achieved[77] and storage of elastic energy during an eccentric contraction,[53] which is then transferred to the ensuing concentric contraction. When the concentric action is intended to be rapid, a prior eccentric contraction allows concentric force to be developed more rapidly.[78] In jumping, SSC potentiation may[79] or may not[80] be associated with increased muscle activation in the concentric phase, raising the possibility of reflex potentiation associated with SSC. Even when neural enhancement (greater activation of muscle) is present in jumping, it plays a smaller role in SSC potentiation than the muscular mechanisms (transfer of high eccentric force, storage of elastic energy).[80] In contrast, when SSC potentiation is assessed on dynamometers, activation may be the same[60] or even less[59] in the concentric phase compared to an isolated concentric action, emphasizing the importance of muscular over neural mechanisms.

A few studies have compared SSC potentiation in women and men. In jumping with low prestretch loads, women have greater relative potentiation than men[81] (Figure 4.6), whereas with high prestretch loads, potentiation may be greater in men.[75] On dynamometers, results have differed. One study found women to have greater SSC potentiation among young but not old adults[59] (Figure 4.7). Another study found women to be superior only in elderly adults.[30]

One possible mechanism for women's greater SSC potentiation is considered to be their greater ability to reutilize elastic energy stored in eccentric actions.[75,81] Another consideration is that relative to isometric or low velocity concentric force, women have relatively greater high velocity eccentric force but relatively smaller high velocity concentric force (Figures 4.3 and 4.4); therefore, it could be argued that in women eccentric contractions have more to give and concentric actions have more to gain when fast eccentric and concentric actions are combined in the SSC. Thus, the possible mechanisms (e.g., greater percent type I fiber area in women) discussed earlier in connection with the larger ECC/CON ratios in women, also may be implicated women's greater SSC potentiation. Finally, if women in fact have more difficulty in developing force rapidly at the onset of isolated isometric or concentric contractions (see section on rate of force development), perhaps due to their greater muscle compliance (elasticity),[82] then this disadvantage would be minimized at the end of the eccentric phase of SSC, where force already would be high and the series-elastic component stretched at the beginning of the concentric phase.[78]

F. Isometric Strength Curves

Strength (force) varies through a range of movement; the pattern of force change is called a strength curve.[83] The shape of a strength curve is determined mainly by the length-tension relation and changes in muscle moment arm. Strength curves have been assessed most often on the basis of isometric contractions at a series of joint angles through the range of movement. The results of three studies comparing strength curves in men and women are shown in Figure 4.8. In the ankle dorsiflexors[82] (Figure 4.8A) and plantarflexors[84] (Figure 4.8B), there was no gender difference in the strength curves. In contrast, the joint angle corresponding to the summit of the elbow flexor strength curve differed in women and men (Figure 4.8C). In this study[39] it was suggested that the men's decline in strength at the smallest (more flexed) joint angles was caused by the bulging of their larger muscles, which may have aligned the muscle fibers so as to impair force development.

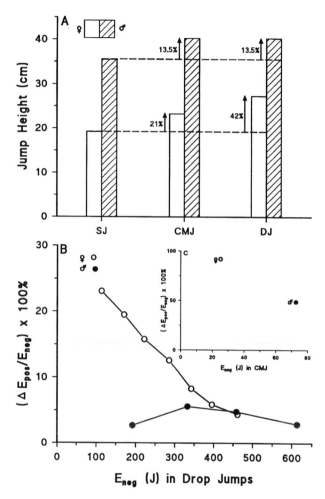

Figure 4.6 Stretch-shorten cycle (SSC) potentiation in jumping. A. The jump heights achieved in squat jumps (SJ) without SSC, countermovement jumps (CMJ) with SSC, and drop jumps (DJ) from a height with SSC. SSC potentiation in CMJ and DJ resulted in greater jump heights compared to no SSC jumps (SJ). Women had greater potentiation than men (percentage values shown). B. The improvement in concentric (positive) work relative to the energy absorbed in the eccentric (negative) phase of DJ ($\Delta E_{pos}/E_{neg} \times 100\%$). The women were able to reutilize a greater percentage of the negative energy (E_{neg}) at lower E_{neg} values. C (inset in B). The improvement in concentric (positive) work relative to the energy absorbed in the eccentric (negative) phase of CMJ ($\Delta E_{pos}/E_{neg} \times 100\%$). The women were able to reutilize a greater percentage of the negative energy (E_{neg}). Based on Komi and Bosco.[81]

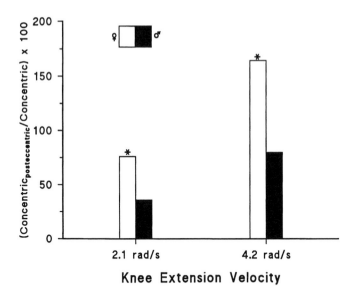

Knee Extension Velocity

Figure 4.7 Stretch-shorten cycle (SSC) potentiation of the knee extensors on an isokinetic dynamometer. Potentiation is expressed as the ratio of concentric force immediately after an eccentric contraction ($Concentric_{posteccentric}$) to the force of an isolated concentric contraction. Women had greater potentiation than men (*$P < 0.05$). Based on Svantesson and Grimby.[59]

III. MUSCLE ENDURANCE

A. Absolute Endurance

Like strength, muscle endurance can be expressed in absolute and relative terms. Absolute endurance can be measured as the duration of maintaining a given isometric force, the number of repetitions that can be done with a given weight, the average force maintained in a sustained maximal isometric contraction over a fixed time period, or, as commonly done on isokinetic dynamometers, the average force maintained over a set number of contractions at a set velocity. Men, because of their greater absolute strength, have greater absolute endurance, particularly when the endurance task requires forces that are a high percentage of women's maximum strength. Men's advantage in absolute endurance is pronounced most in the upper body, where men have close to twice the absolute strength of women. A striking example is shown in Figure 4.9B, which shows, in the arm curl weight-lifting exercise, that the weight that represented 50% of the men's maximal single lift (1 RM) and with which the men on average could do more than 30 repetitions, exceeded the average 1 RM for the women. Thus, many women could not do one repetition with a weight that the men could complete about 35 repetitions.

B. Relative Endurance

Relative endurance tests include the time that a given percentage of maximum isometric force can be sustained, the number of repetitions that can be completed

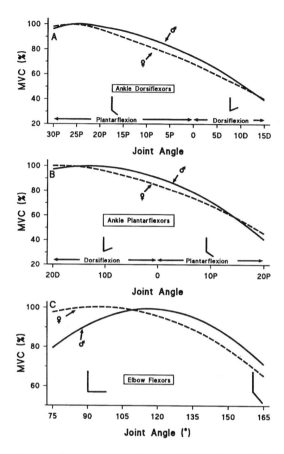

Figure 4.8 Isometric strength curves for ankle dorsiflexion (A) and plantarflexion (B), and elbow flexion (C). Women and men had similar dorsiflexion and plantarflexion strength curves, but differed in the shape of the elbow flexion curve. See text for further discussion. Based on van Schaik et al.[82] (A), Winegard et al.[84] (B), and Tsunoda et al.[39] (C).

with a given percentage of the maximum single lift (1 RM), the relative (%) decline in force during a maximal effort isometric contraction sustained over a fixed time interval, and the relative decline in force over a set number of concentric contractions at a set velocity on an isokinetic dynamometer. In relative endurance tests, women are either equal to or superior to men.

1. Weight Lifting

In some weight-lifting tests, women can do more repetitions than men with a given percentage of the 1 RM.[10,50,85] The gender difference is greater with weights representing smaller percentages of the 1 RM[85] (Figure 4.9A) and may be most evident in muscle groups with the largest gender difference in absolute strength. For example, women who had 52% of the men's absolute elbow flexion 1 RM could do

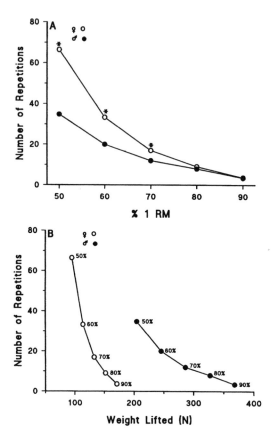

Figure 4.9 Endurance in weight-lifting exercise. A. Relative endurance in the arm curl (elbow flexion) exercise: the number of repetitions completed at various percentages of the one repetition maximum (1 RM). *P < 0.05, women completed more repetitions. B. Absolute endurance: the data in A are plotted in relation to the absolute weight lifted. Men's greater absolute endurance is evident. Based on Maughan et al.[85]

more repetitions with 60% of the 1 RM; in contrast, the women did not do more repetitions with 40 and 60% of the 1 RM in the knee extension exercise, in which they had 62% of the men's 1 RM.[10] On the other hand, female strength athletes who had only 42% of the squat 1 RM of their male counterparts nevertheless had the same (~10%) relative decline in 1 RM performance over 20 successive sets of 1 repetition with the 1 RM.[44]

2. Isometric Contractions

In submaximal isometric relative endurance tests, women can maintain contractions longer than men.[85-87] In the study previously described[44] in which male and female athletes did 20 sets of 1 RM squats, interspersed maximum isometric contractions revealed no gender difference in the decline in peak isometric force during

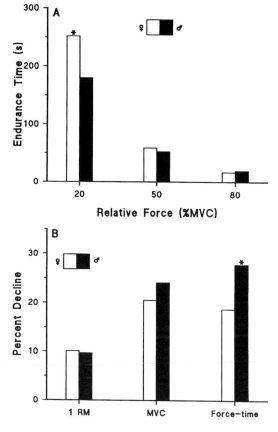

Figure 4.10 A. Relative endurance in isometric knee extension at 20, 50, and 80% of maximal voluntary isometric force (MVC). *P < 0.05, greater relative endurance in women. Based on Maughan et al.[85] B. Male and female strength athletes completed a weight-lifting session comprising 20 sets of 1 repetition maximum (1 RM) in the squat exercise. The percent decline in weight lifting 1 RM, isometric strength (MVC), and isometric rate of force development (Force-time) following the weight-lifting session is shown. The women and men had similar declines in 1 RM and MVC, but men showed a greater decline rate of force development (*P < 0.05). Based on Häkkinen.[44]

the weight lifting session. However, analysis of the force-time curves indicated that the males showed a greater decline in force developed over the first 500 ms of each contraction (Figure 4.10B).

3. Isokinetic Contractions

A common isokinetic relative endurance test consists of 50 consecutive knee extension concentric contractions at a joint angular velocity of 3.14 rad/s (180°/s).[88] No gender difference has been observed in the percent decline in torque over the 50 contractions.[8,33,89]

C. Possible Mechanisms of Observed Gender Difference in Relative Endurance

1. Neural Factors

In submaximal isometric endurance tests, the EMG at the endurance limit is less than that achieved in an unfatigued MVC.[87,90] The EMG deficit in sustained contractions could be the result of decreased motor unit activation[91] or failure of neuromuscular propagation.[90] One study found men to have a greater decline than women in EMG during a fatiguing weight-lifting protocol,[44] suggesting that men may be more susceptible to failure of central activation or neuromuscular propagation. In contrast, women's superior endurance in isometric handgrip exercise was not associated with a difference in the EMG response, suggesting that the mechanism for women's superior endurance was distal to the muscle action potential.[87]

2. Muscle Fiber Type Distribution

Women's superior endurance in submaximal isometric tests might be related to their greater type I/II area ratio[10,17,23,40,47,49-52] and perhaps percent type I fibers,[10,40,52] because type I fibers have greater resistance to fatigue than type II fibers. However, studies of the correlation between isometric endurance and fiber type distribution have been inconsistent. In active physical education students, a positive correlation was found between percent type I fibers in vastus lateralis and isometric endurance at 50% MVC in a leg press action.[92] In contrast, in untrained subjects no correlation was found between percent type I fibers or percent type I fiber area and knee extension endurance at 20, 50, and 80% MVC.[93] Furthermore, if the explanation is a greater percent type I fiber area, one would expect women to show a smaller decline in the previously described isokinetic fatigue test because a smaller decline is correlated with a high percent type I fibers.[88] Instead, no gender difference has been observed.[8,33,89]

3. Fiber Area

Women's smaller mean fiber area[10,17,23-26] may be an advantage in endurance tests because there would be a smaller diffusion distance for oxygen and metabolites. A smaller mean fiber area also might favor a greater capillary density (capillaries/mm^2), which would enhance endurance performance.

4. Stretch-Shorten Cycle

Women's greater ability to reutilize elastic energy stored in eccentric contractions might contribute to their greater endurance in weight-lifting tests,[10,50,85] which consist of coupled eccentric-concentric contractions (i.e., stretch-shorten cycle).

5. Specific Tension and Muscle Blood Flow

There are some reports of smaller specific tension in women's muscles.[20,34] In endurance tests (isometric, weight-lifting) in which muscle blood flow might be compromised because of increased intramuscular tension, a smaller specific tension might favor women, who would be less susceptible to occlusion of blood flow. The data in Figure 4.10A are relevant to this possibility, for they show that at the two highest relative force levels (50 and 80% MVC), in which occlusion would have been present in both women and men, there was no difference in endurance. In contrast, at the lowest intensity (20% MVC), where some blood flow was possible and women's advantage regarding specific tension could be expressed, women indeed had greater endurance. However, another study found women's superior isometric endurance to be greater at 50% than 30% MVC.[87] In relation to occlusion of blood flow in isometric contractions, it is notable that men show a greater elevation of blood pressure than women in sustaining an isometric contraction, perhaps a compensation for a greater specific tension; nevertheless, women could maintain the contraction longer.[86]

6. Muscle Dimensions

Another possible explanation for women's greater relative endurance is based on the concept that whereas force is determined by muscle cross-sectional area (CSA), the metabolic cost of the contraction is determined by muscle volume (CSA × length).[94] Men, by being taller, have longer muscles and therefore may incur a greater metabolic cost in maintaining a given force.[94]

IV. EVOKED MUSCLE CONTRACTILE PROPERTIES

Muscle contractile properties typically are measured under isometric conditions at or close to optimal muscle length for force production. Electrical stimulation of the motor nerve or motor point is used to evoke maximal twitch and tetanic contractions.

A. Twitch

The gender difference in twitch force is generally similar to that for isometric MVC (Figure 4.11); the difference is greater in upper[15,95] than lower[13,42,82,84,96] limb muscles. The ankle plantarflexor muscles are a notable and unexplained exception. In this muscle group, the female/male (F/M) ratio is greater for twitch than MVC and evoked tetanic force.[3,13,84,97] In the most extreme example, the F/M ratio for plantarflexor twitch force was 1.3 (i.e., women actually had significantly greater twitch force), whereas the ratios for MVC and 50 Hz force were 0.75 and 0.8, respectively.[3]

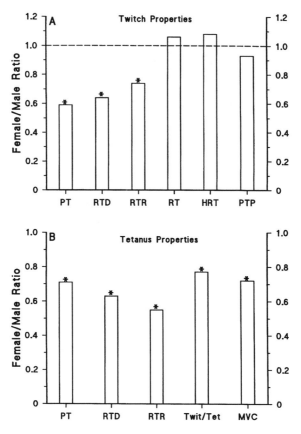

Figure 4.11 Female/male ratios for evoked isometric contractile properties of the ankle dorsiflexors. A. Twitch peak torque (PT), rate of torque development (RTD), rate of
torque relaxation (RTR), rise time (RT, time from 10% to 90% PT), half-relaxation
time (HRT), and potentiated (by 100 Hz tetanic stimulation) twitch torque (PTP).
B. Tetanus peak torque (PT), rate of torque development (RTD), rate of torque
relaxation (RTR), twitch/tetanus ratio (Twit/tet), and voluntary peak torque (MVC).
*P < 0.05, significant gender difference. Based on O'Leary et al.[96,98]

Twitch contraction time (time-to-peak force + half relaxation time) is generally
similar in women and men in upper and lower limb muscles[3,13,15,82,84,95-97] (Figure 4.11),
although there have been some observations of longer contraction times in
women.[13,15,95,97] Owing to generally larger twitches with similar or shorter contraction
times, men have greater rates of twitch absolute force development and relaxation[42,95,96]
(Figure 4.11). On the other hand, rate of force development, normalized to peak force,
is similar in women and men.[42]

B. Tetanus

Men have greater tetanus peak force and rates of absolute force development
and relaxation than women[3,42,82,96] (Figure 4.11), but similar normalized (to peak
tetanic force) rates of force development and relaxation.[42]

C. Twitch/Tetanus Ratio

Only one study has compared twitch/tetanus ratios in women and men; men had a greater ratio in the ankle dorsiflexors[96] (Figure 4.11). There are two other studies of the dorsiflexors that did not report twitch/tetanus ratios; however, ratios could be estimated based on the twitch and tetanus forces reported. In contrast to the study shown in Figure 4.11, these studies suggested greater ratios in women.[42,82] In ankle plantarflexors, women had greater twitch but smaller tetanic force than men, indicating a greater twitch/tetanus ratio in women.[3] Some studies have used MVCs as a substitute for evoked tetanus in calculating the twitch/tetanus ratio. Men have a greater twitch/MVC ratio in ankle dosiflexors[97] and elbow flexors,[95] but there is no gender difference in ankle plantarflexors.[97]

D. Posttetanic Potentiation

The potentiation of twitch force by a preceding tetanic contraction is similar in men and women[98] (Figure 4.11). Twitch force also can be potentiated by a preceding maximal voluntary contraction; similar potentiation is seen in women and men.[13,97]

E. Fatiguability

In the ankle dorsiflexors, men showed more fatigue during a 100 Hz tetanus maintained for seven seconds.[98] In contrast, intermittent stimulation of the ankle plantarflexors at 20 Hz over a 2-min period produced similar fatigue in women and men.[3]

V. SUMMARY

Women have about 70% of the leg and 50% of the upper body absolute strength of men. The gender difference in strength is smaller when expressed relative to body mass, smaller still when expressed relative to fat-free body mass, and all but eliminated when expressed relative to muscle cross-sectional area (CSA). Because there is no evidence of a gender difference in the ability to activate muscles, and a small if any difference in specific tension (force per unit muscle CSA), the gender difference in absolute strength can be attributed almost entirely to differences in muscle CSA. Men's larger muscle CSA is the product mainly of larger muscle fiber area and possibly a greater number of fibers.

Isometric absolute rate of force development is greater in men than women, owing to men's greater peak force; on the other hand, observations on rate of force development normalized to peak force have been inconsistent, showing either similar values, greater values in men, or greater values in women.

The gender difference in absolute strength is apparently smaller for eccentric than isometric contractions but larger for high velocity concentric contractions. It is not known why women do relatively better in eccentric contractions. A possible mechanism may be related to women's greater type I/II fiber area ratio because the longer cross-bridge cycle (and attachment) times in type I fibers may enhance force development in eccentric contractions. Women are also more effective in combining eccentric with concentric contractions; that is, the stretch-shorten cycle. Women are able to reutilize, in a subsequent concentric contraction, greater percentage of the energy absorbed in a preceding eccentric contraction.

The shapes of isometric strength curves are for the most part similar in women and men. However, there may be a difference in the elbow flexion strength curve as a result of men's greater muscle size, which impairs force generation at the most flexed joint angles.

Absolute muscle endurance, the ability to sustain a given absolute force, is greater in men than women. In contrast, women are equal or superior to men in relative endurance, the ability to sustain a given percentage of maximal strength. The mechanism(s) responsible for women's superior relative endurance have not been determined, but factors that have been considered include women's larger type I/II fiber area ratio, smaller fiber area, more effective reutilization of stored elastic energy, smaller specific tension, and its influence on blood flow and the economy of shorter muscles.

The peak force of evoked twitch and tetanic contractions shows the same general pattern of gender differences as in voluntary strength. The similar pattern reinforces the dominant role of muscle size in gender differences in strength. Twitch contraction time is slightly longer in women, whereas twitch and tetanus absolute rates of force development and relaxation are greater in men. Potentiation of twitch force by a preceding evoked tetanus or voluntary contraction is similar in women and men.

REFERENCES

1. Nordgren, B., Anthropometric measures and muscle strength in young women, *Scand. J. Rehab.*, 4, 165, 1972.
2. Cioni, R., Giannini, F., Paradiso, C., Battistini, N., Denoth, F., Navona, C., and Starita, A., Differences between surface EMG in male and female subjects evidenced by automatic analysis, *Electroenceph. Clin. Neurophysiol.*, 70, 306, 1988.
3. Davies, C. T. M., Strength and mechanical properties of muscle in children and young adults, *Scand. J. Sports Sci.*, 7, 11, 1985.
4. Froese, E. A. and Houston, M. E., Torque-velocity characteristics and muscle fiber type in human vastus lateralis, *J. Appl. Physiol.*, 59, 309, 1985.
5. Heyward, V. H., Johannes-Ellis, S. M., and Romer, J. F., Gender differences in strength, *Res. Quart.*, 57, 154, 1986.
6. Hoffman, T., Stauffer, R. W., and Jackson, A. S., Sex difference in strength, *Am. J. Sports Med.*, 7, 265, 1979.
7. Laubach, L., Comparative strength of men and women: a review of the literature, *Aviat. Space Environ. Med.*, 47, 534, 1976.
8. Laforest, S., St. Pierre, D. M., Cyr, J., and Gayton, D., Effects of age and regular exercise on muscle strength and endurance, *Eur. J. Appl. Physiol.*, 60, 104, 1990.
9. Maughan, R. J., Watson, J. S., and Weir, J., Strength and cross-sectional area of human skeletal muscle, *J. Physiol.*, 338, 37, 1983.

10. Miller, A. E. J., MacDougall, J. D., Tarnopolsky, M. A., and Sale, D. G., Gender differences in strength and muscle fiber characteristics, *Eur. J. Appl. Physiol.*, 66, 254, 1993.

11. Murray, M. P., Gardner, G. M., Mollinger, L. A., and Sepic, S. B., Strength of isometric contractions. Knee muscles of men aged 20 to 86, *Phys. Ther.*, 60, 412, 1980.

12. Murray, M. P., Duthie, Jr., E. H., Gambert, S. R., Sepic, S. B., and Mollinger, L. A., Age-related differences in knee muscle strength in normal women, *J. Geront.*, 40, 275, 1985.

13. Vandervoort, A. A. and McComas, A. J., Contractile changes in opposing muscles of the human ankle joint with aging, *J. Appl. Physiol.*, 61, 361, 1986.

14. de Koning, F. L., Binkhorst, R. A., Vos, J. A., and van't Hof, M. A., The force-velocity relationship of arm flexion in untrained males and females and arm-trained athletes, *Eur. J. Appl. Physiol.*, 54, 89, 1985.

15. Doherty, T. J., Vandervoort, A. A., Taylor, A. W., and Brown, W. F., Effects of motor unit losses on strength in older men and women, *J. Appl. Physiol.*, 74, 868, 1993.

16. Montoye, H. J. and Lamphiear, D. E., Grip and arm strength in males and females, age 10 to 69, *Res. Quart.*, 48, 109, 1977.

17. Sale, D. G., MacDougall, J. D., Alway, S. E., and Sutton, J. R., Voluntary strength and muscle characteristics in untrained men and women and male bodybuilders, *J. Appl. Physiol.*, 62, 1786, 1987.

18. Alway, S. E., Stray-Gunderson, J., Grumbt, W. H., and Gonyea, W. J., Muscle cross-sectional area and torque in resistance-trained subjects, *Eur. J. Appl. Physiol.*, 60, 86, 1990.

19. Cureton, K. J., Collins, M. A., Hill, D. W., and McElhannon, Jr., F. M., Muscle hypertrophy in men and women, *Med. Sci. Sports. Exerc.*, 20, 338, 1988.

20. Kanehisa, H., Ikegawa, S., and Fukunaga, T., Comparison of muscle cross-sectional area and strength between untrained women and men, *Eur. J. Appl. Physiol.*, 68, 148, 1994.

21. Nygaard, E., Houston, M., Suzuki, Y., Jorgensen, K., and Saltin, B., Morphology of the brachial biceps muscle and elbow flexion in man, *Acta. Physiol. Scand.*, 117, 287, 1983.

22. O'Hagan, F. T., Sale, D. G., MacDougall, J. D., and Garner, S. H., Response to resistance training in young women and men, *Int. J. Sports Med.*, 16, 314, 1995.

23. Schantz, P., Randall-Fox, E., Hutchison, Tydén, W. A., and Åstrand P.-O., Muscle fibre type distribution, muscle cross-sectional area and maximal voluntary strength in humans, *Acta Physiol. Scand.*, 117, 219, 1983.

24. Alway, S. E., Grumbt, W. H., Gonyea, W. J., and Stray-Gunderson, J., Contrasts in muscle and myofibers of elite male and female bodybuilders, *J. Appl. Physiol.*, 67, 24, 1989.

25. Henriksson-Larsen, K., Distribution, number and size of different types of fibres in whole cross-sections of female m tibialis anterior. An enzyme histochemical study, *Acta Physiol. Scand.*, 123, 229, 1985.

26. Staron, R. S., Karapondo, D. L., Kraemer, W. J., Fry, A. C., Gordon, S. E., Falkel, J. E., Hagerman, F. C., and Hikida, R. S., Skeletal muscle adaptations during early phase of heavy-resistance training in men and women, *J. Appl. Physiol.*, 76, 1247, 1994.

27. Colliander, E. B. and Tesch, P. A., Bilateral eccentric and concentric torque of quad-riceps and hamstring muscles in females and males, *Eur. J. Appl. Physiol.*, 59, 227, 1989.

28. Seger, J. Y. and Thorstensson, A., Muscle strength and myoelectric activity in prepubertal and adult males and females, *Eur. J. Appl. Physiol.*, 69, 81, 1994.

29. Hortobágyi, T., Zheng, D., Weidner, M., Lambert, N. J., Westbrook, S., and Houmard, J. A., The influence of aging on muscle strength and muscle fiber characteristics with special reference to eccentric strength, *J. Gerontol., Biol. Sci.*, 50A, B339, 1995.

30. Lindle, R. S., Metter, E. J., Lynch, N. A., Fleg, J. L., Fozard, J. L., Tobin, J., Roy, T. A., and Hurley, B. F., Age and gender comparisons of muscle strength in 654 women and men aged 20–93 yr, *J. Appl. Physiol.*, 83, 1581, 1997.

31. Castro, M. J., McCann, D. J., Shaffrath, J. D., and Adams, W. C., Peak torque per unit cross-sectional area differs between strength-trained and untrained young adults, *Med. Sci. Sports Exerc.*, 27, 397, 1995.

32. Ikai, M. and Fukunaga, T., Calculation of muscle strength per unit cross-sectional area of human muscle by means of ultrasonic measurement, *Int. Z. Angew. Physiol. Einschl. Arbeitsphysiol.*, 26, 26, 1968.

33. Kanehisa, H., Nemoto, I., Okuyama, H., Ikegawa, S., and Fukunaga, T., Force generation capacity of knee extensor muscles in speed skaters, *Eur. J. Appl. Physiol.*, 73, 544, 1996.

34. Young, A., Stokes, M., and Crowe, M., The size and strength of the quadriceps muscles of old and young men, *Clin. Physiol.*, 5, 145, 1985.

35. Belanger, A. Y. and McComas, A. J., Extent of motor unit activation during effort, *J. Appl. Physiol.*, 51, 160, 1981.

36. Rutherford, O. M., Jones, D. A., and Newham, D. J., Clinical and experimental application of the percutaneous twitch superimposition technique for the study of human muscle activation, *J. Neurol. Neurosurg. Psychiat.*, 49, 1288, 1986.

37. Forsberg, A. M., Nilsson, E., Werneman, J., Bergstrom, J., and Hultman, E., Muscle composition in relation to age and sex, *Clin. Sci.*, 81, 249, 1991.

38. Maughan, R. J., Watson, J. S., and Weir, J., The relative proportions of fat, muscle and bone in the normal human forearm as determined by computed tomography, *Clin. Sci.*, 66, 683, 1984.

39. Tsunoda, N., O'Hagan, F., Sale, D. G., and MacDougall, J. D., Elbow flexion strength curves in untrained men and women and male bodybuilders, *Eur. J. Appl. Physiol.*, 66, 235, 1993.

40. Simoneau, J. A. and Bouchard, C., Human variation in skeletal muscle fiber-type proportion and enzyme activities, *Am. J. Physiol.*, 257, E567, 1989.

41. Young, A., The relative isometric strength of type I and type II muscle fibres in the human quadriceps, *Clin. Physiol.*, 4, 23, 1984.

42. Behm, D. G. and Sale, D. G., Voluntary and evoked muscle contractile characteristics in active men and women, *Can. J. Appl. Physiol.*, 19, 253, 1994.

43. Bell, D. G. and Jacobs, I., Electro-mechanical response times and rate of force development in males and females, *Med. Sci. Sports Exerc.*, 18, 31, 1986.

44. Häkkinen, K., Neuromuscular fatigue and recovery in male and female athletes during heavy resistance exercise, *Int. J. Sports Med.*, 14, 53, 1993.

45. Komi, P. V. and Karlsson, J., Skeletal muscle fiber types, enzyme activities and physical performance in young males and females, *Acta Physiol. Scand.*, 103, 210, 1978.

46. Morris, A. F., Clarke, D. H., and Dainis, A., Time to maximal voluntary isometric contraction (MVC) for five different muscle groups in college adults, *Res. Quart.*, 54, 163, 1983.

47. Clarkson, P. M., Kroll, W., and Melchionda, A. M., Age, isometric strength, rate of tension development and fiber type composition, *J. Geront.* 36, 648, 1981.

48. Essen-Gustavsson, B. and Borges, O., Histochemical and metabolic characteristics of human skeletal muscle in relation to age, *Acta Physiol. Scand.*, 126, 107, 1986.

49. Glenmark, B., Hedberg, G., and Jannson, E., Changes in muscle fibre type from adolescence to adulthood in women and men, *Acta Physiol. Scand.*, 146, 251, 1992.

50. Nygaard, E., Skeletal muscle fiber characteristics in young women, *Acta Physiol. Scand.*, 112, 299, 1981.

51. Saltin, B., Henrikson, Nygaard, J. E., and Andersen, P., Fiber types and metabolic potentials of skeletal muscles in sedentary men and endurance runners, *Ann. N.Y. Acad. Sci.*, 301, 2, 1977.

52. Simoneau, J. A., Lortie, G., Boulay, M. R., Thibault, M. C., Theriault, G., and Bouchard, C., Skeletal muscle histochemical and biochemical characteristics in sedentary male and female subjects, *Can. J. Physiol. Pharmacol.*, 63, 30, 1985.

53. Komi, P. V., Physiological and biomechanical correlates of muscle function: effects of muscle structure and stretch-shortening cycle on force and speed, *Exerc. Sports Sci. Rev.*, 12, 81, 1984.

54. Viitasalo, J. T. and Komi, P. V., Force-time characteristics and fiber composition in human leg extensor muscles, *Eur. J. Appl. Physiol.*, 40, 7, 1978.

55. Colliander, E. B. and Tesch, P. A., Responses to eccentric and concentric resistance training in females and males, *Acta Physiol. Scand.*, 141, 149, 1990.

56. Griffin, J. W., Tooms, R. E., Vander Zwaag, R., Bertorini, T. E., and O'Toole, M. L., Eccentric muscle performance of elbow and knee muscle groups in untrained men and women, *Med. Sci. Sports Exerc.*, 25, 936, 1993.

57. Dudley, G. A., Harris, R. T., Duvoisin, M. R., Hather, B. M., and Buchanan, P., Effect of voluntary vs. artificial activation on the relationship of muscle torque to speed, *J. Appl. Physiol.*, 69, 2215, 1990.

58. Westing, S. H., Seger, J. Y., and Thorstensson, A., Effects of electrical stimulation on eccentric and concentric torque-velocity relationships in man, *Acta Physiol. Scand.*, 140, 17, 1990.

59. Svantesson, U. and Grimby, G., Stretch-shortening cycle during plantar flexion in youing and elderly women and men, *Eur. J. Appl. Physiol.*, 71, 381, 1995.

60. Svantesson, U., Grimby, G., and Thomeé, R., Potentiation of concentric plantar flexion torque following eccentric and isometric actions, *Acta Physiol. Scand.*, 152, 287, 1994.

61. Westing, S. H., Cresswell, A. G., and Thorstensson, A., Muscle activation during maximal voluntary eccentric and concentric knee extension, *Eur. J. Appl. Physiol.*, 62, 104, 1991.

62. Davison, K. S., Ioannidis, G., Tsunoda, N., Sale, D. G., MacDougall, J. D., and Moroz, J., Influence of gender and training on muscle activation in eccentric and concentric actions, *Med. Sci. Sports Exerc.*, 27(Suppl.), S89, 1995.

63. Curtin, N. A. and Edman, K. A. P., Force-velocity relation for frog muscle fibres: effects of moderate fatigue and intracellular acidification, *J. Physiol.*, 474.3, 483, 1994.

64. Houston, M. E., Norman, R. W., and Froese, E. A., Mechanical measures during maximal velocity knee extension exercise and their relation to fibre composition of the human vastus lateralis muscle, *Eur. J. Appl. Physiol.*, 58, 1, 1988.

65. Prince, F. P., Hikida, R. S., and Hagerman, F. C., Human muscle fibre types in powerlifters, distance runners and untrained subjects, *Pflugers Arch.*, 363, 19, 1976.

66. Prince, F. P., Hikida, R. S., and Hagerman, F. C., Muscle fiber types in women athletes and non-athletes, *Pflugers Arch.*, 371, 161, 1977.

67. Ryushi, T., Hakkinen, K., Kauhannen, H., and Komi, P. V., Muscle fiber characteristics, muscle cross-sectional area and force production in strength athletes, physically active males and females, *Scand. J. Sports Sci.*, 10, 7, 1988.

68. Poulin, M. J.,Vandervoort, A. A., Patterson, D. H., Kramer, J. F., and Cunningham, D. A., Eccentric and concentric torques of knee and elbow extension in young and older men, *Can. J. Appl. Sport Sci.*, 17, 3, 1992.

69. Vandervoort, A. A., Kramer, J. F., and Wharram, E. R., Eccentric knee strength of elderly females, *J. Geront.*, 45, B125, 1990.

70. Aniansson, A., Hedberg, M., Henning, G.-B., and Grimby, G., Muscle morphology, enzymatic activity, and muscle strength in elderly men: a follow-up study, *Muscle Nerve*, 9, 585, 1986.

71. Grimby, G., Aniansson, A., Zetterberg, C., and Saltin, B., Is there a change in relative muscle fibre composition with age?, *Clin. Physiol.*, 4, 189, 1984.

72. Jennekens, F. G. I., Tomlinson, B. E., and Walton, J., Histochemical aspects of five limb muscles in old age: an autopsy study, *J. Neurol. Sci.*, 14, 259, 1971.

73. Lexell, J. and Downham, D. Y., What is the effect of ageing on type 2 muscle fibres?, *J. Neurol. Sci.*, 107, 250, 1992.

74. Anderson, M. B., Coté, III, R. W., Coyle, E. F., and Roby, F. B., Leg power, muscle strength, and peak EMG activity in physically active college men and women, *Med. Sci. Sports*, 11, 81, 1979.

75. Aura, O. and Komi, P. V., The mechanical efficiency of locomotion in men and women with special emphasis on stretch-shortening exercises, *Eur. J. Appl. Physiol.*, 55, 37, 1986.

76. Svantesson, U., Ernstoff, B., Bergh, P., and Grimby, G., Use of Kin-Com dynamometer to study the stretch-shortening cycle during plantar flexion, *Eur. J. Appl. Physiol.*, 62, 415, 1991.

77. Enoka, R. M., Eccentric contractions require unique activation strategies by the nervous system, *J. Appl. Physiol.*, 81, 2339, 1996.

78. Van Ingen Schenau, G. J., An alternative view of the concept of utilisation of elastic energy in human movement, *Human Movt. Sci.*, 3, 301, 1984.

79. Bosco, C., Tarkka, I., and Komi, P. V., Effect of elastic energy and myoelectrical potentiation of triceps surae during stretch-shortening cycle exercise, *Int. J. Sports Med.*, 3, 137, 1982.

80. Bosco, C., Viitasalo, J. T., Komi, P. V., and Luhtanen, P., Combined effect of elastic energy myoelectrical potentiation during stretch-shortening cycle exercise, *Acta Physiol. Scand.*, 114, 557, 1982.

81. Komi, P. V. and Bosco, C., Utilization of stored elastic energy in leg extensor muscles by men and women, *Med. Sci. Sports*, 10, 261, 1978.

82. van Schaik, C. S., Hicks, A. L., and McCartney, N., An evaluation of the length-tension relationship in elderly human ankle dorsiflexors, *J. Gerontol.*, 49, B121, 1994.

83. Kulig, K., Andrews, J. G., and Hay, J. G., Human strength curves, *Exerc. Sports Sci. Rev.*, 12, 417, 1984.

84. Winegard, K. J., Hicks, A. L., and Vandervoort, A. A., An evaluation of the length-tension relationship in elderly human plantarflexor muscles, *J. Gerontol., Biol. Sci.*, 52A, B337, 1997.

85. Maughan, R. J., Harmon, M., Leiper, J. B., Sale, D., and Delman, A., Endurance capacity of untrained males and females in isometric and dynamic muscular contractions *Eur. J. Appl. Physiol.*, 55, 395, 1986.

86. Petrofsky, J. S., Burse, R. L., and Lind, A. R., Comparison of physiological responses of women and men to isometric exercise, *J. Appl. Physiol.*, 38, 863, 1975.

87. West, W., Hicks, A., Clements, L., and Dowling, J., The relationship between voluntary electromyogram, endurance time and intensity of effort in isometric handgrip exercise, *Eur. J. Appl. Physiol.*, 71, 301, 1995.

88. Thorstensson, A. and Karlsson, J., Fatiguability and fibre composition of human skeletal muscle, *Acta Physiol. Scand.*, 98, 318, 1976.

89. Kanehisa, H., Okuyama, H., Ikegawa, S., and Fukunaga, T., Sex difference in force generation capacity during repeated maximal knee extensions, *Eur. J. Appl. Physiol.*, 73, 557, 1996.

90. Fugelvand, A. J., Zackowski, K. M., Huey, K. A., and Enoka, R. M., Impairment of neuromuscular propagation during human fatiguing contractions at submaximal forces, *J. Physiol.*, 460, 549, 1993.

91. Löscher, W. N., Cresswell, A. G., and Thorstensson, A., Central fatigue during a long-lasting submaximal contraction of the triceps surae, *Exp. Brain Res.*, 108, 305, 1996.

92. Hultén, B., Thorstensson, A., Sjödin, B., and Karlsson, J., Relationship between isometric endurance and fibre types in human leg muscles, *Acta Physiol. Scand.*, 93, 135, 1975.

93. Maughan, R. J., Nimmo, M. A., and Harmon, M., The relationship between muscle myosin ATP-ase activity and isometric endurance in untrained male subjects, *Eur. J. Appl. Physiol.*, 54, 291, 1985.

94. de Haaan, A., Rexwinkel, R., van Doorn, J. E., Westra, H. G., Hollander, A. P., Huijing, P. A., Woittiez, R. D., and Sargeant, A. J., Influence of muscle dimensions on economy of isometric exercise in rat medial gastrocnemius muscles *in situ, Eur. J. Appl. Physiol.*, 57, 57, 1988.

95. O'Hagan, F., Tsunoda, N., Sale, D. G., and MacDougall, J. D., Elbow flexor evoked twitch contractile properties in untrained men and women and male bodybuilders, *Eur. J. Appl. Physiol.*, 66, 240, 1993.

96. O'Leary, D. D., Hope, K., Sale, D. G., and Moroz, J., Contractile properties of the dorsiflexor muscles in young men and women, *Physiologist*, 39, A-59, 1996.

97. Belanger, A. Y., McComas, A. J., and Elder, G. B. C., Physiological properties of two antagonistic human muscle groups, *Eur. J. Appl. Physiol.*, 51, 381, 1983.

98. O'Leary, D. D., Hope, K., Sale, D. G., and Moroz, J., Post-tetanic potentiation in dorsiflexor muscles of young women and men, *Med. Sci. Sports Exerc.*, 28 (suppl), S168, 1996.

CHAPTER 5

Muscle Sympathetic Nerve Activity During Exercise and Influences of Gender

Steven M. Ettinger, M.D.

CONTENTS

1-8493-8194-0/98/$0.00+$.50
© 1999 by CRC Press LLC

I. INTRODUCTION

Several key cardiovascular physiological responses seen with exercise include increases in heart rate, blood pressure, and myocardial contractility. These adjustments result in part from alterations in the autonomic nervous system. Regulation of both sympathetic and parasympathetic neural outflow are dependent upon input from centers located within the brain and from various baro-, mechano- and chemoreceptors located throughout the body. The enormous volume of work evaluating the exercise response has focused predominately on the regulatory systems as they relate to men. Gender-related differences in maximal aerobic uptake have been demonstrated and explained in part by differences in various physiological variables. Women have a smaller heart size and blood volume, lower arterial O_2 content, and lower hemoglobin concentration.[1-4] Pulmonary volume and ventilatory volume are also lower in women as compared to men during exercise.[5] Preliminary studies suggest that the response of the autonomic nervous system during exercise may differ in men as compared to women.[6,7] In premenopausal women, the ovarian cycle also may modify the response of the chemoreflex during static handgrip exercise. The following chapter serves to review the present understanding of the various regulatory neuropathways involved during static and rhythmic exercise and the potential influences of gender.

II. CARDIOVASCULAR REGULATION

A. Central Command

Stimulation of alpha motor neurons located in the somatomotor regions of the brain results in the activation and recruitment of skeletal muscle fibers that are essential for the performance of physical activity.[8] Increases in sympathetic neural outflow from the cardiovascular center of the medulla (dorsal lateral region) results in increases in heart rate and myocardial contractility along with an increase in vasomotor tone (vasoconstriction) (Figure 5.1). Stimulation of these sympathetic efferent fibers was postulated to occur in parallel with alpha motor neurons.[9] Termed central command, this pathway plays a significant role in regulating blood flow to skin during volitional activity and in controlling heart rate responses.[10-12] The regulation of skin blood flow is essential for maintaining body temperature that has been demonstrated to influence not only the rate at which muscle tension is generated but the relaxation properties of muscle.[13] Recordings of skin sympathetic nerve activity

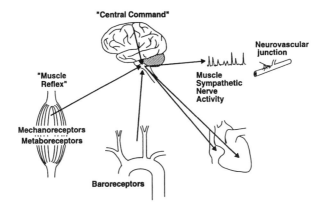

Figure 5.1   Central and Peripheral Reflexes. Central Command refers to the parallel activation
of both alpha motor neurons located in the cerebral cortex and sympathetic neural
fibers located in the cardiovascular center of the medulla (dorsal lateral region).
As a result, increases in heart rate and myocardial contractility are observed along
with increases in vasomotor tone. Muscle Reflex refers to activation of either
metabo- or mechano-receptors located within the skeletal muscle. Stimulation of
these afferent receptors by either specific byproducts of cellular metabolism or by
stretching of the muscle results in increases in heart rate and vasomotor tone.
Baroreceptors located within the walls of the aortic arch and carotid sinus, relay
signals through the tractus solitarius into the medulla and result in reductions in
sympathetic neural outflow and vasomotor tone. The mean voltage neurogram
obtained by microneurographic technique reflects bursts of sympathetic nerve
activity recorded from the efferent limb of the reflex.

reflects activity of both vasoconstricting and vasodilating (sudomotor) neural
fibers.[14,15] Stimulation of sudomotor fibers results in cutaneous vasodilation by causing the release from sweat glands of vasoactive substances. Alterations in the electrical
conductance of the skin are used to measure sweat gland activity and can be used to
assess the efferent limb of the central command reflex.[16] Vissing et al. measured
efferent skin sympathetic nerve activity (SSNA) in response to various volitional
efforts and maneuvers.[17] Changes in SSNA as measured by microneurography were
noted to occur immediately before the onset of the exercise paradigm (voluntary
muscle contractions) and increased as the exercise progressed. At the completion of
the exercise, SSNA returned towards baseline. When a period of postexercise circulatory arrest was introduced, SSNA still returned towards baseline once the voluntary
effort ceased. The critical findings of this study were twofold. First, the study extended
the observations of earlier work in defining the role of central command as it relates
to the regulation of skin blood flow during volitional activity.[18] Secondly, by demonstrating a close link between the onset of muscle contractions and burst activity on
the mean voltage neurogram, it strengthened and supported the theory of parallel
activation involving both alpha-motor neurons and efferent sympathetic neural fibers.
The importance of central command is evident not only during exercise, but in the
moments just before skeletal muscle activation, a period of time that has been referred
to as the anticipatory phase.[10,11,19,20] The teleological significance of an increasing
heart rate immediately prior to the onset of activity relates to the priming effects on
the cardiovascular system. By increasing the heart rate and cardiac output, the antic-

ipatory phase serves to optimize skeletal muscle perfusion and favorably impacts upon the balance between supply (of essential nutrients provided by the circulatory system) and demand (of exercising skeletal muscle).

B. Baroreflex and Resistance Vessels

In addition to central command, impulses originating from pressor-sensitive baroreceptors located within the walls of the aortic arch and carotid sinus relay information to the nucleus tractus solitarius in the medulla (NTS).[21,22] Stimulation of this area inhibits sympathetic neural outflow, which leads to a reduction in vasomotor tone (vasodilation) (Figure 5.1). It has been suggested that the baroreflex serves to maintain homeostasis during exercise by attenuating increases in arterial pressure. This effect serves to limit potential end-organ damage, which could result from uncontrolled elevations in blood pressure. The decrease in heart rate associated with activation of the baroreceptors is mediated by the vagal nuclei in the medulla.

Although reflexes originating within the aortic arch and carotid sinus are critical in adjusting sympathetic neural outflow,[23] the vessels that are ultimately responsible for the regulation of skeletal muscle blood flow and important in the control of arterial pressure are the small arteries and arterioles.[21,22] An increase in sympathetic neural outflow results in the release of norepinephrine by postsynaptic nerve endings. Initially stored in vesicles, the neurotransmitter enters the neurovascular junction. The resulting increase in vasomotor tone (vasoconstriction), leads to an increase in vascular resistance and a reduction in blood flow.[24,25] Sympathetic vasodilation of resistance vessels is achieved by a reduction or withdrawal of pre-existing basal sympathetic tone. Alterations in flow through resistance vessels is achieved by a complex interaction that involves not only the sympathetic nervous system, but the autoregulatory characteristics of the vessel, the generation and release of endothelium-derived relaxing factors, and the interstitial chemical milieu of the vascular bed.

Studies pertaining to the structural characteristics of the arterial resistance vessels demonstrate the presence of both alpha-1 and alpha-2 receptors. Alpha-1 receptors predominately located on the larger resistance vessels are felt to be responsible for the regulation of vascular resistance, and alpha-2 receptors located principally on small terminal arterioles regulate capillary perfusion pressure.[26,27] Studies have demonstrated alpha-1 receptors to be metabolite-insensitive while alpha-2 receptors to be metabolite-sensitive.[26,27] The intrinsic properties of these alpha-receptors allow for the regulation of skeletal muscle blood flow. Seals demonstrated the close link between changes in sympathetic nerve activity and changes in vascular resistance. Using microneurographic techniques and venous occlusion plethysmography — methods to be described in detail later in this chapter — subjects performed static handgrip exercise at increasing workloads. Increases in both leg muscle sympathetic nerve activity and calf vascular resistance were observed during and after arm exercise.[28] These effects were observed to be both time- and intensity-dependent.

The regulation of skeletal muscle blood flow is not only limited to mechanisms that influence the systemic (arterial) circulation. Constriction of large capacitance vessels (veins) results in the redistribution of blood flow from the visceral organs into the central circulation. This leads to an increase in venous return and ventricular preload. Additional adjustments in arterial vasomotor tone by the baroreceptors act in concert with the increasing preload to provide effectively adequate cardiac output to vital organs, which must be maintained during the exercise.[29]

C. Metabo- and Mechano-Reflex

The third pathway involved in regulating the cardiovascular system's response to exercise is termed the exercise pressor reflex. Finely myelinated (group III) and unmyelinated (group IV) nerve fibers serve as sensory receptors within the peripheral organs (i.e. muscle) and provide a source of continuous feedback to the central nervous system.[30,31] During muscle contractions, the resulting mechanical deformation stimulates afferent nerve terminal endings termed mechanoreceptors. Although group III afferents act primarily in response to stretch or compression, these fibers also have been shown to react to chemical changes within the interstitium of the skeletal muscle.[32,33] Group IV afferent nerve fibers respond to changes in concentrations of various byproducts of cellular metabolism and as such have been termed chemo- or metaboreceptors. Group IV fibers also are felt to be polymodal as they have been shown to respond to mechanical stimulation.[32,34] Activation of both group III and IV afferent nerve fibers leads to a rise in systolic blood pressure by increasing sympathetic neural outflow.

1. The Exercise Pressor Reflex

In 1937, Alam and Smirk performed a series of experiments during which time the circulation to the extremities (legs or arms) was occluded (circulatory arrest) prior to the performance of the exercise paradigm.[35] Blood pressure increased during the exercise and fell only a few mmHg when the exercise was stopped. When blood flow to the limb was restored, blood pressure decreased towards baseline. If circulatory arrest was continued for 3 to 4 minutes after the completion of the exercise, a gradual increase in the blood pressure response was demonstrated. These findings were observed to occur independently of muscle mass (i.e., arm or leg exercises). The investigators concluded that the persistent elevation in blood pressure was not attributed to mental or central effects as only restoration of limb blood flow abolished the observed pressor response. These elegant studies were the first to suggest that a reflex originating within the skeletal muscle contributed to the cardiovascular system's response to exercise. This reflex was felt to be triggered by substances liberated by the active muscle and accumulated within the interstitium. Termed the chemo- or metaboreflex, this pathway has been shown to play a critical role in regulating sympathetic neural outflow to both active and inactive muscle during isometric (static) and moderate to heavy levels of isotonic (rhythmic) activity.[33,36-39]

During exercise, skeletal muscle blood flow increases in the active limb in an attempt to match increasing metabolic demands. Sympathetic neural outflow (muscle sympathetic nerve activity — MSNA) plays a critical role in maintaining the balance between supply (cardiac output) and demand (of the exercising skeletal muscle).[36,40,41] Barcroft, Bonnar, Edholm, and Eftron[42] used plethysmography to demonstrate a two- to threefold increase in resting forearm blood flow after the radial, median, and ulnar nerves to the arm were blocked by injections of a local anesthetic (procaine and adrenaline). These results provided evidence that resting human skeletal muscle had a predominance of vasoconstrictor tone. During exercise, the production of vasoactive substances by the contracting skeletal muscle acts directly on the resistance vessels in an effort to decrease vasomotor tone. The subsequent vasodilation leads to an increase in blood flow that is essential in providing the metabolic substrates necessary for skeletal muscle contraction. The reduction in vascular resistance is countered by an increase in sympathetic neural outflow. Increases in vasomotor tone serve to direct blood flow away from less active structures (splanchnic organs and inactive muscle) and to counter the metabolically induced vasodilation. Blood flow to resting skeletal muscle ranges between 1 and 5 ml/min/100 g and accounts for 15 to 20% of the resting cardiac output. With exercise, blood flow to exercising muscle can increase up to 15 to 20 times basal level.[43] If left unchecked the vascular reservoir of the skeletal muscle potentially could exceed the maximal increase in cardiac output.[40,44] Therefore, increases in sympathetic neural outflow directed to the active muscle bed is essential for maintaining systemic arterial pressure and avoiding potential compromises in flow to essential organs.

The concept known as sympatholysis refers to the ability of the muscle to continually increase blood flow (vasodilation forces) in the presence of increasing MSNA (vasoconstriction forces). During exercise, the production and accumulation of metabolic substances result in the stimulation of alpha receptors at the level of the small terminal arterioles. The resulting vasodilatory response serves to counter the effects of the increased sympathetic neural outflow that is directed toward the active muscle bed (i.e., sympatholysis).[45] The mechanism(s) by which sympatholysis is achieved, at what point during exercise it predominates, and whether it fully counteracts the increased vasoconstricting forces are not known fully. Recently, Shoemaker et al. failed to demonstrate the presence of functional sympatholysis during a rhythmic handgrip exercise paradigm.[46] During a graded rhythmic handgrip exercise paradigm, significant reductions in skeletal muscle blood flow were associated with an increased reliance on nonoxidative metabolism. This was demonstrated by use of NMR spectroscopy (increasing development of intracellular acidosis) and measurements of venous lactate (increasing concentrations). In this study, increases in sympathetic neural outflow and vasomotor tone were achieved by lower body negative pressure introduced prior to the onset of the rhythmic exercise. The findings of reduced venous hemoglobin saturations, along with increased plasma lactate levels and intracellular hydrogen ion concentrations throughout the exercise, suggested that the increase in vasomotor tone, regulated by the sympathetic nervous system, was not countered by the vasodilatory effects of the vascular bed, that is, functional sympatholysis did not occur. The results of this study would suggest that if sympatholysis was to occur and be the dominant force acting on the vascular bed, the resulting increase in blood flow directed toward the exercising muscle might surpass maximal cardiac output and cause hemodynamic instability. Therefore it would appear that homeostasis is better served by a partial rather than unrestricted sympatholytic effect. Prior works have provided evidence to suggest that activation of the metaboreflex is important in countering the potential destabilizing effects of an unrestricted metabolically induced vasodilation.[47] The dynamic parameters involved in this response remain in question and will be reviewed later in the chapter. In an effort to study the sympathetic nervous system during rest and in response to exercise, several techniques have been developed that measure various points along the efferent limb. The following section will briefly review two of these mechanisms before focusing on the technique of microneurography.

III. MEASUREMENT TECHNIQUES

A. Venous Plethysmography

Venous occlusion plethysmography initially was used to measure blood flow to internal organs[48] and now is used routinely to measure changes in blood flow to both upper and lower extremities. As described by Brodie and Russell, the objective of the technique is to arrest completely venous return to the organ or limb for several seconds without interfering with arterial inflow.[49] A continuous recording of the change in volume is made using the segment of limb that is distal to the venous occlusion cuff. A portion of the limb also can be studied (forearm) by placing an arterial occlusion cuff distal to the venous occlusion cuff. This maneuver serves to exclude potential confounding effects on changes in volume that result from circulation of the distal appendage (hand or foot).[50] The initial rate of expansion (Δ volume) of the limb during venous occlusion is assumed to represent actual arterial inflow occurring immediately before the venous cuff is inflated. With the limb resting at an angle above the level of heart to maintain free venous drainage, measurements of skeletal muscle blood flow can be made for several minutes following various interventions. Several types of plethysmographs have been used to measure changes in limb volume (displacement using water or air and photo-reflection) and more recently mercury in Silastic strain-gauge (measures changes in limb circumference).[51]

B. Norepinephrine Kinetics

Released from postganglionic sympathetic fibers, norepinephrine (NE) serves as the primary neurotransmitter of the sympathetic nervous system.[52] Depolarization-induced increases in intracellular concentrations of calcium causes release of NE by exocytosis.[53] In humans, the greatest source of NE at rest and during exercises is from skeletal muscle.[54-56] Initially, measurements of plasma NE concentrations were used to assess total body activity of the sympathetic nervous system. Using this noncompartmental model to calculate NE kinetics as a means to assess sympathetic nerve activity has significant limitations. As sympathetic outflow is not generalized or uniform to all organs, this method is limited in its ability to assess sympathetic neural outflow to specific target sites (i.e., kidneys, skin, skeletal muscle).[57-61] In addition, the essential assumption of this model relates to the supposition that all of the hormone is present in a measurable compartment. Due to observations that the predominant NE fraction is located in inaccessible compartments including the neurovascular junction and nerve terminal endings, a two-compartment model was developed (compartment 1 includes accessible circulating NE; compartment 2 includes the inaccessible regions or organs that contain NE). The neurotransmitter is exchanged readily between compartments 1 and 2.[52] During an intravenous infusion of 7[³H]NE, collections of arterialized venous samples are obtained at 30, 40, and 50 minutes and at various intervals following the completion of the infusion. Initial concerns over the use of this model were raised regarding the large dosages of 7[³H]NE that needed to be given intravenously and the effects of such dosages on the steady state of the hormone.[62,63] The development of a three compartment model allowed investigators to estimate organ-specific levels of sympathetic nerve activity (compartment 1 included NE released into the synaptic cleft and entering the plasma; compartment 2 included intraneural and intracellular NE; and compartment 3 included the pool of NE cleared and metabolized by the kidneys and tissues, respectively).[61] Although the use of the three-compartment model allows for a better fit in assessing NE kinetics, plasma concentrations of this neurotransmitter are still dependent upon rates of neuronal reuptake, which can be effected by medications, clearance by tissues, and the presence of local factors that influence NE release from presynaptic nerve terminals.[64] Limitations of this technique include the need to infuse a tracer isotope (³H-NE) and the difficulty in studying changes in sympathetic neural outflow that occur at the onset of exercise.[65]

C. Microneurography

In an effort to study somatosensory and proprioceptive pathways, Vallbo and Hagbarth developed a percutaneous approach to record nerve impulses.[66] Introduced in 1966, direct (intraneural) recordings of postganglionic nerve fascicles served as an indirect measurement of afferent nerve fiber activity. Today, measurements of muscle sympathetic nerve activity (MSNA) by microneurography have provided significant insights and enhanced the understanding of the cardiovascular system's response to exercise. Although predominately large nerves of both upper and lower extremities have been studied (arms: median, radial, ulnar; legs: peroneal, tibial, popliteal) due to the small size of the electrodes, recordings from small nerve branches also have been obtained.

At the start, the nerve to be studied is localized by external palpation and/or electrical stimulation. A resin-coated electrode made of tungsten wire with a diameter of 0.2 mm (1 to 5 µm tip) is advanced through the skin. A reference electrode is placed a few centimeters away in the subcutaneous tissue. The recording electrode is advanced slowly in an attempt to impale a nerve fascicle as a stimulus [1 to 4 volts] is delivered through the electrode. When a muscle fascicle is impaled a twitch is observed or felt by the subject. The electrical stimulus is discontinued and the preamplifier is switched to the recording mode. In an effort to increase the signal-to-noise ratio, the recording is amplified (50,00 to 100,000 times), filtered (700 to 2,000 Hz) and integrated to optimize the resulting mean voltage neurogram.[67] Various maneuvers (i.e., tapping or stretching of the innervated muscle bed, Valsalva, apnea, auditory, and tactile stimuli, mental stress) along with visual inspection of burst morphology (width of base, rate of upstroke, and downstroke) and relationship between burst and QRS complex on ECG (pulse-synchronicity) aid in discerning

MSNA

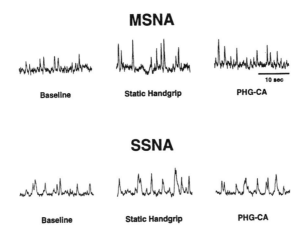

| Baseline | Static Handgrip | PHG-CA |

SSNA

| Baseline | Static Handgrip | PHG-CA |

Figure 5.2 Mean Voltage Neurogram of MSNA and SSNA. Microneurographic recordings demonstrate both muscle and skin sympathetic nerve activity. As reviewed in the text, burst morphology differs between muscle and skin. Muscle bursts are narrow-based and pulse-synchronous. Skin bursts are broad-based and can be visualized following an arousal stimuli, i.e., noise, stroking of the skin. During static exercise and PE-CA (postexercise-circulatory arrest), MSNA increases and remains elevated. During static exercise SSNA increases while during PE-CA, SSNA returns towards baseline. MSNA, muscle sympathetic nerve activity; SSNA, skin sympathetic nerve activity; PHG-CA, post-handgrip circulatory arrest.

whether the recording is from a skin fascicle (a mixture of sudomotor and vasoconstrictor impulses), from a pure muscle fascicle (predominantly vasoconstrictor impulse) or from a mixed site. If an optimal nerve trace is not observed, the recording electrode is repositioned. Bursts of nerve impulses are observed (audio and visual) as a result of the local injury that occurs when the electrode impales the nerve fascicle. Examples of a mean voltage neurogram from a skin and muscle fascicle are shown in Figure 5.2. Burst counts (expressed as bursts/min) or burst amplitude (expressed as mm/min) serve to quantify neural activity. Alternatively, burst counts may be expressed in relation to heart beat (bursts/100 heart beats).

The ability to record nerve activity is dependent not only upon the specific amplification and filtering parameters, but on the size and position of the nerve fascicle with respect to the recording electrode. As the site (limb) must remain relaxed and with minimal movement the technique permits for the measurement of efferent muscle sympathetic nerve activity (MSNA) to inactive skeletal muscle. Although studies have used microneurography to measure MSNA to active muscle groups, the constraints imposed by movement preclude the use of this technique during vigorous levels of exercise. Microneurography also is limited by a technical constraint in that not all muscle nerve fascicles impaled by the microelectrode (as confirmed by a muscle twitch) display measurable bursts on the mean voltage neurogram. Although repositioning and fine adjustments of the recording electrode may increase the strength of the muscle twitch, an optimal signal may not be obtained. This limitation is consistent with the anatomical observation that efferent fibers run in groups throughout a nerve and are not distributed evenly. Typically, the tracing represents a recording from multi and not single motor units. Although increases in MSNA are related to increases in NE spillover, the rate of discharge does not predict the vasomotor response — in other words, the change in burst count and resulting increase in resistance is variable. This may be linked to the fact that the MSNA recording is from a localized site and does not measure all of the sympathetic fibers within the fascicle.[68,69]

In an effort to confirm that the observed signal is from a postganglionic sympathetic fiber (efferent fascicle), several maneuvers were performed initially. The first involved the injection of lidocaine around the nerve site proximal to the recording electrode.[70] Injections also were made around the nerve site distal to the recording electrode. The elimination of the signal following the proximal injections confirmed a site of efferent and not afferent nerve activity. Nerve conduction velocities also were measured and were demonstrated to be on the order of 1 m/sec (average conduction velocity 0.74 to 1.11 m/sec for median and peroneal nerves). This is consistent with conduction velocities of unmyelinated type C (group IV) fibers.[70,71] Finally, transient loss of nerve activity was demonstrated following the intravenous infusion of a ganglion-blocking agent. The recovery of nerve activity was observed to occur several minutes later following the discontinuation of the infusion.[72]

Recordings of resting MSNA at different times within the same individual have demonstrated a relative consistency in burst frequency.[73] Additionally, recordings within an individual from different muscle fascicles reveal a remarkable uniformity in burst count.[73] As a result of these findings, efferent muscle sympathetic nerve activity as measured by microneurography is considered to be relatively uniform throughout the body. This concept is extremely important and allows for inferences to be made regarding sympathetic nerve activity directed toward active skeletal muscle. Simultaneous intraneural recordings from different target organs (skin and muscle) have demonstrated distinctly different and predictable patterns of nerve responses not only during rest but following various maneuvers. This finding supports the concept that sympathetic neural outflow directed to different target organs (i.e., skin, muscle, renal, and splanchnic beds) may not be uniform but instead controlled by various regional centers.[74] In addition, the performance of mental as opposed to physical exercise may influence MSNA uniformity. Anderson et al. demonstrated differences in MSNA responses during the performance of a mental task.[75] As heart rate and blood pressure increased throughout the activity (arithmetic), MSNA to the arm (radial nerve) and leg (peroneal nerve) differed. Although MSNA increased in the leg during both stress and recovery phases, increases in MSNA directed to the arm were observed only during the recovery period. The study also served to demonstrate that increases in muscle sympathetic neural outflow can occur in response to a mental stress.

IV. MUSCLE SYMPATHETIC NERVE ACTIVITY (MSNA)

The effects of the following hemodynamic and physiological parameters on muscle sympathetic nerve activity have been studied in great detail. Before exploring the effects of various types of exercise and gender on MSNA these parameters will be reviewed.

A. Effectors

1. Blood Pressure

Within an individual, burst activity increases during periods of reduced blood pressure and decreases during periods of elevated blood pressure.[72] Recordings during carotid sinus nerve stimulation provided evidence to link MSNA responses to the carotid baroreflex. Impulses originating from these pressor-sensitive receptors relay information to the NTS in the medulla.[8] During diastole, the sympathoinhibitory effects of the arterial baroreceptors on central sympathetic neural outflow are eliminated. Burst activity is observed when the peripheral baroreceptors are in effect unloaded.[23,29] This association is defined as pulse-synchronicity and refers to the effects of the arterial baroreceptors in modifying sympathetic neural outflow. Recent work suggests that changes in vessel area, in addition to changes in pressure, are a key determinant of baroreflex activity.[76] A link between burst activity and the ECG also has been found as a result of the arterial baroreceptors. The time interval between the peak of the R-wave on the ECG and the peak of the recorded burst on the tracing provides a measure of the latency period of the baroreflex.[71] Measurements of this interval are relatively constant throughout a recording and can be used to differentiate bursts from artifact (electrical noise).

In animals, studies have shown that when blood pressure is raised acutely, arterial baroreceptor activity increases.[77,78] This inverse relationship provides investigators with a means to augment baseline sympathetic tone and MSNA. Changes in the ambient pressure at the level of the carotid sinus or of the lower extremities can be used to alter basal MSNA. The ability to increase sympathetic nerve activity allows for the detection of potential effects of various physiological interventions that might otherwise not be observed. Despite the initial decrease in MSNA that is associated with an acute rise in blood pressure, with time arterial baroreceptor activity returns to baseline (resetting of receptor threshold), and subsequent measurements of MSNA demonstrate that the level of activity approaches prehypertensive values.[79,80] Therefore, it is important to consider that the effects of an acute intervention on sympathetic neural outflow may not reflect accurately changes that would occur during continuous or chronic exposure to the intervention.

a. Hypertension

No significant difference in baseline sympathetic neural outflow between hypertensive and normotensive subjects has been observed. The appearance of essential hypertension is related to abnormal tone at the level of the resistance vessels and does not appear to be related to a generalized increase in sympathetic neural outflow. As a result of long-standing hypertension, arterial baroreceptors are reset and higher levels of blood pressure are necessary to inhibit sympathetic neural outflow.[81,82] Although baseline levels of MSNA may be similar, sympathetic neural outflow in response to various interventions may differ between normotensive and hypertensive individuals.[83] This may be related to the assumption that cardiopulmonary baroreflex control of MSNA is heightened in hypertensive individuals. Withdrawal of this controlling influence allows for observed differences in MSNA between normo- and hypertensive subjects.

2. Body Position

Changes in body position affect sympathetic neural outflow. Passive raising of the legs and tilting of the body into a head-down position[84] reduce MSNA responses, while changing to a more upright position increases MSNA responses.[84] Placing the body or limb into a tank or enclosing a limb within a chamber that alters the ambient surrounding forces by creating either negative or positive pressure in an effort to mimic changes in body position affects MSNA. A specially designed cuff placed around the neck can influence both carotid and aortic baroreceptors. With negative pressure (suction), transmural pressure increases and MSNA decreases, although with positive pressure, transmural pressure decreases and MSNA increases. Exposing the lower body to negative pressure (LBNP) simulates the hemodynamic changes that occur with standing, while the subject remains in the supine position. This results in a progressive increase in MSNA. Although earlier works suggested selective disengagement of high and low pressure baroreceptors depending upon the degree of LBNP,[85,86] Taylor et al. recently demonstrated that both cardiopulmonary and aortic baroreceptors are activated at low levels of LBNP.[76]

3. Respirations

In a pattern similar to that seen with changes in arterial pressure, alterations in MSNA are coupled to the phases of the respiratory cycle. Increased activity observed during the expiratory phase appears to be linked to the effects of expiration on blood pressure and the release of the sympathoinhibitory (vagal) lung inflation reflex.[70,87] Experiments also have demonstrated that although periods of hypoxia stimulate resting MSNA, periods of hyperoxia may or may not attenuate resting levels of MSNA.[88,89] One potential difference for this response may be related to the presence of respiratory disorders (i.e., obstructive sleep apnea).

a. Valsalva's Maneuver

The various phases of this baroreflex-mediated maneuver influence MSNA in a predictable manner. The onset of the forced expiration against a closed glottis (phase I), is associated with an initial increase in intrathoracic pressure and an increase in systolic pressure. During the straining stage (phase II), decreased systemic venous return reduces stroke volume and mean arterial pressure while heart rate begins to increase. Phase III occurs when straining stops and is associated with further reductions in arterial pressure and increases in heart rate. Finally, phase IV is associated with an abrupt rise in arterial pressure and bradycardia.[84] At the start of the Valsalva maneuver, MSNA is attenuated due to the initial increase in blood pressure. During the second and third stages of the maneuver as a result of progressive reductions in

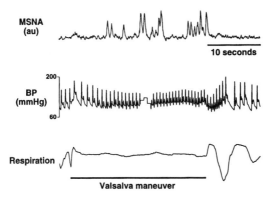

Figure 5.3 Effects of Valsalva's Maneuver on MSNA. Phase I of Valsalva's maneuver is
associated with an increase in systolic blood pressure and an attenuation in MSNA.
Phase II is associated with a decrease in ventricular preload, stroke volume, and
systolic blood pressure. MSNA increases during this phase. As systolic blood
pressure continues to decrease (phase III), MSNA remains elevated. At the end
of the maneuver, the abrupt rise in systolic blood pressure (phase IV) is associated
with a reduction in MSNA. MSNA, muscle sympathetic nerve activity; BP, blood
pressure; Respirations, recorded by pneumograph.

blood pressure, sympathetic neural outflow increases. At the completion of the
maneuver the rise in sympathetic neural outflow is attenuated resulting from the
overshoot in blood pressure. This simple maneuver can be used to confirm the site
of the recording microelectrode. Figure 5.3 demonstrates a Valsalva maneuver and
the expected MSNA responses.

4. Mental Stress (Arousal Stimuli)

Under periods of increased emotion or stress, blood pressure and blood flow to
skin increases. During this time sympathetic neural outflow to muscle is unchanged[84]
or increased.[75] If the recording microelectrode is positioned within a skin fascicle,
sympathetic nerve activity is observed to increase with cognitive stress. Of interest
is the finding that the SSNA response is extinguished with repetition of the stimuli.
The difference in sympathetic neural outflow to muscle and skin in response to
mental stress provides another means of confirming the recording site.

5. Temperature

Barcroft and Edholm evaluated the effects of temperature on forearm blood flow
using venous plethysmography and demonstrated augmentation in flow as temperature increased (increases in flow from 0.5 cc/100 cc forearm/min at 13°C to 17.6
cc/100 cc forearm/min at 45°C).[90] Ray et al. demonstrated an association between
increasing MSNA and muscle temperature. Increase in mechanoreceptor activation
contributed to the increase in MSNA response as sympathetic neural outflow returned
toward baseline during a period of postexercise circulatory arrest.[91]

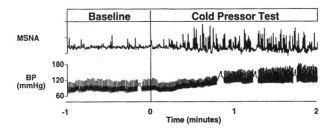

Figure 5.4 Cold Pressor Testing and MSNA. The application of ice water to the skin for
approximately two minutes leads to measurable increases in muscle and skin
sympathetic nerve activity. This maneuver is used to assess sympathetic neural
function. Although increases in arterial blood pressure typically result in decreases
in MSNA, during cold pressor, testing increases in MSNA are associated with
increases in blood pressure. BP, blood pressure; MSNA, muscle sympathetic
nerve activity.

a. Cold Pressor Test (CPT)

This unique and simple maneuver has been used to study the effects of the
sympathetic nervous system on both peripheral and cardiac circulation.[92] The application of ice water to the skin for approximately two minutes leads to measurable
increases in muscle and skin sympathetic nerve activity (Figure 5.4). As mentioned
previously, regulation of MSNA is linked to the arterial baroreflex such that increases
in arterial blood pressure result in decreases in MSNA.[29] During the CPT, however,
increases in MSNA are associated with increases in blood pressure. This relationship
allows CPT to be used to assess sympathetic neural function.[93,94] Increases in skin
sympathetic nerve activity also are observed during CPT and are felt to be related
to exposure to the painful or noxious stimulus. Victor et al. demonstrated that the
increased heart rate observed during CPT is related to the increase in sympathetic
nerve activity and its effects on the sinus node as opposed to withdrawal of parasympathetic tone.[95]

6. Blood Flow to Exercising Muscle

The effects of blood flow on MSNA have been studied using both rhythmic and
static exercise paradigms. During muscle contractions, increased end products act in
a paracrine fashion to reduce the vasomotor tone of resistance vessels (autoregula-
tion). Additionally, these substances stimulate the metaboreceptors and the resulting
increase in sympathetic neural outflow raises blood pressure by increasing vasomotor
tone. Previously, this increase in mean arterial pressure was felt to be important in
increasing perfusion to the exercising muscle.[40,41] The increased flow serves to limit
any potential mismatch between supply and demand. Joyner, however, demonstrated
that the increase in blood pressure following the activation of the metaboreflex did
not improve blood flow to the exercising muscle sufficiently to prevent continuous
reductions in venous O_2 saturations from the exercising arm.[96] This would suggest
that although the metaboreflex contributes to the increase in blood pressure during
exercise, the resulting vasoconstriction limits rather than improves skeletal muscle

blood flow. In an effort to study further the relationship between blood flow and changes in MSNA, Joyner et al. used negative pressure to increase forearm blood flow and demonstrated attenuated MSNA responses during bouts of heavy rhythmic forearm exercise.[97] Therefore, the relationship between MSNA and blood flow appears to be of a reciprocal nature, whereby increases in skeletal muscle blood flow during exercise are associated with attenuated increases in MSNA.

7. Age

Although resting MSNA appears to increase with age,[98,99] some studies have failed to demonstrate a statistically significant effect. Plasma concentrations of NE appear to increase,[100-102] or remain unchanged with age.[7] Esler et al. found that MSNA and cardiac plasma norepinephrine rates increased with age although renal plasma NE spillover did not, suggesting that regional changes in sympathetic outflow may occur with age.[103] A reduction in arterial baroreceptor control of sympathetic neural outflow does not appear to explain the association between increasing MSNA and age.[104] Blood flow to exercising skeletal muscle has been shown to decrease or remain unchanged with age.[105,106] Reductions in blood flow may be related to limitations in the ability to increase heart rate, cardiac output, and stroke volume. Whether this results in increases in baseline MSNA remains to be determined. Physical activity also may influence the effects of aging on MSNA as active older subjects demonstrate greater resting MSNA as compared to sedentary age-matched subjects. Schmidt demonstrated age-related neuraxonal dystrophy — abnormalities in the structural characteristics of terminal axons and synapses.[107] Whether these abnormalities interfere with neurotransmitter release or reuptake at the neurovascular junction remains to be studied.

B. The Exercise Pressor Reflex

Several factors influence not only the level but the rate of change of muscle sympathetic nerve activity during exercise. These include the type of exercise, the duration and intensity of exercise, muscle mass, degree of fatigue, level of training, and the environmental conditions (i.e., temperature, humidity, diet, drugs). In general, MSNA responses are greater during static as compared to rhythmic exercise. For both static and rhythmic exercises there is a threshold intensity after which MSNA increases. This level of work, defined as the percentage of the maximal voluntary contraction (% MVC) varies from person to person. During static exercise, the resulting decrease in tissue perfusion due to the increase in interstitial pressure serves to trap metabolites that stimulate afferent nerve fibers. During rhythmic contractions the reductions in tissue perfusion are transient as a result of intermittent periods of muscle relaxation. Static exercises performed at levels 10 to 15% MVC often do not result in significant increases in MSNA.[108,109] During rhythmic exercise, workload (% MVC) as well as the size of the muscle group (arm vs. leg) are important determinants of MSNA.[110] As the duration of exercise increases, however, MSNA rises regardless of whether static or rhythmic work is being performed. A rhythmic protocol performed at a lower % MVC can increase MSNA if performed for a prolonged period of time.[111-113] Some investigators observed an initial reduction in MSNA at the onset of rhythmic exercise.[114,115] Potential mechanisms relating to this effect will be discussed below. Muscle fatigue also has been observed to influence sympathetic neural outflow. At any given point in time (up to the point of muscle exhaustion), MSNA responses increase as the perception of fatigue increases.[116]

During static exercise, the heart rate increase occurs in a direct relationship to the mass of the exercising muscle.[101,102] An association between muscle mass and MSNA also has been observed.[101,102,117] Additional factors however appear to modify the effects of muscle mass on sympathetic neural outflow. Seals compared MSNA responses during a one- and two-arm static handgrip exercise paradigm.[118] Although increases in MSNA from baseline to end-exercise were greater when performed with two arms as compared to one arm, the results were not additive. This inhibitory interaction postulated by Seals, serves a potential role in preventing an extreme or inappropriate increase in arterial pressure by the sympathetic nervous system that could result from exercising increasingly larger muscle groups.[118]

The relationship between sympathetic neural outflow and the changes that occur with training are complex. Skeletal muscle blood flow is increased during exercise in part by augmentations in cardiac output and by a process that occurs at the cellular level referred to as active hyperemia.[8] The release of vasoactive substances produced by the exercising muscle and vascular endothelium results in dilatation of the arteriole bed. This process is independent of hormonal and neural influences. Reactive hyperemia refers to arteriole dilatation and the marked increase in blood flow that occurs following a period of ischemia (reactive hyperemic blood flow; RHBF).[8] Sinoway et al. demonstrated that although resting blood flow was similar in the forearms of tennis players and a group of age-matched controls, RHBF responses were significantly greater in the dominant forearm of the tennis players as compared to the nondominant forearm.[119] Potential explanations included a localized peripheral response to training within the muscle that resulted in an increase in capillary density and increased flow in the trained as compared to untrained limb. One would therefore anticipate, as suggested by Joyner,[97] that increases in blood flow to the trained arm would result in attenuated increases in MSNA as compared to the response observed during exercise involving the untrained limb. The effects of training on MSNA were evaluated by Sinoway et al. in a group of bodybuilders.[120] During a static handgrip exercise, attenuations in the rise of MSNA were observed in the bodybuilders as compared to the control group. Attenuations in the development of intracellular acidosis as measured by ^{31}P NMR spectroscopy also were observed in the bodybuilders . This was consistent with the hypothesis that training alters cellular metabolism and reduces the development of muscle acidosis. In an attempt to control for potential differences in cellular metabolism a second group of experiments were performed using an ischemic exercise paradigm. Following an initial period of circulatory arrest subjects performed a rhythmic handgrip exercise. Although similar levels of cellular acidosis were achieved in both control and bodybuilder groups, MSNA responses remained attenuated in the bodybuilders as compared to the control group. This elegant body of work suggests that the attenuation in MSNA that is associated with training is in part related to mechanisms that are independent of changes in blood flow or alterations in cellular metabolism. The following section serves to review the basic principles and responses of both central command and the metaboreflex during static and rhythmic exercise.

1. Static Exercise

At the onset of static handgrip exercise, heart rate and blood pressure increase. This response is mediated in part by effects from both central command and the mechanoreflex.[121] Withdrawal of vagal tone at the level of the sinoatrial node is primarily responsible for the initial increase in heart rate.[8] Increases in MSNA are not observed at the onset of exercise but have a one- to two-minute lag time.[39,122] This delay is explained partially by the time required for the accumulation of the various metabolic substances that stimulate the metaboreceptors. Blood flow to the exercising muscle appears to play a critical role in the manifestation of the exercise pressor reflex, as changes effect the washout of metabolites. At the completion of the exercise if the circulation to the limb is interrupted, these substance(s) remain trapped within the interstitium and continuously stimulate the metaboreflex. During this period of postexercise circulatory arrest (PE-CA), the muscle is inactive as volitional activity ceases. The effects of both central command and the mechanoreflex are eliminated. Therefore, PE-CA serves to isolate the effects of the metaboreflex. During PE-CA, increases in heart rate observed during the bout of exercise are no longer noted and the heart rate returns toward baseline. This suggests that the metaboreflex does not participate in adjusting the heart rate response during static exercise.[122]

During oxidative phosphorylation, ATP is converted to ADP and inorganic phosphate. As glycogen is utilized for energy by the exercising muscle (glycolysis), the intracellular concentrations of lactic acid increase. ^{31}P nuclear magnetic resonance spectroscopy (NMR) measures metabolic changes in high energy phosphate compounds at the cellular level and provides an opportunity to isolate potential metaboreceptor-stimulating substances. NMR spectroscopy identifies and quantitates the chemical properties of a specific sample by collecting and recording characteristic signals (resonance) emitted during pulsed low-energy radio-wave exposure.[123] Studies utilizing NMR spectroscopy have demonstrated that the production and accumulation of lactic acid, hydrogen ions, and diprotonated phosphate are associated with increases in MSNA and therefore may serve as substances that stimulate the metaboreceptors.[120,124] Following an infusion of dichloroacetate (DCA), which decreases plasma lactate concentrations, attenuations in MSNA responses were observed during a static handgrip exercise paradigm.[125] DCA increases the activity of pyruvate dehydrogenase, which is the rate-limiting enzyme in the oxidation of lactate to pyruvate.[126,127] Other substances suggested to stimulate metaboreceptors include adenosine,[128,129] bradykinin,[130] prostaglandins,[131] capsaicin,[132] and potassium.[133,134]

2. Rhythmic Exercise

During rhythmic exercise, central and peripheral mechanisms play a critical role in not only ensuring an increase in cardiac output but controlling the distribution of blood flow to active and inactive organs and maintaining systemic arterial pressure.[110] Although increase in heart rate (chronotropic effect) enhances cardiac output, without concomitant adaptations by the peripheral circulation, stroke volume and arterial pressure could not be maintained adequately. While central mechanisms consist of the intrinsic properties of the heart, peripheral mechanisms include three pathways: mechanical, neural, and humoral. Interactions between these three pathways are important in determining ventricular preload and afterload — critical variables that influence cardiac output during rhythmic exercise.

With the onset of upright posture, the pooling of blood in the compliant venous system decreases ventricular preload. To maintain adequate stroke volume, peripheral mechanisms are activated to direct blood flow to the heart. The increase in mechanical pressure generated by contracting skeletal muscle on the deep veins serves to enhance venous return and raise right atrial pressure. This effect is seen immediately at the onset of rhythmic exercise.[135-137] Following the contraction phase, relaxation of the muscle releases the mechanical pressure on the vessel wall and results in the generation of negative transmural forces. This draws blood from the superficial into the deep venous system, further increasing venous return.[110] Contraction of the abdominal muscles during rhythmic exercise raises intra-abdominal pressure, which increases venous return. The increase in intra-abdominal pressure additionally serves to redirect blood flow away from the visceral organs, further increasing the volume of the vascular compartment.[135] The third mechanical pump that works in series with skeletal and abdominal muscles comprises the muscles of respiration. During inspiration, the changing position of the diaphragm causes a decrease in intrathoracic pressure and an increase in intra-abdominal pressure. The flow of blood within the inferior vena cava during this phase is directed toward the heart, thereby increasing venous return. During expiration, the change in position of the diaphragm and increase in intrathoracic pressure acts to decrease venous return. Moreno et al. elegantly demonstrated the interaction between the liver and the diaphragm during the respiratory cycle and the effects on venous return.[138] During inspiration, the diaphragm acts to limit the outflow of blood from the liver while the increase in intra-abdominal pressure causes blood to pool within this organ. With expiration, the increased hepatic blood volume is released and directed toward the heart.

The effects of these three mechanical muscle pumps act in concert with the sympathetic nervous system to maintain adequate cardiac output throughout the period of activity. At the onset of rhythmic exercise, increases in heart rate and cardiac output are related to the withdrawal of parasympathetic (vagal) tone. Following this initial response, the sympathetic nervous system is activated and the increase in vasomotor tone results in constriction of the resistance vessels. This serves to decrease blood flow to inactive organs (splanchnic bed) and optimize circulating blood volume. As with static exercise, increased sympathetic neural outflow has been observed to be directed toward the active muscle bed during rhythmic exercise.[139,140]

C. The Gender Effect

Increasing sympathetic nerve activity has been proposed as a potential mechanism for the increasing prevalence of cardiovascular disorders associated with aging.

Although the cardiovascular system is under continuous regulation by the autonomic nervous system, most of the earlier studies make no distinction with regards to the effects of gender. If differences in sympathetic neural outflow exist between men and women, then it may explain in part why premenopausal women have a lower prevalence of cardiovascular disorders as compared to age-matched males and then catch up once menopause is reached.[141]

Long-term follow-up of the Framingham population demonstrated that the majority of cardiovascular events occurred in men (60%) as compared to women (40%). Although acute myocardial infarction and angina pectoris were the predominant coronary syndromes experienced by men, the predominant syndrome in women was angina pectoris.[141] Gender-related differences in cardiovascular morbidity and mortality also were observed in this study population. In women, significant increases in morbidity were demonstrated in the 55-and-over age group, which may be related to the effects of menopause. Hormone replacement therapy has been demonstrated to reduce cardiovascular morbidity and mortality by as much as 50% in postmenopausal women.[142] Prior to the development of overt cardiac symptoms, mortality rates in women lagged behind those of men by approximately a decade. However, by the time women become symptomatic from their coronary artery disease, their risk of death was greater. The incidence of sudden cardiac death in the Framingham population was 3.1 per 1000 in men and 1.1 per 1000 in women. Differences in autonomic tone may have contributed to this finding. Additional studies involving the Framingham population examined survival rates following the development of congestive heart failure secondary to hypertension, valvular heart disease, or coronary artery disease. Significant survival benefits were observed again in the women as compared to men (one-year survival rates of 57% in men and 64% in women).[143]

One potential explanation of the cardioprotective effect associated with gender relates to the influences of the hormone estrogen. Although a full review of the cardiovascular effects of estrogen is beyond the scope of this chapter studies have demonstrated that this hormone exhibits: calcium channel-blocking activity,[144,145] attenuating affects on the production of catecholamines, alterations in the release of NE[146] and modulation of vascular tone by endothelial-dependent and -independent mechanisms.[147,148] Additionally, *in vitro* analysis of synaptosome activity demonstrated an inhibitory effect of the hormone on the efflux and uptake of ^{3}H-NE.[149] Physiologically, estrogen increases cardiac output, reduces vascular resistance, lowers arterial blood pressure,[150] and dilates coronary arteries.[151] Although estrogen also has been shown to impact favorably upon lipid profiles by increasing HDL and decreasing LDL,[152] the cardioprotective effects of the hormone may relate ultimately to its effects on the vascular wall in altering vasomotor tone. An attenuated-pressor response during stress testing in a group of postmenopausal women who received a six-week course of estrogen supports the vasoactive influence of estrogen.[153] Attenuations in the response to mental stress was observed in a group of men who received a single dose of estrogen, suggesting that the effects may be gender-independent.[154] One potential mechanism by which estrogen may influence sympathetic neural outflow relates to its effects on substrate utilization and cellular metabolism.

1. Cellular Metabolism and Gender

Enzymatic evaluation of muscle samples obtained from the vastus lateralis have demonstrated that sedentary men have a smaller percentage of type I-oxidative, slow-twitch muscle fibers as compared to women (Chapter 3).[155,156] This study revealed a reduced capacity in men to oxidize fatty acid as compared to women as demonstrated by a decreased ratio of 3-hydroxyacyl CoA dehydrogenase : succinic dehydrogenase. The women also demonstrated a reduced capacity to utilize glycogen as compared to men. The effects of estrogen on carbohydrate metabolism may enhance further the observed structural differences (Chapter 6).[157] Prior work in women has demonstrated that plasma lactate production during heavy exercise is reduced during phases of the menstrual cycle associated with increased concentrations of estrogen.[158] In evaluating ovarian hormonal influences in animals, Kendrick et al. demonstrated that estradiol replacement (subcutaneous injections of beta-estradiol 3-benzoate) in previously oophorectomized rats resulted in the decreased utilization of myocardial glycogen during a treadmill exercise paradigm as measured by tissue sampling.[159] The effects were felt to be mediated by the influence of estradiol in increasing both the plasma concentrations of lipid substrates and the activity of enzymes necessary to increase fatty acid oxidation (i.e., lipoprotein lipase) (Chapter 8).[160,161] Tarnopolsky et al. demonstrated that during submaximal exercise, the utilization of lipids in premenopausal women (midfollicular phase) was greater as compared to men while glycogen utilization was attenuated (muscle biopsy specimens).[162,163] Plasma levels of glucose, free fatty acids, and glycerol were similar between the men and women at baseline and at the end of the exercise paradigm. Although these studies support changes in cellular metabolism as a potential mechanism by which estrogen influences sympathetic neural outflow, several works failed to demonstrate similar findings. Herling et al. evaluated the effects of the menstrual cycle on free fatty acid metabolism. During both follicular (days 4 to 10) and luteal (days 18 to 24) phases of the cycle, post absorptive free fatty acid flux was unchanged.[164] An enhanced flux of free fatty acids into muscle potentially could explain the paradoxical findings of increased lipid oxidation in the face of unchanging plasma substrate concentrations in women (Chapter 8).[165-167]

2. MSNA and Gender

Ng et al. observed higher resting burst counts (MSNA) in men as compared to age-matched women.[7] In this report, muscle sympathetic nerve activity was observed to be progressively higher in young women, young men, older women, and older men, supporting the concept that MSNA increases with age. Contrary to the microneurographic findings, however, venous plasma NE concentrations were observed to be similar between the groups. Jones et al. studied the effects of gender on MSNA responses during three maneuvers: handgrip exercise to fatigue, cold pressor testing, and a stress stimuli (mental arithmetic).[168] Baseline levels of MSNA were observed to be lower in women as compared to men. During the static handgrip paradigm MSNA responses in men were greater as compared to women. However, when controlling for differences in absolute workload between the subjects no gender effect was observed. Contrary to these findings, the authors observed attenuated MSNA responses in women (pre- and postmenopausal) as compared to a group of age-matched men during a freely perfused static handgrip exercise paradigm that included a period of postexercise circulatory arrest[6] (Figure 5.5). The attenuation in muscle sympathetic nerve activity was associated with a reduction in the intracellular concentrations of hydrogen ions and diprotonated phosphate as measured by ^{31}P NMR spectroscopy. The effect of gender on MSNA responses was independent of differences in the level of training. Similar attenuations in MSNA responses were observed in the women as compared to the men during a rhythmic thumb exercise (adduction of the adductor pollicus). This confirmed that the gender-related effects were independent of differences in muscle mass and absolute workload. During a rhythmic handgrip exercise performed under ischemic conditions the gender-related effect on MSNA responses was no longer observed. This suggested that blood flow was necessary for the full expression of the gender effect.

In an attempt to further study the effects of estrogen on sympathetic neural outflow, static handgrip exercise was performed in women during two phases of their ovarian cycle: the menstrual phase (days 1 to 4) and the follicular phase (days 10 to 12). These times were selected in an effort to evaluate the effects of high (days 10 to 12) and low (days 1 to 4) estrogen concentrations. The two phases also served to minimize potential confounding effects of progesterone as changes in the level of this hormone are minimal throughout this time (days 1 to 12).[169] Progesterone has been shown to alter cellular metabolism of both lipids and carbohydrates.[170] MSNA responses during the static handgrip exercise paradigm were attenuated during the phase of increased estrogen concentration (follicular phase). The attenuated response in MSNA was not associated with a cycle-related effect on cellular metabolism, as ^{31}P NMR spectroscopy failed to demonstrate differences in hydrogen ion production or changes in diprotonated phosphate concentrations between the two cycle phases. To evaluate the effects of blood flow on MSNA responses during the menstrual cycle, an ischemic rhythmic handgrip exercise paradigm was performed by arresting the circulation to the arm prior to a handgrip exercise. MSNA responses were similar during the early and late phases of the ovarian cycle, suggesting that blood flow is again necessary for the full expression of the gender effect.

Del Rio et al. demonstrated that during an arousal stimuli (mental stress), estradiol blunted the response of the adrenal medulla (smaller increases in heart rate, blood pressure, plasma free fatty acids, and ketones) in men.[154] Additionally, following estradiol therapy, increases in plasma NE concentrations were reduced significantly during the period of mental stress. To evaluate the effects of estrogen on cellular metabolism in men, Tarnopolsky et al.[171] studied a group of men who were treated with a 17-beta estradiol (E2) patch in a cross-over, single-blind design for a period of nine days with a four week washout period (100 mcg per day for three days; 200 mcg per day for three days; 300 mcg per day for three days). Biopsy samples from the vastus lateralis muscle along with plasma samples were obtained prior to and following a cycling exercise paradigm. At the completion of the cycling exercise, subjects performed a static handgrip exercise paradigm followed by a period of post-handgrip circulatory arrest. As previously discussed the period of post-handgrip circulatory arrest serves to isolate the effects of the metaboreflex. Estradiol

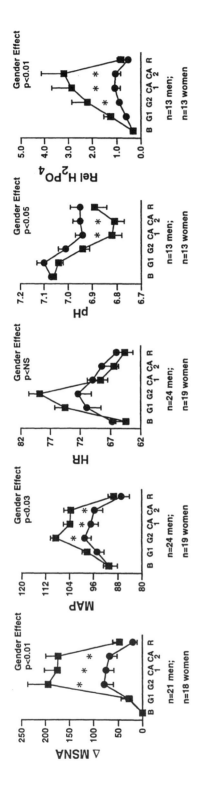

Figure 5.5 Effects of Gender on Various Hemodynamic and Metabolic Parameters. During a static handgrip exercise paradigm performed at 30% MVC, changes in ΔMSNA, MAP, pH and $H_2PO_4^-$ were greater in men as compared to women. ΔMSNA, change in muscle sympathetic nerve activity (in mm/min); HR, heart rate (in beats per min); Rel H_2PO_{4-}, relative concentration of diprotonated phosphate; B, baseline; G1 and G2, static handgrip minutes 1 and 2; CA1 and CA2, post-handgrip circulatory arrest minutes 1 and 2; R, recovery (mean value during 5 minutes). Values are means ± SE. P values, main effects of gender on various exercise parameters; NS, not significant. *P < 0.05. Reproduced from *J. Appl. Physiol.*, 80(1), 245–251, 1996. Influences of gender on sympathetic nerve responses to static exercise. Ettinger et al.

treatment significantly increased plasma estradiol concentrations to female midfollicular levels. Estradiol treatment, however, failed to attenuate glycogen utilization or to increase plasma free fatty acid concentrations during the cycling exercise. Additionally, estrogen failed to attenuate MSNA responses during the static handgrip exercise paradigm as compared to placebo.[172]

3. Gender, Estrogen, and Blood Flow

As reviewed previously, increases in blood flow to exercising muscle can attenuate the anticipated rise in MSNA response.[97] In an attempt to define additional mechanisms by which gender effects sympathetic neural outflow, attention has focused on estrogen and its effects on skeletal muscle blood flow. Recent studies have demonstrated a link between endothelium-dependent flow-mediated vasodilation and the menstrual cycle.[173] Following a maximal vasodilating stimulus (circulatory arrest for five minutes), changes in brachial artery diameter (reactive hyperemia) were observed to be greater during the follicular and luteal phases of the ovarian cycle as compared to the menstrual phase. Serum estradiol levels are lowest during the menstrual phase as compared to the other two phases.[169] The effects of estrogen on arterial reactivity appear to be gender-independent. Genetic males undergoing sex hormone manipulation (long-term high-dose estrogen therapy) were observed to have greater increases in brachial artery diameter (reactive hyperemic responses) as compared to a group of age-matched male controls. Additionally, the reactive hyperemic responses of the men receiving estrogen were found to be similar to a group of age-matched women.[174] A potential mechanism by which gender effects MSNA responses may relate to estrogen and its ability to increase skeletal muscle blood, thereby enhancing the washout of specific substance(s) that have been associated with metaboreceptor activation.

V. CONCLUSION

The integration of the various control systems that influence the cardiovascular system's response to exercise are complex. The development of various noninvasive as well as invasive techniques has allowed investigators to evaluate the various neural pathways. Although preliminary work suggests that gender influences sympathetic neural outflow, specific mechanisms remain to be elucidated. Preliminary studies offer insights into a potential link between changes in estrogen concentrations and MSNA. Whether related to an effect on skeletal muscle metabolism, skeletal muscle blood flow, or on the integration of the exercise pressor reflex, requires further investigation.

REFERENCES

1. Åstrand, P.-O. and Rodaahl, K., *Textbook of Work Physiology. Physiological Bases of Exercise,* 3rd ed., McGraw Hill, New York, NY, 1–756, 1986.

2. Drinkwater, B. L., Women and exercise: physiological aspects, *Exerc. Sports Sci. Rev.,* 12, 21, 1984.

3. Adams, K. F., Vincent, L. M., McAllister, S. M., el-Ashmawy, H., and Sheps, D. S., The influence of age and gender on left ventricular response to supine exercise in asymptomatic normal subjects, *Am. Heart J.,* 113(3), 732, 1987.

4. Lewis, D. A., Kamon, E., and Hodgson, J. L., Physiological differences between genders. Implications for sports conditioning, *Sports Med.,* 3(5), 357, 1986.

5. Mitchell, J. H., Tate, C., Raven, P., Cobb, F., Kraus, W., Moreadith, R., O'Toole, M., Saltin, B., and Wenger, N., Acute response and chronic adaptation to exercise in women, *Med. Sci. Sports Exerc.,* 24(6 Suppl), S258, 1992.

6. Ettinger, S. M., Silber, D. H., Enders, B. G., Gray, K. S., Sutliff, G., Whisler, S. K., McClain, J. M., Smith, M. B., Yang, Q. X., and Sinoway, L. I., Influences of gender on sympathetic nerve responses to static exercise, *J. Appl. Physiol.,* 80(1), 245, 1996.

7. Ng, A. V., Callister, R., Johnson, D. G., and Seals, D. R., Age and gender influence muscle sympathetic nerve activity at rest in healthy humans, *Hypertension,* 21, 498, 1993.

8. McArdle, W. D., Neural control of human movement, in *Exercise Physiology: Energy, Nutrition and Human Performance, 4th ed.,* McArdle, W., Katch, F. I., and Katch, V. L., Eds., Williams & Wilkins, Baltimore, MD, 1996, Chapter 19.

9. Hobbs, S. F., Central command during exercise: parallel activation of the cardiovascular and motor systems by descending command signals, in *Circulation, Neurobiology, and Behavior,* Smith, O. A., Galosy, R. A., and Weiss, S. M., Eds., Elsevier, New York, NY, 1982, 217.

10. Freyschuss, U., Cardiovascular adjustment to somatomotor activation. The elicitation of increments in heart rate, aortic pressure and venomotor tone with the initiation of muscle contraction, *Acta Physiol. Scand.,* 342(Suppl), 1, 1970.

11. Goodwin, G. M., McCloskey, D. I., and Mitchell, J. H., Cardiovascular and respiratory responses to changes in central command during isometric exercise at constant muscle tension, *J. Physiol. (London),* 226(1), 173, 1972.

12. Vallbo, Å. B., Hagbarth, K.-E., Torebjörk, H. E., and Wallin, B. G., Somatosensory, proprioceptive and sympathetic activity in human peripheral nerves, *Physiol Rev.,* 59, 919, 1979.

13. Rall, J. A. and Woledge, R. C., Influence of temperature on mechanics and energetics of muscle contraction, *Am. J. Physiol.,* 259 (Regulatory Integrative Comp. Physiol. 28), R197, 1990.

14. Hagbarth, K.-E., Hallin, R. G., Hongell, A., Torebjörk, H. E., and Wallin, B. G., General characteristics of sympathetic activity in human skin nerves, *Acta Physiol. Scand.,* 84, 164, 1972.

15. Hallin, R. G. and Torebjörk, H. E., Single unit sympathetic activity in human skin nerves during rest and various manoeuvres, *Acta Physiol. Scan.,* 92, 303, 1974.

16. Lloyd, D. P. C., Average behavior of sweat glands as indicated by impedance changes, *Proc. Natl. Acad. Sci. U.S.A.,* 45, 410, 1959.

17. Vissing, S. F., Scherrer, U., and Victor, R. G., Stimulation of skin sympathetic nerve discharge by central command. Differential control of sympathetic outflow to skin and skeletal muscle during static exercise, *Circ. Res.,* 69(1), 228, 1991.

18. Saito, M., Naito, M., and Mano, T., Different responses in skin and muscle sympathetic nerve activity to static muscle contraction, *J. Appl. Physiol.,* 69(6), 2085, 1990.

19. Eldridge, F. L., Millhorn, D. E., and Waldrop, T. G., Exercise hyperpnea and locomotion: parallel activation from the hypothalamus, *Science,* 211, 844, 1981.

20. Krogh, A. and Lindhard, J., The regulation of respiration and circulation during the initial stages of muscular work, *J. Physiol. (London)*, 47, 112, 1913–1914.
21. Berne, R. M. and Levy, M. N., The peripheral circulation and its control, in *Physiology. 2nd ed.*, Berne, R. M. and Levy, M. N., Eds., C V Mosby Company, St. Louis, MO, 1988, Chapter 33.
22. Berne, R. M., and Levy, M. N. Interplay of central and peripheral factors in the control of the circulation, in *Physiology. 2nd ed.*, Berne, R. M. and Levy, M. N., Eds., C V Mosby Company, St. Louis, MO, 1988, Chapter 36.
23. Wallin, B. G., Sundlöf, G., and Delius, W., The effect of carotid sinus nerve stimulation on muscle and skin nerve sympathetic activity in man, *Pflügers Arch.*, 358, 101, 1975.
24. Celander, O. The range of control exercise by a sympathicoadrenal system: a quantitative study on blood vessel and other smooth muscle effectors in the cat, *Acta Physiol. Scand.*, 32(Suppl. 116), 1, 1954.
25. Shepherd, J. T. and Vanhoutte, P. M., *The Human Cardiovascular System: Facts and Concepts*, Raven, New York, NY, 1979.
26. Faber, J. E., *In situ* analysis of alpha-adrenoceptors on arteriolar and venular smooth muscle in rat skeletal muscle microcirculation, *Circ. Res.*, 62(1), 37, 1988.
27. Ohyanagi, M., Faber, J. E., and Nishigaki, K., Differential activation of alpha 1- and alpha 2-adrenoceptors on microvascular smooth muscle during sympathetic nerve stimulation, *Circ. Res.*, 68(1), 232, 1991.
28. Seals, D. R., Sympathetic neural discharge and vascular resistance during exercise in humans, *J. Appl. Physiol.*, 66(5), 2472, 1989.
29. Sundlöf, G. and Wallin, B. G., Human muscle nerve sympathetic activity at rest: Relationship to blood pressure and age, *J. Physiol.*, 274, 621, 1978.
30. Rowell, L. B. and O'Leary, D. S., Reflex control of the circulation during exercise: chemoreflexes and mechanoreflexes, *J. Appl. Physiol.*, 69(2), 407, 1990.
31. Mitchell, J. H., Kaufman, M. P., and Iwamoto, G. A., The exercise pressor reflex: Its cardiovascular effects, afferent mechanism, and central pathways, *Ann. Rev. Physiol.*, 45, 229, 1983.
32. Kaufman, M. P., Waldrop, T. G., Rybicki, K. J., Ordway, G. A., and Mitchell, J. H., Effects of static and rhythmic twitch contractions on the discharge of group III and IV muscle afferents, *Cardiovasc. Res.*, 18(11), 663, 1984.
33. Kaufman, M. P., Longhurst, J. C., Rybicki, K. J., Wallach, J. H., and Mitchell, J. H., Effects of static muscular contraction on impulse activity of group III and IV afferents in cats, *J. Appl. Physiol.*, 55(1), 105, 1983.
34. Mitchell, J. and Schmidt, R., Cardiovascular reflex control by afferent fibers from skeletal muscle receptors, in *Handbook of Physiology. The Cardiovascular System. Peripheral Circulation and Organ Blood Flow. Volume III, Part 1.* Shepherd, J. T. and Abboud, F. M., Eds., American Physiological Society, Bethesda, MD, 1983, 623.
35. Alam, M. and Smirk, F. H., Observations in man upon a blood pressure raising reflex arising from the voluntary muscles, *J. Physiol. (London)*, 89, 372, 1937.
36. Victor, R. G. and Seals, D. R., Reflex stimulation of sympathetic outflow during rhythmic exercise in humans, *Am. J. Physiol.*, 257 (*Heart Circ. Physiol.*, 26), H2017, 1989.
37. Rowell, L. B., How are cardiovascular and metabolic functions matched during exercise: What is the exercise stimulus?, in *Human Circulation. Regulation During Physical Stress.* Rowell, L. B., Ed., Oxford University Press, London, U.K., 1986, Chapter 11.

38. Shepherd, J. T., Blomqvist, C. G., Lind, A. R., Mitchell, J. H., and Saltin, B., Static (isometric) exercise. Retrospection and introspection, *Circ. Res.,* 48(Suppl. I, No. 6), I179, 1981.

39. Victor, R. G., Seals, D. R., and Mark, A. L., Differential control of heart rate and sympathetic nerve activity during dynamic exercise: insight from direct intraneural recordings in humans, *J. Clin. Invest.,* 79, 508, 1987.

40. Rowell, L. B. and Sheriff, D. D., Are muscle "chemoreflexes" functionally important? *News Physiol. Sci.,* 3, 250, 1988.

41. Sheriff, D. D., O'Leary, D. S., Scher, A. M., and Rowell, L. B., Baroreflex attenuates pressor response to graded muscle ischemia in exercising dogs, *Am. J. Physiol.,* 258 (*Heart Circ. Physiol.,* 27), H305, 1990.

42. Barcroft, H., Bonnar, W. M., Edholm, O. G., and Effron, A. S., On sympathetic vasoconstrictor tone in human skeletal muscle, *J. Physiol.,* 102, 21, 1943.

43. Berne, R. M. and Levy, M. N., Special circulations, in *Physiology. 2nd ed.,* Berne, R. M. and Levy, M. N., Eds., C V Mosby Company, St. Louis, MO, 1988, Chapter 35.

44. Andersen, P. and Saltin, B., Maximal perfusion of skeletal muscle in man, *J. Physiol. (London),* 366, 233, 1985.

45. Hansen, J., Thomas, G. D., Harris, S. A., Parsons, W. J., and Victor, R. G., Differential sympathetic neural control of oxygenation in resting and exercising human skeletal muscle, *J. Clin. Invest.,* 98(2), 584, 1996.

46. Shoemaker, J. K., Pandey, P., Herr, M. D., Silber, D. H., Yang, Q. X., Smith, M. B., Gray, K., and Sinoway, L. I., Augmented sympathetic tone alters muscle metabolism during exercise: lack of metabolic evidence for functional sympatholysis, *J. Appl. Physiol.,* 82(6), 1932, 1997.

47. Sinoway, L. and Prophet, S., Skeletal muscle metaboreceptor stimulation opposes peak metabolic vasodilation in humans, *Circ. Res.,* 66(6), 1576, 1990.

48. Roy, C. S., The physiology and pathology of the spleen, *J. Physiol.,* 3, 203, 1881.

49. Brodi, T. G. and Russell, A. E., On the determination of the rate of blood flow through an organ, *J. Physiol. (Proc.),* 32, 1905.

50. Grant, R. T. and Pearson, R. S. E., The blood circulation in the human limb; observations on the difference between the proximal and distal parts and remarks on the regulation of body temperature, *Clin. Sci.,* 3, 119, 1938.

51. Whitney, R. J., The measurements of volume changes in human limbs, *J. Physiol.,* 121, 1, 1953.

52. Linares, O. A., Jacquez, J. A., Zech, L. A., Smith, M. J., Sanfield, J. A., Morrow, L. A., Rosen, S. G., and Halter, J. B., Norepinephrine metabolism in humans. Kinetic analysis and model, *J. Clin. Invest.,* 80(5), 1332, 1987.

53. Langer, S. Z., Presynaptic regulation of the release of catecholamines, *Pharmacol. Rev.,* 32(4), 337, 1980.

54. Hasking, G. J., Esler, M. D., Jennings, G. L., Dewar, E., and Lambert, G., Norepinephrine spillover to plasma during steady-state supine bicycle exercise. Comparison of patients with congestive heart failure and normal subjects, *Circulation,* 78, 516, 1988.

55. Savard, G., Strange, S., Kiens, B., Richter, E. A., Christensen, N. J., and Saltin, B., Noradrenaline spillover during exercise in active versus resting skeletal muscle in man, *Acta Physiol. Scand.,* 131(4), 507, 1987.

56. Savard, G. K., Richter, E. A., Strange, S., Kiens, B., Christensen, N. J., and Saltin, B., Norepinephrine spillover from skeletal muscle during exercise in humans: role of muscle mass, *Am. J. Physiol.,* 257 (*Heart Circ. Physiol.,* 26), H1812, 1989.

57. Esler, M., Assessment of sympathetic nervous function in humans from noradrenaline plasma kinetics, *Clin. Sci. (London)*, 62(3), 247, 1982.
58. Kopin, I. J., Lake, R. C., and Ziegler, M., Plasma levels of norepinephrine, *Ann. Intern. Med.*, 88, 671, 1978.
59. Lake, C. R., Chernow, B., Feuerstein, G., Goldstein, D. S., and Ziegler, M. G., The sympathetic nervous system in man: its evaluation and the measurement of plasma norepinephrine, in *Norepinephrine*, Ziegler, M. G. and Lake, C. R., Eds., Williams and Wilkins, Baltimore, MD, 1984, 70.
60. Lake, C. R., Ziegler, M. G., and Kopin, I. J., Use of plasma norepinephrine for evaluation of sympathetic neuronal function in man, *Life Sci.*, 18(11), 1315, 1976.
61. Esler, M., Willett, I., Leonard, P., Hasking, G., Johns, J., Little, P., and Jennings, G., Plasma noradrenaline kinetics in humans, *J. Auton. Nerv. Syst.*, 11(2), 125, 1984.
62. Bufano, G., Vaona, G., and Starcich, R., Approach to the pharmacokinetics of *dl*-7-3H-noradrenaline, *Eur. J. Clin. Pharmacol.*, 6, 88, 1973.
63. Jacquez, J. A., Kinetics of distribution of tracer labelled materials, in *Compartmental Analysis in Biology and Medicine*, 1st ed., Jacquez, J. A., Ed., Elsevier, New York, NY, 1972, Chapter 7.
64. Esler, M., Jennings, G., Korner, P., Willett, I., Dudley, F., Hasking, G., Anderson, W., and Lambert, G., Assessment of human sympathetic nervous system activity from measurements of norepinephrine turnover, *Hypertension*, 11(1), 3, 1988.
65. Leuenberger, U., Gleeson, K., Wroblewski, K., Prophet, S., Zelis, R., Zwillich, C., and Sinoway, L., Norepinephrine clearance is increased during acute hypoxemia in humans, *Am. J. Physiol.*, 261 (*Heart Circ. Physiol.*, 30), H1659, 1991.
66. Vallbo, Å. B. and Hagbarth, K.-E., Impulses recorded with microelectrodes in human muscle nerves during stimulation of mechanoreceptors and voluntary contractions, *Electroencephalogr. Clin. Neurophysiol.*, 23, 392, 1967.
67. Seals, D. R. and Victor, R. G., Regulation of muscle sympathetic nerve activity during exercise in humans, in *Exercise & Sport Sciences Reviews*, Vol. 19, Holloszy, J. O., Ed., Williams and Wilkins, Baltimore, MD, 1991, Chapter 9.
68. Esler, M., Jennings, G., Lambert, G., Meredith, I., Horne, M., and Eisenhofer, G., Overflow of catecholamine neurotransmitters to the circulation: source, fate and functions, *Physiol. Rev.*, 70(4), 963, 1990.
69. Wennergren, G., Aspects of central integrative and efferent mechanisms in cardiovascular reflex control, *Acta Physiol. Scand. Suppl.*, 428, 1, 1975.
70. Hagbarth, K.-E. and Vallbo, Å. B., Pulse and respiratory grouping of sympathetic impulses in human muscle nerves, *Acta Physiol. Scand.*, 74, 96, 1968.
71. Fagius, J. and Wallin, B. G., Sympathetic reflex latencies and conduction velocities in normal man, *J. Neurol. Sci.*, 47(3), 433, 1980.
72. Delius, W., Hagbarth, K.-E., Hongell, A., and Wallin, B. G., General characteristics of sympathetic activity in human muscle nerves, *Acta Physiol. Scand.*, 84(1), 65, 1972.
73. Sundlöf, G. and Wallin, B. G., The variability of muscle nerve sympathetic activity in resting recumbent man, *J. Physiol. (London)*, 272, 383, 1977.
74. Kenney, M. J., Gebber, G. L., Barman, S. M., and Kocsis, B., Forebrain rhythm generators influence sympathetic activity in anesthetized cats, *Am. J. Physiol.*, 259 (*Regulatory Integrative Comp. Physiol.*, 28), R572, 1990.
75. Anderson, E. A., Wallin, B. G., and Mark, A. L., Dissociation of sympathetic nerve activity in arm and leg muscle during mental stress, *Hypertension*, 9 (Suppl. III), III-114, 1987.

76. Taylor, J. A., Halliwill, J. R., Brown, T. E., Hayano, J., and Eckberg, D. L., 'Non-hypotensive' hypovolaemia reduces ascending aortic dimensions in humans, *J. Physiol.*, 483, 289, 1995.

77. Abboud, F. M. and Thames, M. D., Interaction of cardiovascular reflexes in circulatory control, in *Handbook of Physiology. The Cardiovascular System. Peripheral Circulation and Organ Blood Flow*, Shepherd, J. T. and Francois, F. M., Eds., *Am. Physiol. Soc.*, Bethesda, MD, 1983, Section 2.

78. Thames, M. D. and Abboud, F. M., Interaction of somatic and cardiopulmonary receptors in control of renal circulation, *Am. J. Physiol.*, 237(5), H560, 1979.

79. Kezdi, P., Mechanisms of the carotid sinus in experimental hypertension, *Circulation*, 11, 145, 1962.

80. McCubbin, J. W., Green, J. H., and Page, I. H., Baroreceptor function in chronic renal hypertension, *Circ. Res.*, 18, 205, 1956.

81. Folkow, B., Di Bona, G. F., Hjemdahl, P., Toren, P. H., and Wallin, B. G., Measurements of plasma norepinephrine concentrations in human primary hypertension. A word of caution on their applicability for assessing neurogenic contributions, *Hypertension*, 5(4), 399, 1983.

82. Morlin, C., Wallin, B. G., and Eriksson, B. M., Muscle sympathetic activity and plasma noradrenaline in normotensive and hypertensive man, *Acta Physiol. Scand.*, 119(2), 117, 1983.

83. Rea, R. F. and Hamdan, M., Baroreflex control of muscle sympathetic nerve activity in borderline hypertension, *Circulation*, 82, 856, 1990.

84. Delius, W., Hagbarth, K.-E., Hongell, A., and Wallin, B. G., Manoeuvres affecting sympathetic outflow in human muscle nerves, *Acta Physiol. Scand.*, 84, 82, 1972.

85. Scherrer, U., Vissing, S. F., and Victor, R. G., Effects of lower-body negative pressure on sympathetic nerve responses to static exercise in humans, *Circulation*, 78, 49, 1988.

86. Sundlöf, G. and Wallin, B. G., Effect of lower body negative pressure on human muscle nerve sympathetic activity, *J. Physiol. (London)*, 278, 525, 1978.

87. Eckberg, D. L., Nerhed, C., and Wallin, B. G., Respiratory modulation of muscle sympathetic and vagal cardiac outflow in man, *J. Physiol.*, 365, 181, 1985.

88. Seals, D. R., Johnson, D. G., and Fregosi, R. F., Hypoxia potentiates exercise-induced sympathetic neural activation in humans, *J. Appl. Physiol.*, 71(3), 1032, 1991.

89. Leuenberger, U., Jacob, E., Sweer, L., Waravdekar, N., Zwillich, C., and Sinoway, L., Surges of muscle sympathetic nerve activity during obstructive apnea are linked to hypoxemia, *J. Appl. Physiol.*, 79(2), 581, 1995.

90. Barcroft, H. and Edholm, O. G., The effects of temperature on blood flow and deep temperature in the human forearm, *J. Physiol.*, 102, 5, 1943.

91. Ray, C. A. and Gracey, K. H., Augmentation of exercise-induced muscle sympathetic nerve activity during muscle heating, *J. Appl. Physiol.*, 82(6), 1719, 1997.

92. Greene, M. A., Boltax, A. J., Lustig, G. A., and Rogow, E., Circulatory dynamics during the cold pressor test, *Am. J. Cardiol.*, 16, 54, 1965.

93. Cuddy, R. P., Smulyan, H., Keighley, J. F., Markason, C. R., and Eich, R. H., Hemodynamic and catecholamine changes during a standard cold pressor test, *Am. Heart J.*, 71(4), 446, 1966.

94. Cummings, M. F., Steele, P. M., Mahar, L. J., Frewin, D. B., and Russell, W. J., The role of adrenal medullary catecholamine release in the response to a cold pressor test, *Cardiovasc. Res.*, 17(4), 189, 1983.

95. Victor, R. G., Leimbach, W. N., Jr., Seals, D. R., Wallin, B. G., and Mark, A. L., Effects of the cold pressor test on muscle sympathetic nerve activity in humans, *Hypertension*, 9(5), 429, 1987.

96. Joyner, M. J., Does the pressor response to ischemic exercise improve blood flow to contracting muscles in humans? *J. Appl. Physiol.,* 71(4), 1496, 1991.

97. Joyner, M. J. and Wieling, W., Increased muscle perfusion reduces muscle sympathetic nerve activity during handgripping, *J. Appl. Physiol.,* 75(6), 2450, 1993.

98. Wallin, B. G., Delius, W., and Hagbarth, K.-E., Comparison of sympathetic nerve activity in normotensive and hypertensive subjects, *Circ. Res.,* XXXIII, 9, 1973.

99. Jones, P. P., Davy, K. P., Alexander, S., and Seals, D. R., Age-related increase in muscle sympathetic nerve activity is associated with abdominal adiposity, *Am. J. Physiol.,* 272, E976, 1997.

100. Goldstein, D. S., Lake, C. R., Chernow, B., Ziegler, M. G., Coleman, M. D., Taylor, A. A., Mitchell, J. R., Kopin, I. J., and Keiser, H. R., Age-dependence of hypertensive-normotensive differences in plasma norepinephrine, *Hypertension,* 5(1), 100, 1983.

101. Mitchell, J. H., Payne, F. C., Saltin, B., and Schibye, B., The role of muscle mass in the cardiovascular response to static contractions, *J. Physiol.,* 309, 45, 1980.

102. Seals, D. R., Washburn, R. A., Hanson, P. G., Painter, P. L., and Nagle, F. J., Increased cardiovascular response to static contraction of larger muscle groups, *J. Appl. Physiol.,* 54(2), 434, 1983.

103. Esler, M. D., Turner, A. G., Kaye, D. M., Thompson, J. M., Kingwell, B. A., Morris, M., Lambert, G. W., Jennings, G. L., Cox, H. S., and Seals, D. R., Aging effects on human sympathetic neuronal function, *Am. J. Physiol.,* 268, R278, 1995.

104. Ng, A. V., Johnson, D. G., Callister, R., and Seals, D. R., Muscle sympathetic nerve activity during postural change in healthy young and older adults, *Clin. Auton. Res.,* 5(1), 57, 1995.

105. Wahren, J., Saltin, B., Jorfeldt, L., and Pernow, B., Influence of age on the local circulatory adaptation to leg exercise, *Scand. J. Clin. Lab Invest.,* 33(1), 79, 1974.

106. Jasperse, J. L., Seals, D. R., and Callister, R., Active forearm blood flow adjustments to handgrip exercise in young and older healthy men, *J. Physiol.,* 474(2), 353, 1994.

107. Schmidt, R. E., Dorsey, D., Parvin, C. A., Beaudet, L. N., Plurad, S. B., and Roth, K. A., Dystrophic axonal swellings develop as a function of age and diabetes in human dorsal root ganglia, *J. Neuropathol. Exp. Neurol.,* 56(9), 1028, 1997.

108. Victor, R. G., Pryor, S. L., Secher, N. H., and Mitchell, J. H., Effects of partial neuromuscular blockade on sympathetic nerve responses to static exercise in humans, *Circ. Res.,* 65(2), 468, 1989.

109. Seals, D. R., Cardiopulmonary baroreflexes do not modulate exercise-induced sympathoexcitation, *J. Appl. Physiol.,* 64(5), 2197, 1988.

110. Rowell, L. B., O'Leary, D. S., and Kellogg, D. L., Jr., Integration of cardiovascular control systems in dynamic exercise, in *Handbook of Physiology, Section 12, Exercise: Regulation and Integration of Multiple Systems,* Rowell, L. B. and Shepherd, J. T., Eds., Oxford University Press, New York, NY, 1996, Chapter 17.

111. Seals, D. R., Chase, P. B., and Taylor, J. A., Autonomic mediation of the pressor responses to isometric exercise in humans, *J. Appl. Physiol.,* 64, 2190, 1988.

112. Saito, M., Mano, T., Abe, H., and Iwase, S., Responses in muscle sympathetic nerve activity to sustained hand-grips of different tensions in humans, *Eur. J. Appl. Physiol.,* 55, 493, 1986.

113. Seals, D. R., Chase, P. B., and Taylor, J. A., Autonomic mediation of the pressor responses to isometric exercise in humans, *J. Appl. Physiol.,* 64(5), 2190, 1988.

114. Ray, C. A., Rea, R. F., Clary, M. P., and Mark, A. L., Muscle sympathetic nerve responses to dynamic one-legged exercise: Effect of body posture, *Am. J. Physiol.,* 264 (*Heart Circ. Physiol.,* 33), H1, 1993.

115. Saito, M., Tsukanaka, A., Yanagihara, D., and Mano, T., Muscle sympathetic nerve responses to graded leg cycling, *J. Appl. Physiol.,* 75(2), 663, 1993.

116. Seals, D. R., Reiling, M. J., and Johnson, D. G., Peak sympathetic nerve activity during fatiguing isometric exercse in humans, *Soc. Neurosci. Abstr.,* 16, 862, 1990.

117. Buck, J. A., Amundsen, L. R., and Nielsen, D. H., Systolic blood pressure responses during isometric contractions of large and small muscle groups, *Med. Sci. Sports Exerc.,* 12(3), 145, 1980.

118. Seals, D. R., Influence of muscle mass on sympathetic neural activation during isometric exercise, *J. Appl. Physiol.,* 67(5), 1801, 1989.

119. Sinoway, L. I., Musch, T. I., Minotti, J. R., and Zelis, R., Enhanced maximal metabolic vasodilation in the dominant forearms of tennis players, *J. Appl. Physiol.,* 61(2), 673, 1986.

120. Sinoway, L. I., Rea, R. F., Mosher, T. J., Smith, M. B., and Mark, A. L., Hydrogen ion concentration is not the sole determinant of muscle metaboreceptor responses in humans, *J. Clin. Invest.,* 89, 1875, 1992.

121. Hollander, A. P. and Bouman, L. N., Cardiac acceleration in man elicited by a muscle-heart reflex, *J. Appl. Physiol.,* 38(2), 272, 1975.

122. Mark, A. L., Victor, R. G., Nerhed, C., and Wallin, B. G., Microneurographic studies of the mechanisms of sympathetic nerve responses to static exercise in humans, *Circ. Res.,* 57, 461, 1985.

123. Miller, R. G., Boska, M. D., Moussavi, R. S., Carson, P. J., and Weiner, M. W., ^{31}P nuclear magnetic resonance studies of high energy phosphates and pH in human muscle fatigue. Comparison of aerobic and anaerobic exercise, *J. Clin. Invest.,* 81(4), 1190, 1988.

124. Victor, R. G., Bertocci, L., Pryor, S., and Nunnally, R., Sympathetic nerve discharge is coupled to muscle cell pH during exercise in humans, *J. Clin. Invest.,* 82, 1301, 1988.

125. Ettinger, S., Gray, K., Whisler, S., and Sinoway, L., Dichloroacetate reduces sympathetic nerve responses to static exercise, *Am. J. Physiol.,* 261 (*Heart Circ. Physiol.,* 30), H1653, 1991.

126. Evans, O. B. and Stacpoole, P. W., Prolonged hypolactatemia and increased total pyruvate dehydrogenase activity by dichloroacetate, *Biochem. Pharmacol.,* 31(7), 1295, 1982.

127. Whitehouse, S. and Randle, P. J., Activation of pyruvate dehydrogenase in perfused rat heart by dichloroacetate, *Biochem. J.,* 134, 651, 1973.

128. Biaggioni, I., Killian, T. J., Mosqueda-Garcia, R., Robertson, R. M., and Robertson, D., Adenosine increases sympathetic nerve traffic in humans, *Circulation,* 83(5), 1668, 1991.

129. Costa, F. and Biaggioni, I., Role of adenosine in the sympathetic activation produced by isometric exercise in humans, *J. Clin. Invest.,* 93(4), 1654, 1994.

130. Stebbins, C. L. and Longhurst, J. C., Bradykinin-induced chemoreflexes from skeletal muscle: implications for the exercise reflex, *J. Appl. Physiol.,* 59(1), 56, 1985.

131. Stebbins, C. L., Maruoka, Y., and Longhurst, J. C., Prostaglandins contribute to cardiovascular reflexes evoked by static muscular contraction, *Circ. Res.,* 59(6), 645, 1986.

132. Kaufman, M. P., Iwamoto, G. A., Longhurst, J. C., and Mitchell, J. H., Effects of capsaicin and bradykinin on afferent fibers with endings in skeletal muscle, *Circ. Res.,* 50, 133, 1982.

133. Fallentin, N., Jensen, B. R., Byström, S., and Sjøgaard, G., Role of potassium in the reflex regulation of blood pressure during static exercise in man, *J. Physiol. (London)*, 451, 643, 1992.

134. Rybicki, K. J., Waldrop, T. G., and Kaufman, M. P. Increasing gracilis muscle interstitial potassium concentrations stimulate group III and IV afferents, *J. Appl. Physiol.*, 58(3), 936, 1985.

135. Guyton, A. C., Douglas, B. H., Langston, J. B., and Richardson, T. Q., Instantaneous increase in mean circulatory pressure and cardiac output at onset of muscular activity, *Circ. Res.*, 11, 431, 1962.

136. Sheriff, D. D., Rowell, L. B., and Scher, A. M., Is rapid rise in vascular conductance at onset of dynamic exercise due to muscle pump? *Am. J. Physiol.*, 265 (*Heart Circ. Physiol.*, 34), H1227, 1993.

137. Sheriff, D. D., Zhou, X. P., Scher, A. M., and Rowell, L. B., Dependence of cardiac filling pressure on cardiac output during rest and dynamic exercise in dogs, *Am. J. Physiol.*, 265 (*Heart Circ. Physiol.*, 34), H316, 1993.

138. Moreno, A. H., Burchell, A. R., Van der Woude, R., and Burke, J. H., Respiratory regulation of splanchnic and systemic venous return, *Am. J. Physiol.*, 213(2), 455, 1967.

139. Klabunde, R. E., Attenuation of reactive and active hyperemia by sympathetic stimulation in dog gracilis muscle, *Am. J. Physiol.*, 251 (*Heart Circ. Physiol.*, 20), H1183, 1986.

140. Thompson, L. P. and Mohrman, D. E., Blood flow and oxygen consumption in skeletal muscle during sympathetic stimulation, *Am. J. Physiol.*, 245 (*Heart Circ. Physiol.*, 14), H66, 1983.

141. Lerner, D. J. and Kannel, W. B., Patterns of coronary heart disease morbidity and mortality in the sexes: a 26-year follow-up of the Framingham population, *Am. Heart J.*, 111(2), 383, 1986.

142. Wolf, P. H., Madans, J. H., Finucane, F. F., Higgins, M., and Kleinman, J. C., Reduction of cardiovascular disease-related mortality among postmenopausal women who use hormones: evidence from a national cohort, *Am. J. Obstet. Gynecol.*, 164(2), 489, 1991.

143. Ho, K. K. L., Anderson, K. M., Kannel, W. B., Grossman, W., and Levy, D., Survival after the onset of congestive heart failure in Framingham Heart Study subjects, *Circulation*, 88(1), 107, 1993.

144. Collins, P., Rosano, G. M. C., Jiang, C., Lindsay, D., Sarrel, P. M., and Poole-Wilson, P. A., Cardiovascular protection by oestrogen-a calcium antagonist effect?, *Lancet*, 341, 1264, 1993.

145. Jiang, C., Poole-Wilson, P. A., Sarrel, P. M., Mochizuki, S., Collins, P., and MacLeod, K. T., Effect of 17β-oestradiol on contraction, Ca^{2+} current and intracellular free Ca^{2+} in guinea-pig isolated cardiac myocytes. *Br. J. Pharmacol.* 106: 739, 1992.

146. Du, X. J., Dart, A. M., Riemersma, R. A., and Oliver, M. F., Sex difference in presynaptic adrenergic inhibition of norepinephrine release during normoxia and ischemia in the rat heart, *Circ. Res.*, 68(3), 827, 1991.

147. Furchgott, R. F. and Zawadzki, J. V., The obligatory role of endothelial cells in the relaxation of arterial smooth muscle by acetylcholine, *Nature (London)*, 288, 373, 1980.

148. Ignarro, L. J., Byrns, R. E., Buga, G. M., and Wood, K. S., Endothelium-derived relaxing factor (EDRF) released from artery and vein appears to be nitric oxide (NO) or a closely related radical species, *Fed. Proc.*, 46(1), 644 (Abstract), 1987.

149. Janowsky, D. S. and Davis, J. M., Progesterone-estrogen effects on uptake and release of norepinephrine by synaptosomes, *Life Sci.,* 9(9), 525, 1970.

150. Rosano, G. M. C., Sarrel, P. M., Poole-Wilson, P. A., and Collins, P., Beneficial effect of oestrogen on exercise-induced myocardial ischaemia in women with coronary artery disease, *Lancet,* 342, 133, 1993.

151. Jiang, C., Sarrel, P. M., Poole-Wilson, P. A., and Collins, P., Acute effect of 17β-estradiol on rabbit coronary artery contractile responses to endothelin-1, *Am. J. Physiol.,* 263, H271, 1992.

152. Bush, T. L. and Miller, V. T., Effects of pharmacologic agents used during menopause: impact on lipids and lipoproteins, in *Menopause: Physiology and Pharmacology,* Mishell, D. R., Ed., Year Book Medical Publishers Inc., Chicago, IL, 1987, 187.

153. Lindheim, S. R., Legro, R. S., Bernstein, L., Stanczyk, F. Z., Vijod, M. A., Presser, S. C., and Lobo, R. A., Behavioral stress responses in premenopausal and postmenopausal women and the effects of estrogen, *Am. J. Obstet. Gynecol.,* 167(6), 1831, 1992.

154. Del Rio, G., Velardo, A., Zizzo, G., Avogaro, A., Cipolli, C., Della Casa, L., Marrama, P., and MacDonald, I. A., Effect of estradiol on the sympathoadrenal response to mental stress in normal men, *J. Clin. Endocrinol. Metab.,* 79(3), 836, 1994.

155. Green, H. J., Fraser, I. G., and Ranney, D. A., Male and female differences in enzyme activities of energy metabolism in vastus lateralis muscle, *J. Neurol. Sci.,* 65, 323, 1984.

156. Komi, P. V. and Karlsson, J., Skeletal muscle fibre types, enzyme activities and physical performance in young males and females, *Acta Physiol. Scand.,* 103, 210, 1978.

157. Kalkhoff, R. K., Effects of oral contraceptive agents on carbohydrate metabolism, *J. Steroid Biochem.,* 6(6), 949, 1975.

158. Jurkowski, J. E. H., Jones, N. L., Toews, C. J., and Sutton, J. R., Effects of menstrual cycle on blood lactate, O_2 delivery, and performance during exercise, *J. Appl. Physiol., Respirat. Environ. Exercise Physiol.,* 51(6), 1493, 1981.

159. Kendrick, Z. V., Steffen, C. A., Rumsey, W. L., and Goldberg, D. I., Effect of estradiol on tissue glycogen metabolism in exercised oophorectomized female rats, *J. Appl. Physiol.,* 63(2), 492, 1987.

160. Kendrick, Z. V. and Ellis, G. S., Effect of estradiol on tissue glycogen metabolism and lipid availability in exercised male rats, *J. Appl. Physiol.,* 71, 1694, 1991.

161. Rooney, T. P., Kendrick, Z. V., Carlson, J., Ellis, G. S., Matakevich, B., Lorusso, S. M., and McCall, J. A., Effect of estradiol on the temporal pattern of exercise-induced tissue glycogen depletion in male rats, *J. Appl. Physiol.,* 75(4), 1502, 1993.

162. Tarnopolsky, M. A., Atkinson, S. A., Phillips, S. M., and MacDougall, J. D., Carbohydrate loading and metabolism during exercise in men and women, *J. Appl. Physiol.,* 78(4), 1360, 1995.

163. Tarnopolsky, L. J., MacDougall, J. D., Atkinson, S. A., Tarnopolsky, M. A., and Sutton, J. R., Gender differences in substrate for endurance exercise, *J. Appl. Physiol.,* 68(1), 302, 1990.

164. Heiling, V. J. and Jensen, M. D., Free fatty acid metabolism in the follicular and luteal phases of the menstrual cycle, *J. Clin. Endocrinol. Metab.,* 74(4), 806, 1992.

165. Blatchford, F. K., Knowlton, R. G., and Schneider, D. A., Plasma FFA responses to prolonged walking in untrained men and women, *Eur. J. Appl. Physiol. Occup. Physiol.,* 53, 343, 1985.

166. Costill, D. L., Fink, W. J., Getchell, L. H., Ivy, J. L., and Witzmann, F. A., Lipid metabolism in skeletal muscle of endurance-trained men and women, *J. Appl. Physiol.,* 47, 787, 1979.

167. Friedmann, B. and Kindermann, W., Energy metabolism and regulatory hormones in women and men during endurance exercise, *Eur. J. Appl. Physiol. Occup. Physiol.,* 59, 1, 1989.

168. Jones, P. P., Spraul, M., Matt, K. S., Seals, D. R., Skinner, J. S., and Ravussin, E., Gender does not influence sympathetic neural reactivity to stress in healthy humans, *Am. J. Physiol.,* 270 (*Heart Circ. Physiol.,* 39), H350, 1996.

169. Wilson, J. D. and Foster, D. W., *Textbook of Endocrinology,* 7th ed., W B Saunders Company, Philadelphia, PA, 1985, pp. 214.

170. Hatta, H., Atomi, Y., Shinohara, S., Yamamoto, Y., and Yamada, S., The effects of ovarian hormones on glucose and fatty acid oxidation during exercise in female ovariectomized rats, *Horm. Metabol. Res.,* 20(10), 609, 1988.

171. Tarnopolsky, M. A., Ettinger, S., MacDonald, J. R., Roy, B. D., and MacKenzie, S., 17-β estradiol (E2) does not affect muscle metabolism in males, *Med. Sci. Sports Exerc.,* 29(5), S93, 1997.

172. Ettinger, S. M., MacDonald, J. R., and Tarnopolsky, M. A., Effects of estrogen on muscle sympathetic nerve activity (MSNA) during static exercise in men, *Med. Sci. Sports Exerc,* in press, (abstract), 1997.

173. Hashimoto, M., Akishita, M., Eto, M., Ishikawa, M., Kozaki, K., Toba, K., Sagara, Y., Taketani, Y., Orimo, H., and Ouchi, Y., Modulation of endothelium-dependent flow-mediated dilatation of the brachial artery by sex and menstrual cycle, *Circulation,* 92(12), 3431, 1995.

174. New, G., Timmins, K. L., Duffy, S. J., Tran, B. T., O'Brien, R. C., Harper, R. W., and Meredith, I. T., Long-term estrogen therapy improves vascular function in male to female transsexuals, *J. Am. Coll. Cardiol.,* 29, 1437, 1997.

CHAPTER 6

Gender Differences in Carbohydrate Metabolism: Rest, Exercise, and Post Exercise

Brent C. Ruby, Ph.D.

CONTENTS

1-8493-8194-0/98/$0.00+$.50

I. INTRODUCTION

Exercise participation among males and females has risen consistently during the last two decades. It is also likely that the 1996 U.S. Surgeon General report regarding physical activity and health will increase the growing number of both male and female participants. Seemingly, as rapid as the increase in regular exercise participation is the increase in sport nutritional marketing. Strategic marketing has targeted a broad audience of males and females ranging from recreational exercisers to competitive athletes. However, much of the evidence that supports the advancement and exposure of sports nutrition is based on previous or ongoing research conducted on male subjects. For example, it is accepted widely that carbohydrate (CHO) ingestion during endurance exercise has the potential to enhance performance during endurance activities. However, females have been grossly underrepresented in the CHO feeding research and are rarely included as subjects in such studies.[1,2,3]

The assumption that the CHO demand is the same for males and females may be erroneous and further emphasizes the under representation of females in exercise physiology-related research. An assumption based on limited research is synonymous with committing a type II error in the statistical testing of scientific data (i.e., accepting the null hypotheses when it is, in fact, false). Given the tremendous variation in the hormonal milieu, the disparity in skeletal muscle mass and enzyme activity, the biological significance of each gender, and the gender specific demand to support metabolism in nonskeletal muscle tissues (i.e., uterine and placental), it is difficult to assume homogeneity among male and female exercisers throughout the entire life cycle.

The purpose of this chapter is to describe the previous research related to CHO metabolism in males and females. It is the intent to represent research collected at rest, during exercise, and post-exercise to describe the presence or absence of gender specific CHO metabolism. In addition, previous research attempting to describe gender differences in CHO metabolism has varied dramatically with respect to research design, statistical analyses, subject fitness level, and the physiological measures used to establish conclusions. Each of these factors will be discussed as a potentially confounding variable that may work in concert to mask or cloud true physiological observations. Although the metabolic variation between males and females may translate to differences in event or occupation-specific performance, an increased understanding of the underlying biological significance is the main intent of this chapter.

II. EARLY RESEARCH AND RATIONALE

Using a simple searching engine available on the internet (Internet Grateful Med), a quick scan of exercise physiology research was conducted. Searching the literature on Medline from 1966 to 1979, using the key term of exercise physiology (as a subject) yielded the following results as listed in Table 6.1. Because this search was performed only using the Internet Grateful Med search engine, some articles may exist that are not included or cited by this search engine.

Table 6.1 Internet Grateful Med Search Results Performed
Using the Keyword "Exercise" and/or "Gender
Differences" Subject Listing Specifying Either
Human Males or Females as Research Subjects

Publication Year	Females	Males	Gender Differences
1966–1979	2495	4005	0
1980–1989	6972	10649	41
1990–1998	6642	8193	129

Although the total number of studies related to exercise physiology showed a tendency to increase in the 1980s, there has been a more recent increase in studies of a comparative nature (gender differences). However, when the variation in substrate utilization between genders is considered, only a handful of studies can be located. In addition, it is difficult to form conclusions based on these few papers as the methodologies vary considerably.

It is important to recognize that the rationale for research in this area has not been well-focused in the past. Historically, the anecdotal thinking relates to the concept that because females tend to have a higher percent body fat compared to males, females preferentially use fat more effectively as a fuel source. If this is true, there must be a concomitant and observable overall decrease in the demand for CHO in females. Although anecdotal thoughts are discounted by the scientific community they often are embraced by the lay community. It is the intent of this chapter to discuss how substrate utilization can affect exercise performance while considering the biological significance of gender-specific carbohydrate metabolism.

The rationale for research in this area certainly extends the boundaries of exercise physiology as a discipline. However, to better understand and explain the variations between genders, it is imperative that other studies using various methodologies and nonhuman and *in vitro* models be considered. Although the underlying intent of most of these studies was not likely to solve the gender-metabolism puzzle, the studies provide basic clues to important mechanisms that may help better design future *in vivo,* applied human studies.

III. PROBLEMS SURROUNDING PRIOR RESEARCH

The differences in CHO metabolism between males and females can be described as inconclusive at best. This is primarily a function of the heterogeneity of past research. Although Table 6.2 highlights physiological factors that can influence the selection and utilization of fuels at rest and during exercise, it also includes methodological issues related to study design. An important question for consideration is whether the observed difference between groups (genders) is due to physiology or methodology. When the heterogeneity of past research is considered, it is apparent that both factors can have an influence on the observed conclusions. For this reason, a meta-analysis of gender differences and CHO metabolism would be a complex and futile undertaking. Each of these factors (physiological and methodological) will be discussed as potential mechanisms that may contribute to an observed

Table 6.2   **Physiological and Methodological Factors that May Contribute to Gender Differences in Carbohydrate Metabolism**

Physiological Factors	Methodological Factors
Muscle morphology and histology Fiber type distribution	Subject fitness level
Enzyme activity	Testing protocol (intensity/duration) absolute vs. relative intensity
Hormonal	

Stress
    catecholamines
    growth hormone
	Pre-experiment/study diet glycogen status (liver/muscle)

Gonadotrophins
    estradiol
	Menstrual status of female subjects phase of cycle at time
	  of testing

progesterone	Matching of subjects
Cellular mechanisms	
Insulin receptor	Measurement techniques
Glucose transporters	Statistical analyses, prevalence of type I errors, statistical power

difference in CHO metabolism between males and females at rest, during exercise, and following exercise.

IV. COMMON MEASUREMENT TECHNIQUES

To adequately and accurately identify whether there are observable differences in CHO metabolism between males and females, it is critical to consider the various measurement techniques that have been used in prior research. CHO metabolism often is measured under a variety of specific physiological conditions (i.e., during rest or exercise in a fasted or fed state). Similarly, the specificity of measurement techniques ranges from whole body metabolism to tissue-specific release and uptake. Table 6.3 includes those measurement techniques that have been used to determine carbohydrate metabolism in human subjects. Although these techniques all have been used to quantify CHO metabolism in humans, not all of them have been used with the intent of determining a gender-specific response during rest or exercise. These techniques will be incorporated throughout this chapter during the discussion of previous research during rest, exercise, and post-exercise recovery. However, to better understand the mechanisms that may explain variations between genders, additional *in vitro* methods and animal models will be discussed.

V. EFFECTS OF GENDER ON CARBOHYDRATE METABOLISM IN THE RESTED STATE

It is difficult to study gender differences in CHO metabolism in a rested state when glucose homeostasis is maintained more easily. However, in the rested state, glucose homeostasis can be challenged by a period of fasting or following the ingestion of a high CHO meal. In either situation, glucose concentration requires

Table 6.3   Basic and Applied Measurement Techniques Used to Quantify Carbohydrate
Metabolism in Human Subjects

Measurement Tool	Site of Metabolism
Noninvasive	
Respiratory exchange ratio (RER)*	Whole body CHO oxidation
Positron emission tomography (PET)*	Cerebral glucose uptake
Invasive	
Tissue Sampling	
Blood glucose concentration*	Whole body — glucose homeostasis
Muscle biopsy*	Skeletal muscle glycogen utilization
Insulin clamp*	Insulin stimulated glucose uptake
mRNA expression (glucose transporters)	Variable (+ glucose uptake at brain, liver, skeletal muscle, adipose tissue)
Stable Isotope Tracer Methodology	
[6,6 ^{2}H] glucose infusion*	Hepatic glucose production (Ra)
	Glucose uptake by tissues (Rd)
[^{13}C] bicarbonate infusion	Rate of gluconeogenesis

Note: Ra — rate of appearance; Rd — rate of disposal.
* Previously used to determine gender differences in CHO metabolism.

homeostatic normalization. When hyperglycemic conditions arise, glucose uptake in the rested state is a function of both insulin release and insulin stimulated uptake by a host of tissues (mainly adipose, skeletal muscle, and liver). When hypoglycemic conditions persist, the maintenance of glucose homeostasis also is challenged. When blood glucose is in short supply, the rates of hepatic glycogenolysis and gluconeogenesis need to be sufficient enough to support the constant CHO needs of various tissues (i.e., CNS). Therefore, to consider the extent of gender specific responses to resting CHO metabolism, the biological role of each gender needs to be recognized.

VI. HORMONAL EFFECTS ON INSULIN SENSITIVITY

The unique and obvious difference between males and females is the hormonal milieu surrounding the reproductive process. This is especially true in the eumenorrheic female. Therefore, several studies have focused their attention on how the various reproductive hormones alter the metabolic actions of insulin. The reproductive hormones 17β-estradiol (E_2) and progesterone (P) have somewhat antagonistic roles related to insulin-stimulated glucose uptake. Although P alone has been shown to decrease insulin mediated uptake in adipocyctes[4,5] and skeletal muscle,[6] E_2 alone tends to promote an opposite effect by increasing insulin sensitivity and glucose uptake at the adipose tissue[4,7] and skeletal muscle.[6,7] However, in the eumenorrheic female, concentrations of E_2 and P fluctuate during the course of the normal menstrual cycle. Therefore, when both E_2 and P are administered in concert, the antagonist actions are somewhat offset, suggesting that the E_2:P ratio may be more influential in dictating the metabolic response.[4,6,8] Spellacy[8] has suggested that the result of the changing ratio may be to divert glucose utilization away from the skeletal muscle and adipose tissue in the fed state. This diversion then likely would promote increased hepatic stores of glycogen and perhaps an increased glucose availability to other tissues (i.e., uterine).

Mandour et al.[9] has suggested that E_2 has the potential to decrease the rates of gluconeogenesis and glycogenolysis by increasing the insulin:glucagon ratio. Similarly, if the insulin:glucagon ratio is elevated chronically, insulin sensitivity becomes compromised, resulting in a decreased glucose tolerance and diabetic-like symptoms, a situation common in gestational diabetes. Stevenson et al.[10] also have suggested that E_2 and P enhance the release of insulin from the pancreas. However, although E_2 tends to reduce insulin resistance, P increases it. This increase in E_2-mediated insulin sensitivity has been documented as a significant increase in circulating insulin when postmenopausal women have been provided with low doses of transdermal 17β-estradiol. Additional studies also have documented that elevated E_2 may lead to increased insulin sensitivity in heart and skeletal muscle tissues.[11,12] Nuutila et al.[11] used a positron emission tomography technique to determine glucose uptake under hyperinsulinemic normoglycemic conditions. Whole body insulin sensitivity was 41% higher in the females compared to the males and was attributed to a 47% greater rate of uptake by the femoral muscles. However, Faulkner et al.[13] demonstrated that insulin stimulated glucose uptake during an insulin clamp [during oral glucose tolerance test (OGTT)] was significantly lower in female subjects. Although these results cannot link directly the differences in insulin sensitivity to circulating levels of E_2, they provide strong support for such a mechanism. When the data of Faulkner[13] and Nuutila[11] are considered together, the precise mechanism for alterations in insulin sensitivity is unclear, but may relate to the E_2:P ratio variability between these investigations.

Cagnacci et al.[14] provided postmenopausal females with 50 μg/day of 17β-estradiol (Estraderm) for a period of three months. In response to the transdermal replacement, resting insulin concentrations were significantly lower (90.7 ± 7.7 and 70.2 ± 5.4 pmol/L for pre- and post-treatment, respectively). Similarly, in response to a OGTT, the integrated area under the curve for insulin was significantly less following the treatment (35.3 ± 3.3 and 28.7 ± 2.6 for pre- and post-treatment, respectively). The important component of this study is that, in contrast to traditional forms of hormone replacement therapy, transdermal estrogen administration delivers E_2 directly into the peripheral circulation. This approach removes the nonphysiological effect of first pass, hepatic metabolism thereby exhibiting a response physiologically similar to endogenous E_2.

Kumagai et al.[15] studied the effects of E_2 and P administration during euglycaemic hyperinsulinaemic clamp studies in oophorectomized (OVX) rats. Interestingly, OVX tended to cause a decrease in insulin sensitivity and glucose uptake by the skeletal muscle. Glycogen synthesis by the skeletal muscle also was compromised. However, when OVX animals were supplemented with either E_2 or E_2 and P, insulin sensitivity and rates of glucose uptake were restored to pre-OVX values (Figure 6.1). Therefore, under controlled situations, it is apparent that E_2 and P have the potential to alter the metabolic actions of insulin by inhibiting or facilitating rates

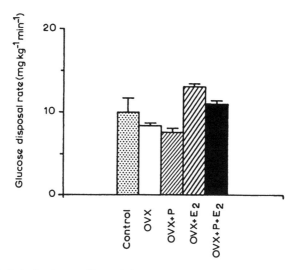

Figure 6.1   Whole-body glucose disposal during hyperinsulinaemic, euglycaemic clamp measurements in rats. (From Kumagai et al., *Acta Physiologica Scandinavica,* 149, 91, 1993. With permission.)

of glucose uptake. These results are similar to those reported by Puah and Bailey[16] who noted that in OVX mice, total muscle (soleus) insulin binding was reduced by 32% following OVX. However, when E_2 was administered, a twofold increase in insulin stimulated glucose uptake at the soleus occurred.

Armoni et al.[17] examined the effects of insulin on glucose transport and subcellular glucose transporter distribution in isolated adipose cells from men and women. Adipocytes from males had a 2.5-fold higher glucose transport rate (relative to cell surface area) under both basal or insulin stimulated conditions. Similarly, the calculated glucose transporter activity in basal plasma membranes (prepared from adipocytes), was 2.7-fold higher in cells from males. Therefore, the potential for glucose uptake by adipose cells is more pronounced in adipocyte cells obtained from males. However, glucose uptake by adipose cells was studied only under basal- and insulin-stimulated conditions. Whether the addition of E_2, in the presence or absence of insulin, would further alter glucose transport is not clear.

VII. HORMONAL INFLUENCE ON GLUCOSE UPTAKE

Thus far, the gender specific responses to resting glucose metabolism have been related to the variation in the hormonal milieu across genders. Prior research suggests that the variation in elevated levels of E_2 and P in females and the relative proportion of each partly explains the subtle differences in resting CHO metabolism between men and women. However, the location of the E_2 mediated increase in insulin sensitivity is inconclusive. As glucose uptake can occur across a variety of tissues, it is uncertain at this time which tissues are maximally and minimally influenced by the changes in the ever-changing reproductive hormone milieu during rest. Meyer and Rapp[18] examined the skeletal muscle of veal calfs for the presence of E_2 receptors. It was found that, although the presence of E_2 receptors was 1,000 times less in skeletal muscle compared to uterine tissue, the properties of the receptors were identical. Therefore, the anabolic and perhaps metabolic effects of E_2 appear to extend beyond what are traditionally considered target tissues.

In regards to tissue-specific glucose uptake, glucose uptake in the female occurs in the same tissue sites (liver, skeletal muscle, CNS) as compared to the male. As previously mentioned, under hyperinsulinemic, euglycaemic clamp, the higher insulin-stimulated glucose uptake seen in females has been associated with enhanced uptake at the femoral muscles.[11] However, the female has the potential for additional glucose uptake by tissues that are solely female (i.e., uterine and placental tissues). Under the assumption that the reproductive hormones E_2 and P have a role in altering a tissues response to insulin, depending on menstrual status and pregnancy, females appear to have more overall avenues for glucose uptake compared to males.

Misra et al.[19] studied the incorporation of [U-C^{14}] glucose by the ampullary and isthmic segments of the fallopian tube and uterus in intact, OVX, OVX + E_2, and OVX + E_2 + P rabbits. Interestingly, OVX reduced the incorporation of [U-C^{14}] glucose in all tissues. However when E_2 was provided the rate of incorporation was increased. Similar to the studies previously mentioned, administration of P antagonized the effects of E_2. In a similar investigation by Shinkarenko et al.,[20] uterine glucose uptake was studied under control and E_2-stimulated conditions. Within 60 minutes of E_2 administration, glucose consumption by the uterus increased by 80%. In addition, lactate production and glycogen formation increased by 150%. Baquer et al.[21] demonstrated a similar E_2-dependent increase in glycolytic flux and in the majority of glycolytic intermediates in rat uterine tissue. Within 48 hours of E_2 administration, key enzymes of glycolysis and the pentose phosphate pathway showed an increase in activity. Therefore the metabolic actions of E_2 are both potent and relatively fast acting in female-specific target tissues such as the uterus. Although these investigations determined the effects of glucose uptake in a tissue unique to the female, the metabolic effects of the reproductive hormones appear to be identical to previously mentioned tissues and whole body glucose metabolism.

Although glucose is primarily considered a fuel at the level of the CNS and skeletal muscle, Boland et al.[22] discovered that glucose exhibits an anabolic effect during development and steroidogenesis in the murine ovarian follicles. Murine follicles were cultured in media containing glucose at concentration between 1 and 5.5 mM. All of the glucose incorporated by the follicles was converted to lactate, indicating a metabolic preference for glycolysis. In addition, growth and steroidogenesis was dependent on available glucose. Those follicles cultured with glucose concentrations less than 2 mM were underdeveloped. This investigation suggests that the gonadotrophins stimulate glycolysis and promote follicle development when adequate glucose is provided. Therefore, it is apparent that glucose availability is critical for the development and normal function of specific tissues in the female.

A tissue that is unique to the female during pregnancy is the placenta. Hay[23] has suggested that some of the key roles of the placenta are related to transfer of nutrients to the developing fetus, consumption of nutrients, and the conversion of nutrients to other usable substrates. What is phenomenal is that the rates of glucose uptake

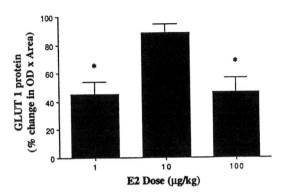

Figure 6.2 Effects of E_2 on GLUT-1 protein in rat brain microvessels. (From Shi and Simpkins, *American Journal of Physiology,* 272, E1016, 1997. With permission.)

by the placenta may exceed those of the brain and tumor tissues. Therefore, gender differences in carbohydrate metabolism are specific to variations in the life cycle. At times, there may be no appreciable difference between males and females in terms of the absolute glucose uptake by the liver or by the skeletal muscle. However, when the regular changes in circulating levels of E_2 and P and the potential for pregnancy in the female are considered, it is less likely that the patterns of CHO metabolism in the male and female are similar.

Yet another avenue for gender specific CHO metabolism has been studied in cerebral tissue. Baxter et al.[24] used positron emission tomography (PET) to study the metabolic rates of seven males and females. The females were studied in the early- to midfollicular phase of the menstrual cycle (days 5 and 15, day 1 considered the first day of menstruation). The female subjects exhibited glucose metabolic rates 19% higher than those of the males. The investigators stated that the observed differences may have been caused by the relatively high levels of estrogen in the female subjects although these values were not reported. Similar results have been reported by Volkow et al.[25] in 15 male and 13 female subjects over two different trials to assess test-retest reliability. Following the first evaluation, glucose metabolism was higher in the females (temporal lobes and cerebellum). Following the second testing session, glucose metabolism was higher in the females (only in the cerebellum). Looking specifically at the expression of glucose transporter 1 (GLUT 1) expression in the blood-brain barrier, Shi and Simpkins[26] discovered that when E_2 was injected in OVX rats, patterns of glucose metabolism were altered significantly. E_2 caused an increase in glucose uptake and GLUT 1 protein expression (Figure 6.2). From these studies it is interesting to note that the metabolic properties of the cerebral tissue also may be altered by varying levels of gonadotrophins, particularly E_2.

VIII. HORMONAL INFLUENCE ON REGULATORY ENZYMES AND GLUCONEOGENESIS

Additional studies have demonstrated that E_2 may alter the activities of glucose-6-phosphate dehydrogenase (G-6PDH)[27] and rates of gluconeogenesis.[28,29] Hansen et al.[27] showed that adult female rats had hepatic G-6PDH activities that were two-fold higher that adult males. When hepatocytes from both males and females were cultured for 48 hours, G-6PDH activities across gender were similar. However, the enzyme activity was increased two- to three-fold with insulin alone, 1.5-fold with E_2 alone, and four- to five-fold with insulin plus E_2. Therefore, the potential of the pentose phosphate pathway and the overall oxidation of glucose appears to be influenced by both circulating levels of insulin and elevated levels of E_2.

Washburn et al.[28] investigated the effects of implanted E_2 on gluconeogenesis in male rainbow trout. Compared to control fish, the glucose synthesis from physio-logical concentrations of alanine was significantly lower in the E_2-treated fish (0.2 and 0.08 $\mu mol \cdot g^{-1} \cdot hr^{-1}$ for the control and E_2-treated fish, respectively). A similar reduction in the rate of glucose synthesis from lactate also was noticed. Similarly, using OVX mice, Ahmed-Sorour and Bailey[29] demonstrated that, with replacement doses of E_2, rates of gluconeogenesis were suppressed and that this was antagonized by elevated levels of P. Treatment with either E_2 or $E_2 + P$ also was shown to increase glycogen deposition.

Under resting conditions, prior data suggests that the presence of gender differences in CHO metabolism are dependent on variations in the circulating levels of E_2 and P (consistently higher in the eumenorrheic female). Fluctuations in the E_2:P appears to exert control of carbohydrate metabolism by altering the insulin-stimulated and insulin-independent (GLUT 1 at blood brain barrier) glucose uptake by different tissues (hepatic and skeletal muscle). Whether these differences are diminished in the amenorrheic female (due to suppressed levels of gonadotrophins) is uncertain. Although it is apparent that the metabolic effects of insulin (the promotion of glucose uptake) are influenced by gender-specific reproductive hormones, the metabolic effects of insulin are diminished considerably during exercise. Therefore, the physiological factors that explain gender differences in substrate utilization at rest may not explain variations during exercise.

IX. EFFECTS OF GENDER ON CARBOHYDRATE METABOLISM DURING EXERCISE

When the differences in CHO metabolism are shifted from a rested state to an exercise situation, the number of confounding variables increases exponentially. Unfortunately, it is nearly impossible to formulate substantial conclusions due to the heterogeneity of past research (subject fitness level, exercise protocol, measurement techniques). Similarly, the potential physiological mechanisms that contribute to any gender-specific response to exercise are even more difficult to ascertain given the disparity of past research. The differences (or the lack thereof) in substrate utilization during exercise between men and women has been the topic of several review articles.[30,31,32,33]

One of the intriguing questions surrounding the issue of fuel selection patterns during exercise is perhaps why study it? The motivation for designing investigations, organizing colloquia at national meetings, and discussing this issue is perhaps as heterogeneous as the past research. As far as this author can interpret, the motivation for research in this area includes but may not be limited to the following: 1) to increase exercise science research on females as it is limited, 2) to determine if there is a difference in exercise performance or perhaps tolerance to exercise across gender, 3) to find ways to improve performance in each gender, 4) to determine whether there are gender-specific nutritional concerns relative to macronutrient intake, 5) to better understand the biological significance of any metabolic differences between genders, and 6) to potentially increase funding if a "comparative" slant is included in the grant proposal. Regardless of the motivation for research in this area, past research has provided a limited number of studies from which to formulate conclusions about CHO metabolism in males and females.

X. GENDER COMPARATIVE HUMAN STUDIES

The exercise protocols used in prior research have differed from intermittent bouts of cycling exercise[34,35] to continuous bouts of either cycling or running.[36,37,38,39,40,41] A variety of measurement tools also have been used in gender comparative research including the respiratory exchange ratio (RER),[36,37,34,35,39,40,41] analyses of blood metabolites,[36,37,38,34,35,40] analyses of muscle biopsies,[37,49] and the use of stable isotopic tracer methodologies.[42] There is also variation in the exercise duration and in the exercise intensity used for testing. Most often the exercise intensity is set relative to the subject's max VO_2 ($\%VO_{2max}$), which may present problems if subjects are not matched on lactate thresholds (LT). (The difference may be due to methodological error rather than gender.) Assume an investigation concludes that females rely less on CHO sources during exercise than males at an exercise intensity of 70% VO_{2max}. However, it is later determined that the LT values were different between genders (73% and 68% of VO_{2max} for the females and males, respectively). If this were the case, the females actually were exercising below LT whereas the males were exercising slightly above. This methodological error may alter the interpretation of the results, thereby leading to either type I (concluding there is a difference, when in reality there is not) or type II errors (concluding there is no difference, when in reality there is). Issues related to gender comparative studies have been discussed in Chapter 1.

Table 6.4 summarizes a select number of investigations that have studied the effects of gender on substrate utilization. Figure 6.3 from Ruby and Robergs[33] incorporates the RER data from five previous studies. Although it is cluttered and represents data from studies using a variety of exercise intensities, the gender-specific lines of best fit collectively indicate a lower RER for females. However, this does not conclusively represent a decreased dependency on CHOs in females during exercise. Rather, it has been included to demonstrate the variation of past research.

In some of the earliest work by Nygaard et al.,[43] muscle biopsies were obtained from males and females before and after a day of downhill skiing. Although exercise intensity was not controlled, it was observed that muscle glycogen was depleted approximately 50% less in females. There were, however, no statistics performed on this comparison. In a more controlled laboratory study, Costill et al.[37] tested trained males and females during a 60-minute treadmill run at a speed equivalent

Table 6.4 Summary of Investigations into Gender Differences in Substrate Utilization During Exercise

Reference	Subjects	Protocol	Results	Conclusions
Tarnopolsky et al., 1990	6 M T 6 F T eumenorrheic & midfollicular	~65% VO_{2max} run for 15.5 km; matched for VO_{2max} LBW & training logs	F RER < M F blood glucose > M F IM glycogen use < M F epinephrine < M F insulin > M	Females use relatively more fat and less carbohydrates during prolonged exercise than males with similar VO_{2max} per LBW and training histories.
Tarnopolsky et al., 1995	7 M T 8 F T midfollicular	70% VO_{2peak} cycle ergometer	F RER < M under both diets M > glycogen use w/ high CHO diet	Males rely more on muscle glycogen when fed a high CHO diet compared to similarly trained females.
Tarnopolsky et al., 1997	8 M T 8 F T	65% VO_{2peak} cycle ergometer	F RER < M during exercise in response to all diets	Males rely more on carbohydrate sources during exercise compared to similarly trained females.
Mendenhall et al., 1995	4 M UT 4 F UT follicular	Cycling @ 50% VO_{2peak}	No differences in RER No difference in IM triglyceride use F IM glycogen use < M F epinephrine < M	Females in the follicular phase rely more on plasma glucose than males for carbohydrate oxidation during moderate intensity exercise.
Froberg & Pedersen, 1984	7 M Active 6 M Active	Cycling @ 80% and 90% VO_{2max} to exhaustion similar VO_{2max} LBW	F lasted longer @ 80% VO_{2max} No differences in times to exhaustion @ 90% VO_{2max} F RER < M @ 80% VO_{2max}	Females use relatively more fat @ 80% VO_{2max}. Differences in times to exhaustion due to > IM glycogen depletion in males as indicated by RER. No differences @ 90% because of similar lactate. No differences in lactate @ 90% responses.
Graham et al., 1986	6 amenorrheic F 6 eumenorrheic F 6 M	30% VO_{2max} for 20 min, 60% VO_{2max} for 20 min, then cycle to exhaustion @ 90% VO_{2max}	Ameno F FFA > M @ 30% VO_{2max} No differences in FFA between eumenorrheic F & M status. No differences in RER Lactate & noradrenaline all F < M	Metabolic sexual dimorphism exists as well as distinct differences in female subgroups identified by menstrual.

Study	Subjects	Protocol	Results	Conclusions
Friedmann & Kinderman, 1989	12 M T 12 F T 12 M UT 12 M UT	T group ran @ 80% VO_{2max} for 14–17 km UT ran @ 75% VO_{2max} for 10 km	UT F FFA > M UT F blood glucose > M No exercise differences in T F & M At rest, UT & T F hGH > M	In untrained subjects there is a difference between F & M in glucose and FFA metabolism. There were no gender differences in substrate responses to exercise in trained subjects.
Costill et al., 1979	12 F T 12 M T	60 min run @ 70% VO_{2max}; matched on VO_{2max}, BW & training	No differences in RER No differences in FFA, glycerol responses during exercise	There are no differences in lipid metabolism in trained males and females during submaximal exercise.
Wallace et al., 1980	10 F T	120 min run @ ~66% VO_{2max} (89% of lactate threshold)	No differences in blood glucose, lactate, glycerol, FFA, ketones during exercise	Trained males and females metabolize fats and carbos similarly during prolonged exercise at comparable relative intensities.
Powers et al., 1980	4 F T 4 M T	90 min run @ 65% VO_{2max} matched on VO_{2max} BW & training	No differences in RER No differences in lactate responses	This data does not support a gender difference in fat metabolism when subjects are matched by VO_{2max} per kg body weight and training volume.

Note: BW = body weight; F = females; FFA = free fatty acids; hGH = human growth hormone; LBW = lean body weight; M = males; IM = intramuscular; RER = respiratory exchange ratio (VCO_2/VO_2); T = trained; UT = untrained; VO_{2max} = maximum O_2 uptake; VO_{2peak} = exercise specific maximal O_2 uptake.

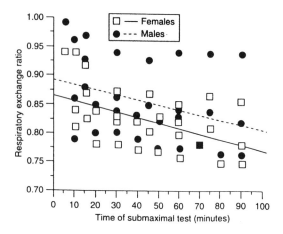

Figure 6.3 Summary of gender differences in the RER response to exercise. (From Ruby and Robergs, *Sports Medicine,* 17, 393, 1994. With permission.)

to 70% of VO_{2max}. Blood samples and expired air samples were collected during the treadmill run. There were no gender differences for the variables RER, FFA, or glycerol during exercise. However, at minute 60, females had a higher blood lactate concentration compared to males. However, it cannot be concluded that the variations in the blood lactate response were the result of gender or simply due to individual differences in the LT. If the mean LT for the female subjects was less than 70% VO_{2max}, 60 minutes of exercise above the LT likely would contribute to an elevated lactate concentration. It also was not mentioned whether the females were eumenorrheic or amenorrheic or at what point in their menstrual cycle testing commenced.

The conclusions of Powers et al.[39] and Wallace et al.[41] were based on differences in the RER response or changes in blood concentrations of metabolic substrates across gender. Powers et al.[39] tested four males and four females matched on values of relative VO_{2max} (ml · kg^{-1} · min^{-1}). Subjects completed a 90-minute treadmill run at a speed equivalent to 65% of relative VO_{2max}. Although there was no statistical significance between males and females, RER was consistently lower in the females for most of the exercise trial (by approximately 0.02). Unfortunately, this, like several studies in exercise science-related research, suffers from a lack of statistical power (small sample size and/or large within group variance). The menstrual status or phase of the menstrual cycle when testing occurred also was not mentioned in this study.

Wallace et al.[41] extended Powers' et al.[39] work by obtaining blood samples during a 120-minute treadmill run at approximately 66% VO_{2max} (11 to 12% below anaerobic threshold) in ten male and ten female subjects (64.0 ± 7.6 and 56.6 ± 6.1 ml · kg^{-1} · min^{-1} for the male and female subjects, respectively). However, the menstrual activity of the female subjects was not mentioned. No differences in RER or blood metabolites (lactate, glucose, glycerol, free fatty acids, ketones) were noted between genders. Wallace concluded that "assuming venous blood concentrations provide some indication of metabolic events," there are no differences in substrate metabolism between well-trained males and females below the anaerobic threshold. Unfortunately, static concentrations of blood metabolites provide no information regarding the rates of appearance and disposal of metabolic nutrients.

Froberg and Pedersen[34] tested physically active males (n = 7) and females (n = 6) matched based on physical activity patterns interpreted from personal interviews (regarding amount and intensity of leisure activities). Although males had a significantly higher VO2 max relative to total body weight (60 ± 4 and 50 ± 4 ml · kg^{-1} · min^{-1}, for the males and females, respectively), there was no difference between genders when VO_{2max} was expressed relative to lean body mass (69 ± 4 and 65 ± 4 max ml · kg^{-1} LBW · min^{-1} for the males and females, respectively). Subjects performed exercise to volitional exhaustion on two separate occasions at both 80 and 90% of VO_{2max}. During exercise at 80% VO_{2max} (minutes 19 to 20), females had a significantly lower RER compared to males (0.97 ± 0.01 and 0.92 ± 0.01 for the males and females, respectively), indicating a decreased dependence on CHO sources during exercise. This difference also was apparent near exhaustion during the 80% VO_{2max} trial. However, there were no differences in the RER response during exercise to exhaustion at 90% VO_{2max}. Blood lactate concentrations were not significantly different between genders at either exercise intensity. Therefore, it was concluded that gender differences in substrate utilization appear to be intensity-related. Unfortunately and similar to prior work, the menstrual activity of the female subjects was not discussed and it is unclear whether testing occurred in the follicular or luteal phase of the menstrual cycle.

This work was later extended by Friedmann and Kindermann[38] during a study testing groups of untrained and endurance-trained males and females. Although this study mentions the inconsistency with past research, these authors do not mention any control for the menstrual phase in the female subjects. One of the concepts that is established in the introduction is that gender differences seem to occur only in untrained subjects[34] and that these differences diminish as subjects become more endurance trained.[37,41] In the present investigation, only the untrained subjects demonstrated a gender difference. Blood glucose concentrations were sporadically higher in the untrained females compared to the untrained males (Figure 6.4). Freidmann and Kindermann[38] concluded that variations in metabolism between genders are minimal and only apparent in untrained individuals. Interestingly, this study did not incorporate RER measurements during exercise to evaluate overall patterns of substrate oxidation.

In a study conducted by Tarnopolsky et al.,[40] a new level of experimental control was established in terms of subject selection (matched on weekly training distance, training bout duration, years of training, most frequent racing event, and frequency of competition). Unlike previous research, menstrual activity was controlled in that female subjects were eumenorrheic, were not currently taking oral contraceptives, and were tested during the midfollicular phase. As a result of the experimental control built into the design, this study can be regarded as a pivotal experiment in the attempt to understand gender differences in substrate utilization. Throughout the 15 Km (~90 min.) treadmill exercise period at approximately 63% of VO_{2max}, females had significantly lower RER values, indicating a decrease in total CHO oxidation (Table 6.5). Consistent with the RER data, muscle glycogen utilization (vastus lateralis)

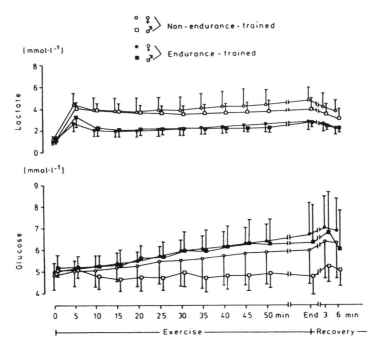

Figure 6.4 Changes in blood lactate and glucose in trained and untrained males and females. (From Friedmann and Kindermann, *European Journal of Applied Physiology,* 59, 1, 1989. With permission.)

was significantly lower in the female runners (approximately 68 and 41% decrease from pre- to post-exercise samples for the males and females, respectively) (Figure 6.5). Blood glucose was significantly higher for the females at 30 minutes and all time points thereafter (Figure 6.5). Insulin showed a main effect for gender indicating an overall higher concentration in females. Although the authors conclude that similarly trained females (relatively high level of fitness, $VO_{2max} = 57.8 \pm 1.8$ ml · kg^{-1} · min^{-1}) rely less on CHO during exercise compared to males, the authors state that the possibility that the females may have had a proportionately higher percentage of oxidative fibers cannot be dismissed (although, as stated in Chapter 3, this may

Table 6.5 Calculated Fuel Consumption During Exercise

	Male (n = 6)	Female (n = 6)
Energy expenditure		
kcal	1,236 ± 53*	1,012 ± 44
kcal/kg BW	18.5 ± 0.8	17.3 ± 0.7
kcal/kg LBW	21.6 ± 0.9	22.1 ± 0.9
Lipid utilization, g	26.9 ± 1.2*	47.6 ± 2.1
Carbohydrate utilization, g	239.7 ± 10.3*	137.3 ± 6.0

Note: Values are means ± SE. BW, body weight; LBW, lean body weight. * P < 0.01.

From Tarnopolsky et al., *Journal of Applied Physiology,* 68, 302, 1990. With permission.

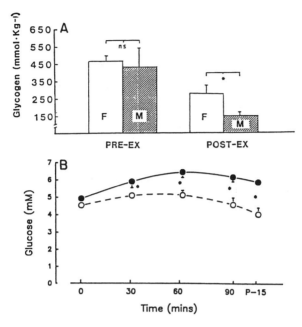

Figure 6.5 Intramuscular glycogen utilization and blood glucose response to exercise in males and females. (From Tarnopolsky et al., *Journal of Applied Physiology*, 68, 302, 1990. With permission.)

be a sex-linked gender difference). Given the extensive matching between the genders and the moderate exercise intensity, it was likely that both groups were below their respective LT. However, future studies should report LT information across genders to demonstrate that the observed difference is due to gender rather than the underlying fitness level.

In a similar study, Tarnopolsky et al.[44] studied the effects of gender on CHO loading and substrate use during exercise. The CHO loading component of this study will be discussed later in the chapter. Again, well-trained males and females were matched on the training characteristics previously mentioned.[40] Subjects exercised at a workload equivalent to 75% VO_{2max} on a cycle ergometer for 60 minutes. This was followed by a rest period (approximately 20 minutes) and exercise to exhaustion at a workload equivalent to 85% VO_{2max}. This exercise protocol was repeated in response to a high (~75% CHO) and low (~59% CHO) CHO diet that was consumed during the five days prior to the exercise trial. Similar to their previous study, the main effect of gender was significant, indicating that regardless of diet the RER was consistently higher for the males, indicating an increased reliance on CHO sources (0.92 and 0.89 for the males and females, respectively). At this higher exercise intensity (75% VO_{2max}), the depletion of muscle glycogen was similar between the genders (during the midfollicular phase). The equivalence of intramuscular lactate concentrations postexercise provided further support for LT equivalence (Table 6.6).

Tarnopolsky et al.[45] again demonstrated this gender-specific response in a recent study attempting to quantify the effects of postexercise dietary supplements on

Table 6.6 Intramuscular Glycogen and Lactate Concentrations

Diet	Men		Women	
	Pre	Post*	Pre	Post*
Glycogen, mmol glycogen/kg dry wt				
Low CHO	401.5 ± 76.8	106.8 ± 25.7	407.3 ± 78.2	78.7 ± 43.7
High CHO	565.4 ± 88.1†	135.2 ± 41.9‡	407.8 ± 57.1	63.5 ± 36.6
Lactate, mmol lactate/kg dry wt				
Low CHO	6.2 ± 1.1	13.3 ± 7.8	5.1 ± 1.1	18.4 ± 3.7
High CHO	6.5 ± 1.8	21.5 ± 9.1	5.3 ± 1.2	16.8 ± 10.7

Note: Values are means ± SD. * Significant change Pre vs. Post ($P < 0.001$). † Significantly greater preglycogen for men on High vs. Low CHO diet ($P < 0.01$). ‡ Significantly greater glycogen use for men on High CHO diet ($P < 0.05$).

From Tarnopolsky et al., *Journal of Applied Physiology,* 75, 2134, 1995. With permission.

muscle glycogen repletion. Using a similar technique for matching subjects, males and females (tested during the midfollicular phase) exercised for 90 minutes at 65% VO_{2max} on a cycle ergometer. Similar to their past work, the main effect for gender was significant for the variable of RER showing an elevated RER in males regardless of diet (0.99 and 0.93 for the males and females, respectively) (Table 6.7).

Therefore, to date, Tarnopolsky and his group at McMaster University have in a sense formulated some of the strongest conclusions regarding gender and substrate utilization. Compared to other past research, the amount of internal validity of Tarnopolsky's work (a direct result of careful matching) has been well-maintained. The moderate exercise intensity (usually ~65% VO_{2max}), the lack of postexercise intramuscular lactate gender differences provided some support that differences in LT between genders were minimal. Furthermore, this same group also found iden-

Table 6.7 Substrate Utilization and Oxygen Consumption During Exercise Trials

Trial Diet	RER	Urea Nitrogen/Creatinine, g/day		%VO$_{2max}$	Heart Rate, beats/min
		Rest	Exercise		
CHO/Pro/Fat					
Men	0.934 ± 0.03	9.05 ± 1.6	9.3 ± 3.2	66.9 ± 0.3	153 ± 2
Women	0.902 ± 0.03*	8.5 ± 2.6	9.86 ± 3.2	64.6 ± 0.6	155 ± 2
CHO					
Men	0.902 ± 0.03	8.9 ± 2.8	10.1 ± 2.8	63.1 ± 0.8	160 ± 5
Women	0.882 ± 0.04*	9.7 ± 3.2	9.3 ± 1.9	63.8 ± 1.1	154 ± 2
Placebo					
Men	0.918 ± 0.02	9.2 ± 3.1	9.7 ± 4.5	63.1 ± 1.7	159 ± 3
Women	0.896 ± 0.03*	9.5 ± 3.1	10.1 ± 3.4	63.5 ± 1.7	153 ± 4

Note: Values are means ± SD. Exercise data [respiratory exchange ratio (RER), maximal O_2 consumption (VO_{2max}), heart rate] are collapsed across 90 min of exercise. * Values are significantly lower for women compared with men; $P < 0.005$.

From Tarnopolsky et al., *Journal of Applied Physiology,* in press, 1997. With permission.

tical LTs in males and females matched on the aforementioned criteria.[46] However, because so few studies have been conducted that either match subjects or control for variations in LT between genders, additional research is warranted. It is also unclear if extensive matching is necessary if subjects are exercised at a percentage relative to their respective LT.

Due to the disparity of past research, it is difficult to establish firm conclusions based on RER and static blood metabolite data. Therefore, it is critical that additional, perhaps more specific, measurement techniques be included in future research (i.e., stable isotope tracer methodology). To this author's knowledge, Mendenhall et al.[42] was the first to use stable isotope tracers to study gender differences in CHO metabolism. Four males and four females exercised for 60 minutes at 50% VO_{2max} on a cycle ergometer. Plasma glucose and free fatty acid (FFA) kinetics were determined by an infusion of $[^2H_2]$ glucose and $[^2H_2]$ palmitate. Overall substrate oxidation was calculated using calculated rates of appearance (Ra) and disposal (Rd) and RER data. Values for Ra and Rd glucose and FFA were similar for males and females. There were also no differences in RER across genders. Interestingly, the relative contribution of blood glucose and muscle glycogen to total CHO oxidation was significantly different between genders (glucose contribution = 20 ± 2 and 28 ± 3% for males and females, respectively; glycogen contribution = 80 ± 2 and 72 ± 3% for males and females, respectively). Plasma epinephrine levels were also higher in males. It was concluded that although males and females oxidize similar amounts of total fat and CHO during exercise, females may rely more heavily on plasma glucose to maintain total CHO oxidation compared to males. Although this study had a small sample size and did not establish the matching criteria of Tarnopolsky's group, it was the first to apply stable isotope methodology to the gender difference question.

XI. ANIMAL MODELS

Thus far, this section has been limited to alterations in substrate utilization in human subjects. However, the gender-specific response to CHO metabolism during exercise also has included several animal studies. Although the ability to extend the conclusions from these studies to humans is difficult, they help establish an understanding of the physiological mechanisms that may contribute to variations in CHO metabolism across gender. The most compelling evidence that supports the concept that the female gonadotrophins influence metabolic activity at rest and during exercise has been developed by Kendrick et al. and his laboratory.[47,48,49] In response to varied doses of E_2, male rats showed an increase in the time to exhaustion during treadmill run exercise. The overall patterns of glycogen depletion during a standardized exercise protocol (120 minutes) was also less following E_2 treatment.[47] The most pronounced E_2 effect was demonstrated by the preservation of liver glycogen, indicating suppression of hepatic glycogenolysis (Table 6.8).

Kendrick et al.[48] provided supplemental E_2 to male rats for a period of five days. Rats were then subjected to a two-hour treadmill exercise protocol. Glycogenolysis was suppressed in all tissues examined (liver, red vastus, white vastus, heart) as a

Table 6.8 Effects of Estradiol on Tissue Glycogen Content After a Submaximal 120 Minute Treadmill Run

Variable	Drug	Rest	2 h
Body wt, g			
Resting	Oil	216 ± 9	
	5-day estradiol	218 ± 12	
Exercise	Oil	220 ± 3	
	5-day estradiol	213 ± 4	
Rectal temperature, °C	Oil	36.4 ± 0.2	38.8 ± 0.4*
	5-day estradiol	36.2 ± 0.5	38.6 ± 0.2*
Tissue glycogen content			
Liver	Oil	66.4 ± 2.1	21.2 ± 2.1*
	5-day estradiol	65.9 ± 3.1	34.6 ± 2.1*‡
Red vastus	Oil	8.1 ± 0.1	3.5 ± 0.2*
	5-day estradiol	8.0 ± 0.3	5.7 ± 0.1*‡
White vastus	Oil	8.0 ± 0.3	3.6 ± 0.2*
	5-day estradiol	8.0 ± 0.5	6.9 ± 0.4†‡
Heart	Oil	5.5 ± 0.4	3.4 ± 0.4*
	5-day estradiol	5.6 ± 0.3	4.2 ± 0.4*‡

Note: Values are means ± SE for 10 animals. Body wt values represent animals killed at rest and preexercise body wt for animals killed at 2 h of exercise. Rectal temperature values are for animals exercised for 2 h. * Significant difference ($P < 0.05$) from resting condition. † Significant difference ($P < 0.05$) from resting oil control. ‡ Significant difference ($P < 0.05$) from oil exercise condition.

From Kendrick et al., *Journal of Applied Physiology,* 63, 492, 1987. With permission.

result of the E_2 treatment (Table 6.9). However, both treatments (E_2 and control) caused a similar increase in plasma glycerol concentration (a generic marker of lipolysis) during exercise. It was concluded that E_2 suppresses glycogenolysis during exercise and thereby must increase the exercising muscles ability to rely on lipid sources.

Rooney et al.[49] provided a similar five-day dose of E_2 to male rats to determine the effects on tissue glycogenolysis and alterations in the skeletal muscle triacyglycerol content. In concert with Kendrick's previous work, Rooney et al.[49] found that E_2 treatment suppresses glycogenolysis in the liver, red vastus, white vastus, and soleus (Figure 6.6). It also was discovered that E_2 treatment increased the resting concentration of triacylglycerol in the red vastus muscle, thus, increasing the potential for elevated fat metabolism due to enhanced intramuscular storage. Therefore, it is unclear whether the dominant action of E_2 is to simply suppress tissue glycogenolysis or to increase the availability of lipid sources. Presumably, an increase in available lipid substrates (enhanced lipolysis and/or increased intramuscular stores) would suppress the dependency on CHO sources during exercise.

Although the effects of gender on lipid metabolism are discussed in another chapter, the potential for E_2 to suppress CHO metabolism by enhancing lipid metabolism warrants some discussion. Hatta et al.[50] provided E_2 and E_2 + P to OVX rats for a period of eight days. Rats were provided with [U-14C] glucose or [1-14C]

Table 6.9 Effects of 5-Day Administration of 17β-Estradiol 3-Benzoate and 120 Minutes of Treadmill Run Exercise on Tissue Glycogen Content

Tissue	Group	Resting	120 Min
Myocardium	Estradiol	5.53 ± 0.20 (8)	5.39 ± 0.82* (5)
	Sham injected	5.63 ± 0.22 (7)	3.22 ± 0.51† (3)
Red vastus	Estradiol	7.32 ± 0.76 (4)	5.74 ± 0.05*† (4)
	Sham injected	7.56 ± 0.84 (4)	2.24 ± 0.33‡ (4)
White vastus	Estradiol	7.52 ± 0.42 (5)	5.65 ± 0.57*† (6)
	Sham injected	7.89 ± 0.36 (5)	3.05 ± 0.44‡ (3)
Liver	Estradiol	72.36 ± 2.82 (4)	33.45 ± 5.05‡§ (4)
	Sham injected	67.62 ± 5.48 (4)	6.39 ± 1.73‡ (3)

Note: Values are means ± SD. Number in parentheses is no. of animals for each group. Estradiol dosage was 2 μg/100 g body wt. * Significantly different between estradiol-replaced and sham-injected animals ($P < 0.05$). † Significantly different between exercise and rest ($P < 0.05$). ‡ Significantly different between exercise and rest ($P < 0.01$). § Significantly different between estradiol-replaced and sham-injected animals ($P < 0.01$).

From Kendrick et al., *Journal of Applied Physiology,* 71, 1694, 1991. With permission.

palmitate prior to exercise. During 60 minutes of treadmill exercise, there were no differences between E_2-treated and control animals for glucose, lactate, plasma FFA, catecholamine, and insulin concentrations. Percentages of [U-^{14}C] glucose recovered as $^{14}CO_2$ were similar between the groups but slightly higher for the control versus E_2-treated animals. Similarly, percentages of [1-^{14}C] palmitate recovered as $^{14}CO_2$

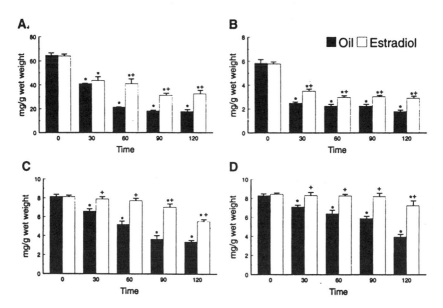

Figure 6.6 Effects of 17β-estradiol 3-benzoate on tissue-specific glycogen deposition and utilization during exercise. (From Rooney, *Journal of Applied Physiology,* 75, 1502, 1993. With permission.)

were higher for the E_2-treated animals early in exercise, indicating an increase in lipid availability. Interestingly, there were no differences in exercise metabolism between the control and the E_2 + P-treated animals. Therefore, the metabolic effects of E_2 appear to alter both CHO and lipid metabolism during exercise. The question remains whether E_2 acts specifically to influence CHO metabolism or causes a secondary suppression in CHO metabolism by enhancing lipid availability and metabolism.

XII. ADDITIONAL EVIDENCE FROM OTHER STUDIES

Additional models discussed in this section will include the use of repeated measure designs that study females during the menstrual cycle and the effects of supplemental E_2 in humans. These areas have been included in that they may contribute to an understanding of the mechanisms associated with gender-specific CHO metabolism. Although early gender comparative studies often ignored the phase of the menstrual cycle, the alterations in the circulating concentrations of reproductive hormones are pronounced between the follicular (pre-ovulatory) and luteal (post-ovulatory) cycles (See Chapter 2).

At the same time as some of the early gender comparative studies were being conducted, Jurkowski et al.[51] studied the effects of the menstrual cycle on the blood lactate response to exercise. Subjects were tested during the follicular (6 to 9 days after the onset of menstruation) and luteal (6 to 9 days following ovulation) phases of the menstrual cycle. Subjects completed two randomly ordered exercise sessions consisting of 20 minutes of cycle ergometry at one-third maximal power output (light), followed by 20 minutes at two-thirds (heavy), followed by exercise to exhaustion at 90% maximal power output (exhaustive). During the follicular phase, lactate concentrations were significantly higher compared to the luteal phase (approximately 30% higher), presumably the result of decreased lactate production. It is also interesting to note that the time to exhaustion was significantly greater during the luteal phase (2.97 ± 0.63 and 1.57 ± 0.32 minutes for the luteal and follicular phases, respectively).

McCracken et al.[52] demonstrated a similar blood lactate response during the luteal phase in response to a graded exercise treadmill run protocol. Although resting lactate concentrations were similar for each phase, the blood lactate concentrations obtained at 3 (5.4 ± 1.2 and 8.7 ± 1.8 mmol/L for the luteal and follicular phase) and 30 minutes (2.4 ± 0.4 and 4.0 ± 1.3 mmol/L for the luteal and follicular phase) post-exercise were significantly lower during the luteal phase. In contrast to Jurkowski et al.,[51] exercise times to exhaustion were not different across the menstrual cycle. It was concluded that the blunted lactate response noted in the luteal phase was likely the result of an overall decrease in CHO metabolism.

Hackney et al.[53] tested female subjects during the follicular and luteal phases using a three stage treadmill exercise protocol (minutes 1 to 10 at 35% VO_{2max}, minutes 10 to 20 at 60% VO_{2max}, minutes 20 to 30 at 75% VO_{2max}). During exercise at 35 and 60% VO_{2max}, RER was significantly lower for the luteal phase (Figure 6.7). However, there was no difference between the phases for the 75% VO_{2max}

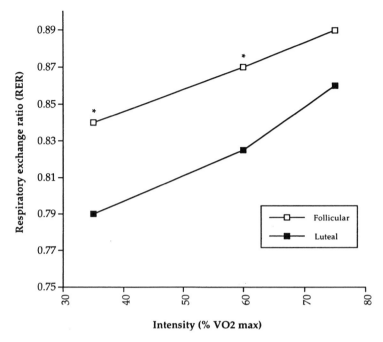

Figure 6.7   Respiratory exchange ratio during exercise in females during the midfollicular and luteal phases of the menstrual cycle, * p < 0.05 vs. luteal phase. (Adapted from Hackney et al., 1994).

exercise period. Values for RER and VO_2 during each stage were used to quantify rates of CHO and lipid oxidation. During exercise at 35 and 60% VO_{2max}, CHO metabolism was significantly lower during the luteal phase of the menstrual cycle (Figure 6.8). These results suggest that during moderate intensity exercise (presumably below the lactate threshold), the luteal phase is associated with a decreased dependency on CHO metabolism.

In contrast, Bonen et al.[54] studied the metabolic response to exercise during the menstrual cycle. Fasted, glucose-loaded and control subjects completed a two stage exercise test (30 minutes at ~38% VO_{2max} followed by 30 minutes at ~80% VO_{2max}) during the follicular and luteal phases of the menstrual cycle. Although there were subtle differences between the three groups, CHO metabolism did not differ between the luteal and follicular phases (based on respiratory and blood metabolite concentration data). Bonen concluded that the selection and utilization of metabolic substrates during exercise are similar in the follicular and luteal phases of the menstrual cycle and that the nutritional state (fasted or fed) is likely to have a more profound effect on metabolism.

Data from Hackney et al.[53] and Nicklas et al.[55] suggested that the storage of CHO, specifically muscle glycogen, differs between the luteal and follicular phases of the menstrual cycle. These results will be discussed in the following section. Nicklas et al.[55] exercised six females to exhaustion (at 70% VO_{2max}) during the luteal and follicular phases. Each exercise test was preceded by a depletion exercise session

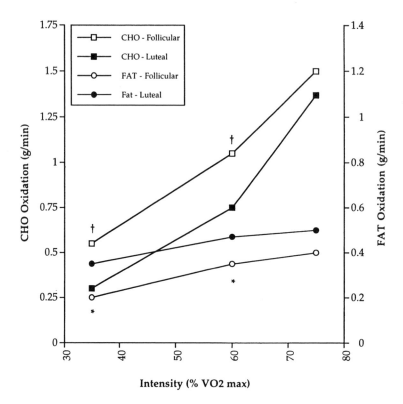

Figure 6.8 Calculated rates of substrate utilization during exercise in females during the midfollicular and luteal phases of the menstrual cycle, *p < 0.05 vs. luteal phase FAT oxidation, † P < 0.05 vs. luteal phase CHO oxidation. (Adapted from Hackney et al., 1994.)

(90 minutes, 60 to 70% VO_{2max} and 4 × 1 minutes at 100% VO_{2max}). There were no differences between the phases in blood glucose, lactate, and FFA. Similarly, muscle glycogen utilization during exercise was similar (although slightly higher during the luteal phase) between the phases of the cycle (55 and 34 μmol/kg wet weight).

In an attempt to study the metabolic actions of E_2 using an *in vivo* human model, Ruby et al.[56] studied the effects of supplemental E_2 treatment on substrate turnover rates during exercise in amenorrheic females. Six amenorrheic females performed treadmill run exercise for 90 minutes at 65% VO_{2max} after 72 hours of placebo and E_2 treatment (Estraderm transdermal E_2). A primed constant infusion of [6,6²H] glucose was used to determine the effects of E_2 on glucose turnover. Overall, exercise rates of glucose Ra and Rd were suppressed significantly following E_2 treatment (Ra – 21.9 ± 7.7 and 18.9 ± 6.2 μmol/kg/min for the control and E_2 trials, respectively, Rd – 21.3 ± 7.8 and 18.5 ± 6.4 μmol/kg/min for the control and E_2 trials, respectively). Although not statistically significant, resting insulin concentrations were slightly lower in response to 72 hours of E_2 treatment (28.1 ± 7.6 and 22.0 ± 4.1 pmol/L for the placebo and E_2 treatment periods, respectively). In contrast, resting FFA concentration was elevated significantly following 72 hours of E_2 treatment

(0.28 ± 0.16 and 0.41 ± 0.27 mmol/L for the placebo and E_2 treatment periods, respectively). The decrease in glucose Ra was attributed to an overall reduction in gluconeogenesis in concert with prior research done on E_2 treated animals.[9,28] As previously mentioned, E_2 tends to promote glucose uptake by the resting muscle under resting conditions when insulin levels are elevated. However, the potential interactions of elevated E_2, exercise-induced insulin suppression and the GLUT-4 transporter activity are unclear. Therefore, in the present study, the E_2-mediated decrease in glucose Rd may be due in part to an exercise-induced suppression of glucose uptake by the exercising skeletal muscles. It may be that skeletal muscle uptake of plasma glucose is suppressed in an effort to provide adequate CHO to other tissues in the female (i.e., uterine). This may be especially important in preparation for and during the early stages of pregnancy. Although the studies that would provide evidence to support this assumption have not been conducted yet, this may be the biological significance at the center of gender variations in CHO metabolism.

Collectively, the combination of gender-comparative animal models and other human models (menstrual comparison and E_2 treatment in amenorrheics) suggest that CHO metabolism during exercise is somewhat gender-specific. However, it is important to note that CHO metabolism during exercise can refer to 1) total oxidation, 2) hepatic glycogenolysis, 3) glycogenolysis in the skeletal muscle, and 4) glucose uptake by the exercising skeletal. Also, one or more of these may be influenced by alterations in the hormonal milieu of the eumenorrheic female. Therefore, it is difficult to conclude that the alteration in CHO metabolism is not simply a function of gender but rather a combination of factors (physiological and methodological) cited in Table 6.2.

XIII. CARBOHYDRATE METABOLISM POST-EXERCISE: GLYCOGEN STORAGE AND RESYNTHESIS

Previous work on the potential for gender-specific CHO metabolism post-exercise has been difficult to recover. However, studies have been conducted on human subjects (male and female comparisons: CHO loading and resynthesis, female-menstrual cycle comparisons) and on animal models (potential for gonadotrophin induced glycogen storage).

Kuipers et al.[57] studied patterns of glycogen resynthesis in endurance-trained subjects (n = 7 males, n = 9 females) following a depletion exercise period (cycle ergometry). Females were tested during the early follicular phase of the menstrual cycle. Immediately post-exhaustive exercise, muscle biopsies were obtained from the vastus lateralis. During a 2.5 hour recovery session, subjects consumed a 25% maltodextrin-fructose solution (total CHO consumed 471 ± 56 and 407 ± 57 g for the males and females, respectively). Both males and females demonstrated a significant increase in muscle glycogen as a result of the refeeding with no differences between gender. (Total resynthesis was 106 and 94 mmol/kg dry weight for the males and females, respectively.)

Tarnopolsky et al.[44] tested similarly trained subjects (n = 7 males, n = 8 females) during a diet-controlled period of four days. Females were tested during the midfollicular phase of the menstrual cycle. Subjects were fed two diets varying in total CHO (55 to 60 and 75% of total energy intake) for a period of four days followed by a 60-minute cycling exercise session (75% VO_{2peak}). Only the males responded favorably to the high CHO diet, demonstrating a significant increase in resting muscle glycogen concentration. The females showed no significant increase in muscle glycogen deposition following the high CHO feeding period. It is interesting to note that because the females were tested in the early- to mid-follicular phase of the menstrual cycle, gonadotrophin levels were likely low. If prior work on other populations is considered (less endurance-trained humans and animal models), it may be that at the onset of ovulation and/or during the luteal phase of the cycle, the potential for glycogen deposition may increase. However, recent work by Gibala et al.,[58] showed only a trivial CHO-loading response in females tested during the luteal phase.

Later work by Tarnopolsky et al.[45] showed no differences between males and females in terms of glycogen deposition during the initial four hours postexercise (90 minutes, 65% VO_{2peak}). Similarly trained males (n = 8) and females (n = 8, during the midfollicular phase) completed three exercise trials followed by isoenergetic CHO, CHO/protein/fat, and placebo supplements. Diets were controlled rigidly for the five days prior to each exercise session. The rates of postexercise glycogen resynthesis were significantly higher for both the CHO and the CHO/protein/fat diet compared to the placebo trial. However, there were no differences between the CHO and the CHO/protein/fat trials. There were also no differences in the rates of post-exercise glycogen resynthesis between males and females (Figure 6.9). These results show that early rates of glycogen resynthesis are similar between the genders, but that the ability to CHO load (super-compensate) may be gender di-morphic.

When the data of Nuutilla et al.[11] is considered, it is feasible to assume that the patterns of glycogen deposition may change in the female as a function of the menstrual cycle. Under hyperinsulinaemic, normoglycaemic conditions, whole body insulin sensitivity was 41% higher in females, with a 47% greater glucose uptake by the skeletal (femoral) muscle. Therefore, immediately postexercise (increased GLUT-4 availability at the skeletal muscle), in a well-fed state (high CHO ingestion), the female (with elevated levels of E_2 at the luteal phase) may demonstrate enhanced glycogen deposition. However, this model has not been developed yet.

XIV. MENSTRUAL CYCLE VARIATIONS IN MUSCLE GLYCOGEN STORAGE/RESYNTHESIS

Data from Hackney et al.[53] and Nicklas et al.[55] suggest that the storage of CHO, specifically muscle glycogen, differ between the luteal and follicular phases of the menstrual cycle. Hackney et al.[53] obtained needle biopsies from 13 females during the luteal and follicular phases. Diet and physical activity were controlled for the 36 hours prior to each biopsy. Muscle (*vastus lateralis*) glycogen was significantly higher during the luteal phase (102.05 ± 4.97 μmol/g wet weight) compared to the

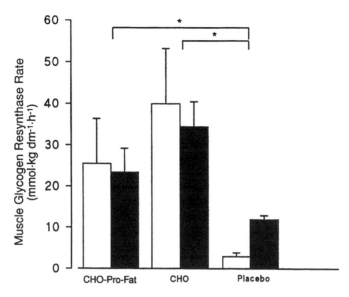

Figure 6.9 Rate of glycogen resynthesis for each trial over the first four hours postexercise. Open bars — males; filled bars — females * $p < 0.05$ (compared to placebo). (From Tarnopolsky et al., *Journal of Applied Physiology,* in press, 1997. With permission.)

follicular phase (90.76 ± 3.56 μmol/g wet weight). Similarly, Nicklas et al.[55] exercised six females to exhaustion (at 70% VO_{2max}) during the luteal and follicular phases. Each exercise test was preceded by an exercise session (90 minutes, 60 to 70% VO_{2max} and 4×1 minutes at 100% VO_{2max}) designed to result in near glycogen depletion. Although there were no differences during exercise between the phases (muscle glycogen utilization, blood glucose, lactate, and FFA), after three days postexercise, total muscle glycogen resynthesis was significantly greater for the luteal phase (88.2 ± 4.7 and 72.1 ± 5.7 μmol/g wet weight for the luteal and follicular phase, respectively). However, because samples were obtained three days postexercise, it is not possible to evaluate the underlying rate of glycogen resynthesis specific to each phase. These results are similar to those from previous animal models that indicate an increased potential for glycogen deposition during periods of elevated E_2.

XV. ANIMAL MODELS: POSTEXERCISE GLYCOGEN RESYNTHESIS

When some of the more compelling animal studies are considered in concert with prior work on human subjects, gender- and the gonadotrophin- (especially E_2) specific glycogen deposition patterns can be explained better. However, the mechanism for these differences has not been established clearly by past research.

Ivey and Gaesser[59] studied the effects of gender on rates of glycogen resynthesis following a five-minute treadmill run in male and female rats. Although exercise resulted in a significant depletion of muscle glycogen in both sexes, the males utilized approximately 50% more muscle glycogen compared to the females. However, the authors attribute this in part to a body weight-dependent (approximately 20% higher in males) increase in total work. During a postexercise (4 hours) recovery period (food was not supplied), there were no differences in postexercise rates of glycogen resynthesis between genders (red vastus: 1.6 and 2.3 mg/hr/g muscle for the males and females, respectively). However, it is important to note that the exercise protocol was only five minutes in duration and that feeding was restricted. It may be that the combination of an extended bout of exercise and CHO supplements postexercise may result in a gender-specific response. Conlee et al.[60] demonstrated a pronounced gender difference in glycogen resynthesis to postexercise stomach tube feeding with CHO (0.6 and 2.9 mg/hr/g muscle for the males and females, respectively).

Ahmed-Sorour and Bailey[29] studied the effects of circulating ovarian hormones on the glycogen deposition patterns in adult female mice. As a result of OVX procedures, glycogen deposition was decreased in all tissues studied. However, when OVX mice were treated with either E_2 or P, glycogen deposition patterns were altered in different tissues (Figure 6.10). It is interesting to note that E_2 had a pronounced effect on glycogen deposition in all tissues. However, treatment with E_2 and P only altered hepatic glycogen deposition compared with OVX animals. Therefore, the gonadotrophin effects on patterns of glycogen deposition are pronounced and apparently tissue-specific.

In the data by Rooney et al.[49] whose procedures and results have been discussed above, the patterns of glycogen depletion during exercise were blunted significantly by five days of E_2 treatment in all tissues studied (hepatic tissue and skeletal muscle). However, what is interesting to note is the concept that increased glycogen depletion may, in some way, enhance total glycogen resynthesis.[61] If males were prone to

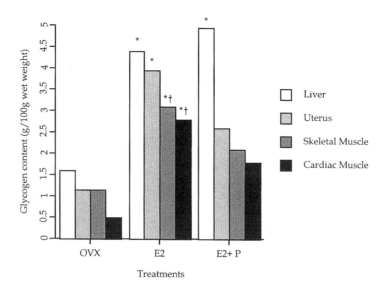

Figure 6.10 Tissue specific glycogen content in response to OVX, E_2 replacement, and E_2 + P replacement in mice. * $p < 0.05$ vs. OVX mice, † $p < 0.05$ vs. E_2 + P treatment. (Adapted from Ahmed-Sorour and Bailey, *Annals of Nutrition & Metabolism*, 25, 208, 1981.)

increased glycogen utilization during exercise, the overall rates of glycogen depletion would be higher, thereby altering the rates of glycogen resynthesis (similar to the concept associated with the classical model for glycogen loading). Therefore, it is uncertain whether the rates of resynthesis are more likely to be affected by overall depletion patterns or by the female-specific gonadotrophin hormones. Certainly, it appears that if a female were to deplete muscle glycogen fully, the gonadotrophin effects may enhance repletion in a variety of tissues. From a biological viewpoint, this may serve as a protective effect for the female during the time she is most likely to become pregnant or in the pregnant female currently supporting a developing fetus.

XVI. PRACTICAL CONSIDERATIONS

Unfortunately, the implications of gender-specific CHO metabolism often are misinterpreted and certainly misrepresented by the lay community. At the same time, the biological significance has been disregarded. Concepts and theories have been developed by coaches and athletes under the assumption that if females rely less on CHO, they may outperform males in ultraendurance events (i.e., ultramarathons and the Ironman triathlon). This also has been suggested by the model created by Whipp and Ward.[62]

This concept also was addressed by Speechly et al.[63] studying similarly trained males (n = 10) and females (n = 10). Subjects were matched based on training histories and completed a 42.2 and 90 km road race. Although there were no differences between males and females for the 42.2 km event, females outperformed males in the 90 km event with average running speeds of 155.2 ± 14.7 and 171.0 ± 11.7 m/min for the male and females, respectively. Females also performed at a higher fraction of VO_{2max} for both the 42.2 and 90 km events. However, dietary intake prior and during the event and menstrual activity were not recorded or controlled, the latter for practical reasons.

If gender comparative research progresses in the direction of performance-related conclusions, it should do so by focusing additional attention to the increasing number of females placed in arduous occupations that require long hours and high levels of exercise intensity (i.e., military operations, wildland firefighting). If a gender differ- ence in CHO metabolism is apparent, the nutritional concerns for females involved in regular intense occupational and/or exercise training may require modification. Ideally, the bulk of the research done in this area should attempt to establish macro- nutrient demands for females (prior to, during, and after exercise). These recom- mendations also should consider variations in CHO metabolism that may occur relative to the menstrual cycle and during pregnancy.

XVII. DIRECTIONS FOR FUTURE RESEARCH

Unfortunately, past research related to gender differences in CHO metabolism has had problems with statistical power and low effect sizes (due to large between group variance and/or small sample size). Although it is difficult to attain large samples because of subject availability and the expense of some measurement techniques (particularly stable isotope tracer methodology), attempts should be made to maximize statistical power and minimize variance within groups.

Other areas that require strict control include but may not be limited to 1) the selection of subjects (sedentary, untrained but gifted, moderately trained, highly trained), 2) controlling for menstrual status/cycle phase and including trials performed in the luteal phase, 3) exercise intensity (relative to LT, VO_{2max}, or absolute workloads). Additional measurement techniques should be incorporated into gender-comparative CHO metabolism studies as they become available. These include the use of stable isotope tracer methodology, which provides kinetic information rather than simply the static concentration of blood metabolites. Similarly, the search for the underlying mechanisms that explain gender differences in CHO metabolism should continue (GLUT-4 activity at rest and during exercise and the variations between genders, the menstrual cycle, and during pregnancy). Regardless, future research should reconsider the biological significance of gender-specific CHO metabolism as a means to understand potential variations in occupational/sport performance and nutritional demands in men and women.

REFERENCES

1. Davis, J. M., Jackson, D. A., Broadwell, M. S., Queary, J. L., and Lambert, C. L., Carbohydrate drinks delay fatigue during intermittent, high intensity cycling in active men and women, *International Journal of Sports Nutrition,* 7, 261, 1997.
2. Fallowfield, J. L. and Williams, C., The influence of a high carbohydrate intake during recovery from prolonged, constant-pace running, *International Journal of Sports Medicine,* 7, 10, 1997.
3. Jeukendrup, A., Brouns, F., Wagonmakers, A. J., and Saris, W. H., Carbohydrate-electrolyte feedings improve 1 h time trial cycling performance, *International Journal of Sports Medicine,* 18, 125, 1997.
4. Salans, L. B., Influence of progestin and estrogen on fat cell size, number, glucose metabolism and insulin sensitivity, *Proceedings of the 53rd Meeting, Endocrine Society,* San Francisco, CA, A59, 1971.
5. Sutter-Dub, M. Th. and Dazey, B., Progesterone and insulin-resistance: studies of progesterone action on glucose transport, lipogenesis and lipolysis in isolated fat cells of the female rat, *Journal of Endocrinology,* 88, 1971.
6. Rushakoff, R. J. and Kalkoff, R. K., Effects of pregnancy and sex steroid administration on skeletal muscle metabolism in the rat, *Diabetes,* 30, 545, 1981.
7. McKerns, K. W. and Bell, P. H., The mechanism of action of estrogenic hormones on metabolism, *Recent Progress in Hormone Research,* 16, 97, 1960.
8. Spellacy, W. N., Carbohydrate metabolism during treatment with estrogen, progesterone, and low-dose oral contraceptives, *American Journal of Obstetrics and Gynecology,* 142, 732, 1982.
9. Mandour, T. A., Kissebah, A. H., and Wynn, V., Mechanism of oestrogen and progeterone effects on lipid and carbohydrate metabolism: alteration in the insulin:glucagon molar ratio and hepatic enzyme activity, *European Journal of Clinical Investigation,* 7, 181, 1977.

10. Stevenson, J. C., Proudler, A. J., Walton, C., and Godsland, I. F., HRT mechanisms of action: carbohydrates, *International Journal of Menopausal Studies,* 39 Supplement, 50, 1994.

11. Nuutila, P., Knuuti, M. J., Miaki, M., Laine H, Ruotsalainen U., Terias, M., Haaparanta, M., Solin, O., and Yki-Jiarvinen, H., Gender and insulin sensitivity in the heart and in skeletal muscles. Studies using positron emission tomography, *Diabetes,* 44, 31, 1995.

12. Donahue, R. P., Prineas, R. J., DeCarlo, D. R., Bean, J. A., and Skyler, J. S., The female 'insulin advantage' in biracial cohort: results from the Miami Community Health Study, *International Journal of Obesity Related Metabolic Disorders,* 20, 76, 1996.

13. Faulkner, B., Hulman, S., and Kushner, H., Gender differences in insulin-stimulated glucose utilization among African-Americans, *American Journal of Hypertension,* 7, 948, 1994.

14. Cagnacci, A., Soldani, R., Carriero, P. L., Paoletti, A. M., Fioretti, P., and Melis, G. B., Effects of low doses of transdermal 17β-estradiol on carbohydrate metabolism in postmenopausal women, *Journal of Clinical Endocrinology and Metabolism,* 74, 1396, 1992.

15. Kumagai, S., Holmang, A., and Bjorntorp, P., The effects of oestrogen and progesterone on insulin sensitivity in female rats, *Acta Physiologica Scandinavica,* 149, 91, 1993.

16. Puah, J. A. and Bailey, C. J., Effects of ovarian hormones on glucose metabolism in mouse soleus muscle, *Endocrinology,* 117, 1336, 1985.

17. Armoni, M., Rafaeloff, R., Barzilai, A., Eitan, A., and Karnieli, E., Sex differences in insulin action on glucose transport and transporters in human omental adipocytes, *Journal of Clinical Endocrinology and Metabolism,* 65, 1141, 1987.

18. Meyer, H. H. and Rapp, M., Estrogen receptor in bovine skeletal muscle, *Journal of Animal Science,* 60, 294, 1985.

19. Misra, D., Roy, S., Gupta, D. N., and Karkun, J. N., Incorporation of [U-C^{14}]-glucose *in vitro* by different parts of the rabbit fallopian tube and uterus, *Endokrinologie,* 69, 21, 1977.

20. Shinkarenko, L., Kay, A. M., and Degani, H., ^{13}C NMR kinetic studies of the rapid stimulation of glucose metabolism by estrogen in immature rat uterus, *NMR-Biomedicine,* 7, 209, 1994.

21. Baquer, N. Z., Sochor, M., Kunjara, S., and McLean, P., Effect of oestradiol on the carbohydrate metabolism of immature rat uterus: the role of fructos-2, 6-bisphosphate and of phosphoribosyl pyrophosphate, *Biochemistry and Molecular Biology International,* 31, 509, 1993.

22. Boland, N. I., Humpherson, P. G., Leese, H.J., and Gosden, R. G., The effect of glucose metabolism on murine follicle development and steroidogenesis *in vitro, Human Reproduction,* 9, 617, 1994.

23. Hay, W. W., The placenta. Not just a conduit for maternal fuels, *Diabetes,* 40 Supplement 2, 44, 1991.

24. Baxter, L. R., Mazziotta, J. C., Phelps, M. E., Selin, C. E., Guze, B. H., and Fairbankes, L., Cerebral glucose metabolic rates in normal human females versus normal males, *Psychiatry Research,* 21, 237, 1987.

25. Volkow, N. D., Wang, G. J., Fowler, J. S., Hitzemann, R., Pappas, N., Pascani, K., and Wong, C., Gender differences in cerebellar metabolism: test-retest reproducibility, *American Journal of Psychiatry,* 154, 119, 1997.

26. Shi, J. and Simpkins, J. W., 17 beta-estradiol modulation of glucose transporter 1 expression in blood-brain barrier, *American Journal of Physiology,* 272, E1016, 1997.

27. Hansen, R. J. and Jngermann, K., Sex differences in the control of glucose-6-phosphate dehydrogenase and 6-phospholuconate dehydrogenase. Interaction of estrogen, testosterone and insulin in the regulation of enzyme levels *in vivo* and in cultured hepatocytes, *Biol. Chem. Hoppe-Seyler,* 368, 955, 1987.

28. Washburn, B. S., Krantz, J. S., Avery, E. H., and Freedland, R. A., Effects of estrogen on gluconeogenesis and related parameters in male rainbow trout, *American Journal of Physiology,* 264, R720, 1993.

29. Ahmed-Sorour, H. and Bailey, C. J., Role of ovarian hormones in the long-term control of glucose homeostasis, glycogen formation and gluconeogenesis, *Annals of Nutrition and Metabolism,* 25, 208, 1981.

30. Ruby, B. C. and Roberds, R. A., Gender differences in substrate utilization during exercise, *Sports Medicine,* 17, 393, 1994.

31. Nygaard, E., Women and exercise — with special reference to muscle morphology and metabolism, in *Biochemistry of Exercise IV B,* Poortmans, J., Ed., University Park, Baltimore, 161, 1981.

32. Chen, J. D. and Bouchard, C., Sex differences in metabolic adaptation to exercise, in *Biochemistry of Exercise VI,* Saltin, B., Ed., Human Kinetics, Champaign, 16, 227, 1986.

33. Aulin, K. P., Gender Specific Issues, *Journal of Sports Sciences,* 13, S35, 1995.

34. Froberg, K. and Pedersen, P. K., Sex differences in endurance capacity and metabolic response to prolonged, heavy exercise, *European Journal of Applied Physiology,* 52, 446, 1984.

35. Graham, T. E., Van Dijk, J. P., Viswanathan, M., Giles, K. A., Bonen, A., and George, J. C., Exercise metabolic responses in men and eumenorrheic and amenorrheic women, in *Biochemistry of Exercise VI,* Saltin, B., Ed., Human Kinetics, Champaign, 16, 227, 1986.

36. Blatchford, F. K., Knowlton, R. G., and Schneider, D., Plasma FFA responses to prolonged walking in untrained men and women, *European Journal of Applied Physiology,* 53, 343, 1985.

37. Costill, D. L., Fink, W. J., Getchell, L. H., Ivy, J. L., and Witzman, F. A., Lipid metabolism in skeletal muscle of endurance-trained males and females, *Journal of Applied Physiology,* 47, 787, 1979.

38. Friedmann, B. and Kinderman, W., Energy metabolism and regulatory hormones in women and men during endurance exercise, *European Journal of Applied Physiology,* 59, 1, 1989.

39. Powers, S. K., Riley, W., and Howley, E. T., Comparison of fat metabolism between trained men and women during prolonged aerobic work, *Research Quarterly for Exercise and Sport,* 51, 427, 1980.

40. Tarnopolsky, L. J., MacDougall, J. D., Atkinson, S. A., Tarnopolsky, M. A., and Sutton, J. R., Gender differences in substrate for endurance exercise, *Journal of Applied Physiology,* 68, 302, 1990.

41. Wallace, J. P., Hamill, C. L., Druckenmiller, M., Hodgson, J. L., and Mendez, J., Concentrations of metabolic substrates during prolonged exercise in men and women, *Medicine and Science in Sports and Exercise,* 12, S101, 1980.

42. Mendenhall, L. A., Sial, S., Coggan, A. R., and K'ein, S., Gender differences in substrate metabolism during moderate intensity cycling, *Medicine and Science in Sports and Exercise,* 27, S213, 1995.

43. Nygaard, E., Andersen, P., Nilsson, P., Eriksson, E., and Kjessel, T., Glycogen depletion pattern and lactate accumulation in leg muscles during recreational downhill skiing, *European Journal of Applied Physiology and Occupational Physiology,* 38, 261, 1978.

44. Tarnopolsky, M. A., Atkinson, S. A., Phillips, S. M., and MacDougall, J. D., Carbohydrate loading and metabolism during exercise in men and women, *Journal of Applied Physiology,* 78, 1360, 1995.

45. Tarnopolsky, M. A., Bosman, M., MacDonald, J. R., Vandeputte, D., Martin, J., and Roy, B. D., Post-exercise protein-carbohydrate and carbohydrate supplements increase muscle glycogen in males and females, *Journal of Applied Physiology,* 83, 1877, 1977.

46. Phillips, S. M., Atkinson, S. A., Tarnopolsky, M. A., and MacDougall, J. D., Gender differences in leucine kinetics and nitrogen balance in endurance athletes, *Journal of Applied Physiology,* 75, 2134, 1993.

47. Kendrick, Z. V., Steffen, C. A., Rumsey, W. L., and Goldberg, D. I., Effect of estradiol on tissue glycogen metabolism in exercised oophorectomized rats, *Journal of Applied Physiology,* 63, 492, 1987.

48. Kendrick, Z. V. and Ellis, G. S., Effect of estradiol on tissue glycogen metabolism and lipid availability in exercised male rats, *Jourrnal of Applied Physiology,* 71, 1694, 1991.

49. Rooney, T. P., Kendrick, Z. V., Carlson, J., Ellis, G. S., Matakevich, B., Lorusso, S. M., and McCall, J. A., Effect of estradiol on the temporal pattern of exercise-induced tissue glycogen depletion in male rats, *Journal of Applied Physiology,* 75, 1502, 1993.

50. Hatta, H., Atomi, Y., Shinohara, S., Yamamoto, Y., and Yamada, S., The effects of ovarian hormones on glucose and fatty acid oxidation during exercise in female ovariectomized rats, *Hormone and Metabolism Research,* 20, 609, 1988.

51. Jurkowski, J. E. H., Jones, N. L., Toews, C. J., and Sutton, J. R., Effects of menstrual cycle on blood lactate, 02 delivery, and performance during exercise, *Journal of Applied Physiology,* 51, 1493, 1981.

52. McCracken, M., Ainsworth, B., and Hackney, A. C., Effects of the menstrual cycle phase on the blood lactate responses to exercise, *European Journal of Applied Physiology,* 69, 174, 1994.

53. Hackney, A. C., McCracken-Compton, M. A., and Ainsworth, B., Substrate responses to submaximal exercise in the midfollicular and midluteal phases of the menstrual cycle, *International Journal of Sport Nutrition,* 4, 299, 1994.

54. Bonen, A., Haynes, F. J., Watson-Wright, W., Sopper, M. M., Pierce, G. N., Low, M. P., and Graham, T. E., Effects of menstrual cycle on metabolic responses to exercise, *Journal of Applied Physiology,* 55, 1506, 1983.

55. Nicklas, B. J., Hackney, A. C., and Sharp, R. L., The menstrual cycle and exercise: performance, muscle glycogen, and substrate responses, *International Journal of Sports Medicine,* 10, 264, 1989.

56. Ruby, B. C., Robergs, R. A., Waters, D. L., Burge, M., Mermier, C., and Stolarczyk, L., Effects of estradiol on substrate turnover during exercise in amenorrheic females, *Medicine and Science in Sports and Exercise,* 29, 1160, 1997.

57. Kuipers, H., Saris, W. H. M., Brouns, F., Keizer, H. A., and ten Bosch, C., Glycogen synthesis during exercise and rest with carbohydrate feeding in males and females, *International Journal of Sports Medicine,* 10, S63, 1989.

58. Gibala, M. J., Walker, J. L., Heigenhauser, G. J. F., and Spriet, L. L., Muscle tricarboxylic acid cycle intermediates in trained females after exhaustive cycle exercise, *Medicine and Science in Sports and Exercise,* 29, S247, 1997.

59. Ivey, P. A. and Gaesser, G. A., Postexercise muscle and liver glycogen metabolism in male and female rats, *Journal of Applied Physiology,* 62, 1250, 1987.

60. Conlee, R. K., Hickson, R. C., Winder, W. W., Hagberg, J. M., and Holloszy, J. O., Regulation of glycogen resynthesis in muscles of rats following exercise, *American Journal of Physiology,* 235, R145, 1978.

61. Zachwieja, J. J., Costill, D. L., Pascoe, D. D., Robergs, R. A., and Fink, W. J., *Medicine and Science in Sports and Exercise,* 23, 44, 1991.

62. Whipp, B. J. and Ward, S. A., Will women soon outrun men?, *Nature*, 2, 25, 1992.

63. Speechley, D. P., Taylor, S. R., and Rogers, G. G., Differences in ultra-endurance exercise in performance-matched male and female runners, *Medicine and Science in Sports and Exercise,* 28, 359, 1996.

CHAPTER 7

Protein Metabolism and Exercise: Potential Sex-Based Differences

Stuart M. Phillips, Ph.D.

CONTENTS

I. INTRODUCTION

The main substrates oxidized during endurance exercise are fat and carbohydrate (CHOs). The proportional oxidation of these fuels during exercise follows an inverse relationship, with the contribution of CHO increasing with high intensities and the contribution of fat being proportionately greater at lower intensities.[1] The overall contribution of protein oxidation to the energy cost of exercise is relatively small. Indirect estimates of its contribution to the energy cost of exercise can be made from urea excretion (sweat and urine), although direct measurements of protein oxidation are possible using amino acid tracers.[2-7] Although there is some degree of variation in these estimates, the contribution of protein to exercising energy generally is considered to be somewhere between 3 and 6% of total exercise energy expenditure.[2,3] What is important to realize, however, is that even a small contribution to a large expenditure of energy could result in a biologically significant amount of protein being oxidized. For example, if protein contributes 5% to an athlete's 4200 kJ/d exercising energy expenditure, this would result in almost 13 g of protein being degraded and oxidized. When one considers that in habitually exercising individuals this additional protein oxidation would occur on a daily basis, it becomes apparent that these individuals may have an increased requirement for dietary protein.[5,7-9] Several studies have concluded that the protein requirements for certain athletic individuals are greater than those for otherwise comparable sedentary persons.[3,5,7-9] In spite of these studies, there is still no consensus as to whether habitual physical activity increases protein requirements.[10] The lack of agreement among researchers in the area of protein requirements for athletes likely arises from a number of confounding issues including variability in the intensity, duration, and mode of exercise, and in the period of adaptation to different (nonhabitual) protein and energy intakes. In addition, it is unclear what is the best method to use in estimating protein requirements.[11,12]

Studies examining the responses of male and female athletes to controlled exercise bouts have provided evidence that exercise elicits a different metabolic and hormonal response in females versus males.[2-4] Of relevance to this chapter is the evidence that suggests there may be sex-based differences in protein metabolism as a result of exercise.[2-4] Support for a sex-related difference in protein metabolism also comes from studies of starvation, a situation in which the metabolic and hormonal response is similar to that during exercise.[13]

This chapter reviews the available data regarding protein and amino acid metabolism that occurs during and following endurance and resistance exercise in both men and women. Where data is available, differences between the sexes with respect to protein metabolism also will be discussed. In addition, the impact of potential differences in protein metabolism between athletes and sedentary controls on protein requirements also will be addressed.

II. AMINO ACID AND PROTEIN METABOLISM IN MUSCLE AND WHOLE BODY DURING EXERCISE

A. Biochemical Aspects of Amino Acid Muscle and Whole-Body Oxidation

Human muscle is recognized to have the capacity to oxidize at least seven amino acids (leucine, isoleucine, valine, glutamate, asparagine, aspartate, and alanine).[14]

Of these amino acids, the oxidation of the branched chain amino acids (BCAA) — leucine, valine, and isoleucine — appears to be increased during catabolic states.[14] The other amino acids that arise due to intramuscular proteolysis are simply exported from muscle.[15,16] In humans, almost 65% of the amino acids exported from exercising muscle are in the form of alanine and glutamine.[17,18] The export of alanine and glutamine is proportionally far greater than their abundance in skeletal muscle (generally 8 to 10% of muscle protein).[19] Of particular importance to amino acid flux during exercise is that the oxidation of BCAA is accelerated relative to the oxidation of other amino acids.[3,6,20,21] This is due to the fact that the BCAA are in high abundance in skeletal muscle (~20% of all muscle protein, by content) and to the fact that the activity of the enzymes responsible for the transamination (branched-chain aminotransferases, BCAAT) and subsequent oxidation (branched-chain keto-acid dehydrogenase, BCKAD) are also high in muscle.[22,23] The result of this compartmentalization of the capacity to oxidize BCAA is that amino nitrogen from the BCAAT reaction in skeletal muscle has two main fates, either transamination with pyruvate to form alanine[19] or transamination with α-ketoglutarate to form glutamate and subsequently glutamine.[24] Another fate for the BCAA-derived nitrogen is the formation of ammonia although, unless BCAA concentrations are somewhat elevated, this is a minor fate for these amino groups.[25,26] The resultant branched-chain keto acids (BCKA), formed from the transamination of BCAA, then can be oxidized by the mitochondrial BCKAD enzyme.[22]

The enzymes for BCAA transamination are present in both glycolytic and oxidative skeletal muscle,[27] and the affinity of the BCAAT enzyme appears to be greatest for leucine followed by isoleucine and then valine.[22] The overall capacity to transaminate BCAA in human skeletal muscle cannot be much greater than the activity of the BCKAD enzyme because, at moderate exercise intensities, BCKA are not released to any significant degree from human skeletal muscle.[28] It appears that at higher intensities of exercise the rate of transamination of amino acids exceeds the capacity for oxidation, for the concentration of BCKA in muscle increases, followed by a delayed release of some keto acids into the blood.[29]

The BCKAD enzyme is a mitochondrial multisubunit enzyme similar in nature to pyruvate dehydrogenase in that it is inactivated by phosphorylation and activated by dephosphorylation.[22] Exercise stimulates BCKAD activation, due possibly to a decrease in the ATP/ADP ratio or an increase in intramuscular acidity.[22,30] In addition, during exercise, BCKAD is activated to a degree that is inversely proportional to the concentration of muscle glycogen.[31,32] The results of Wagenmakers et al.[31] showed that the maximal activity of the BCKAD complex was ~25 μmol $\cdot$ kg wet muscle^{-1} $\cdot$ min^{-1} in humans, and that enzyme was found to be, at most, 20% active. The oxidation of leucine via BCKAD results in the release of CO_2, which has been taken advantage of by a number of investigators to estimate leucine oxidation during exercise.[3,6,20,33-36] Once decarboxylated, leucine then can be metabolized fully to yield acetoacetate (ketogenic).

One of the earliest studies of amino acid flux across exercising muscle reported that muscle was a consumer of BCAA.[17] Since this study, however, such an observation, using a variety of forms of exercise, has not been replicated.[18,25,26,37] In fact, the only amino acid that muscle appears to taken up during exercise on a quantitatively important basis is glutamate.[17,18,38] At the same time that BCAA oxidation is increased during exercise;[3,6,20,21,33-36,39] however, there is a large efflux from the muscle of α-amino nitrogen in the form of ammonia, alanine, and glutamine.[17,19,40] Because it appears that muscle does not take up BCAA during exercise, BCAA oxidation occurring during exercise must result from an increase in intramuscular protein breakdown, to supply BCAA to the free amino acid pool. Relevant to this point is the observation that supplementation with BCAA results in a reduction of protein breakdown, measured as amino acid released from the legs during exercise.[25] However, even the most liberal estimates of protein turnover in muscle (i.e., that 20% of all amino acids released from protein breakdown are BCAA and that protein synthesis is completely suppressed during exercise), combined with negligible BCAA uptake by muscle during exercise, result in a large deficit of BCAA supply to account for all α-amino nitrogen leaving muscle during exercise.[40] Even if muscle proteolysis were elevated markedly (i.e., ten-fold) during exercise, which does not appear to be the case,[6] there is a shortfall of BCAA supply to account for even half of the α-amino nitrogen released from muscle.[40,41] The only other reasonable candidate amino acid, which might supply a source of nitrogen to account for the efflux from muscle, would be glutamine. At present, however, no evidence in humans exists to support this idea.

Many studies have been conducted examining the oxidation of leucine during exercise;[3,6,20,21,33-36,39] however, observations on the oxidation of other amino acids, let alone other BCAA, during exercise is lacking. Wolfe et al.[20,42] have examined lysine oxidation during exercise and observed that the exercise-induced increase in lysine oxidation was almost three-fold lower than the exercise-induced increase in leucine oxidation. Moreover, the data of Wolfe et al.[20,42] also highlight one of the most troublesome incongruities in using leucine oxidation to imply changes in protein metabolism during exercise because urea production was not increased concomitantly. The fact that leucine oxidation increased to such a great extent during exercise without a simultaneous increase in urea production[20,42,43] was somewhat surprising. Studies that have reported urea excretion in urine and sweat have concluded that exercise induced an increase in protein turnover based upon an increase in urea excretion.[44-46] In addition, direct measurements of hepatic urea production in dogs have shown that release of urea by the liver is increased significantly during exercise, although not to the extent expected given the delivery of α-amino nitrogen to the liver.[47] One criticism of the earlier studies of Wolfe et al.[20,42] was that the exercise intensity used to study urea kinetics was quite modest (40% VO_{2peak}) and that the studies reporting increases in urea excretion were at higher intensities.[44] However, application of the same methodology to study urea kinetics at 70% of VO_{2peak} also showed no change in urea production.[43] These authors did conclude that there was an increased reincorporation of urea nitrogen back into body proteins during exercise,[43] which may allow some of the nitrogen from BCAA and other amino acids, liberated by muscle or other tissue proteolysis, to be reused.

It is apparent that BCAA oxidation increases during endurance exercise,[3,6,20,33-35] likely due to an increase in BCKAD activity in the exercising skeletal muscle.[31,32] Oxidation of the BCAA is preceded, however, by transamination via BCAAT, which provides a source of α-amino nitrogen for transamination with pyruvate to form

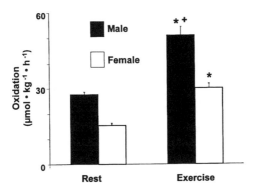

Figure 7.1   Leucine oxidation at rest and during exercise (90 min at ~65% VO$_{2peak}$) in male (N = 6) and female (N = 6) endurance athletes. *, significantly (P < 0.01) different from rest; +, significantly different from corresponding values for females (P < 0.01). Values are means ± standard error (SE). From reference 3, with permission.

alanine or with α-ketoglutarate to form glutamate and subsequently glutamine. Calculation of the total efflux of α-amino nitrogen leaving the muscle primarily as ammonia, alanine, and glutamine is greater than the supply of BCAA from protein breakdown and BCAA uptake by the muscle. It may be that muscle is able to take up sufficient quantities of glutamate, which may also act as a source of nitrogen for formation of alanine and glutamine. Of particular interest is that the nitrogen from leucine transamination does not appear to be incorporated into urea.[42] The other possible fate of the nitrogen from BCAA transamination occurring in the muscle may be incorporated back into liver proteins.[48]

B. Sex Specific Responses

A study by Phillips et al.[3] found that exercise of 90 minutes in duration at ~65% of VO$_{2peak}$ resulted in exercise leucine oxidation values that were 70% greater in trained male athletes versus training-matched female counterparts (Figure 7.1).[4] In spite of subjects consuming the Canadian-recommended nutrient intake (RNI) for protein (0.86 g protein · kg^{-1} · day^{-1}), they were in negative nitrogen balance during the measurements.[3] Assuming a leucine content of body tissues of 590 μmol · g^{-1} [20] and that other amino acids were not recycled, it was calculated that leucine oxidation during exercise could account for at most ~90% of the negative nitrogen balance seen in both groups of athletes.[3] The sex-based difference in leucine oxidation was a main effect; however, and a higher leucine oxidation was evident at rest in the male athletes.[3] In addition, the actual increase in leucine oxidation from rest was 95% in the females and 84% in the males. When the leucine oxidation data of Phillips et al.[3] are expressed as μmol leucine oxidized · kg lean (muscle) mass^{-1} · h^{-1}, which may correct for the amount of muscle and hence the activity of BCKAD, the differences in leucine oxidation persist, but exercising leucine oxidation was only 60% greater in males. Unfortunately, no measurements of muscle BCKAD enzyme activity or activation were made in the two groups to assess why the

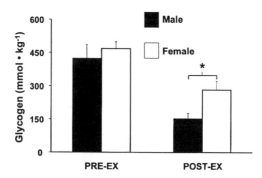

Figure 7.2   Muscle glycogen pre- and post-exercise (15.5 km at ~63% of VO_{2peak}) in males (N = 6) and females (N = 6). *, significant difference between groups (P < 0.05). Values are means ± SE. From reference 4, with permission.

differences in leucine oxidation occurred. In addition, it is not known whether the results[3] can be generalized to include conditions when adequate protein intakes are consumed because the aforementioned subjects were in negative nitrogen balance. It should be emphasized that the protein intake was at the Canadian RNI for protein.

The observations of BCKAD activation and CHO availability made by Wagenmakers et al.[31,49] may shed some insight into why males had a greater leucine oxidation during exercise than their female counterparts.[3] When diet was controlled and training status was matched, a number of studies have reported that females have a lower relative CHO oxidation and higher fat oxidation as compared to males.[2-4] The result is that endurance-trained females, when compared to trained males, utilize less muscle glycogen (Figure 7.2).[4] Because there is an inverse correlation between muscle glycogen content and BCKAD activation,[31] one might predict that the activation of BCKAD in females would be lower than that of males by virtue of the higher muscle glycogen. The result of the reduced exercise-induced increase in BCKAD in the female athletes might result in females oxidizing less BCAA.[3]

A puzzling finding, which serves to illustrate one of the pitfalls of simply using a single indicator of protein metabolism during exercise, is that despite a doubling of leucine oxidation during exercise in both male and female athletes there was no change in urea (sweat plus urinary) excretion,[3] despite adequate rehydration to compensate for exercise-induced dehydration, which may have reduced urea excretion.[50] Based on the findings of Wolfe et al.,[20,42] it is not surprising that increases in leucine oxidation data did not lead to an increase in urea production because nitrogen from BCAA and other amino acids may be reincorporated back into plasma proteins in the liver.[48] Given that the subjects of Phillips et al.[3] were in negative nitrogen balance, it may be that the efficiency of nitrogen reutilization had increased and that as much nitrogen as possible was being recycled.

Earlier observations of sex-based differences in protein metabolism were made by Tarnopolsky et al.[4] In this study male and female subjects were matched for training status, which resulted in an equivalent aerobic capacity per kilogram of lean mass ($VO_2 \cdot kg^{-1} \cdot$ lean body weight^{-1}), and age. In comparison to a day during which subjects rested, it was observed that males had a ~40% increase in urea excretion on

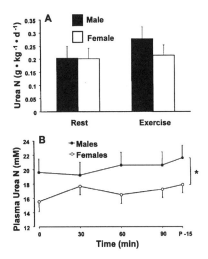

Figure 7.3 **A**. Urinary urea nitrogen (N) excretion expressed relative to body weight on a rest day, prior to exercise, and on the day of exercise (see Figure 7.2 for exercise description), in males (N = 6) and females (N = 6). **B**. Plasma urea N concentration in males and females during exercise and at 15 min post-exercise. *, significant difference between groups (P < 0.05). Values are means ± SE. From reference 4, with permission.

a day when they ran 16 km at ~63% of their VO_{2peak} (Figure 7.3A). In contrast, the training-matched female athletes showed no exercise-induced increase in 24 h-urea excretion, when compared to the rest day. Furthermore, the male athletes had a higher blood urea concentration at rest and during exercise than did their training-matched female counterparts (Figure 7.3B). In support of the previous protein conservation observed in female athletes,[4] a similar observation of increased urinary urea excretion in males was made in a later study that examined age and training-matched male and female athletes (Figure 7.4).[2] In support of these findings,[2,4] studies of urea excretion in rats have shown that female rats excrete less urinary urea following exercise than male rats.[51] Moreover, investigations of sex-based differences during starvation in both animals[52] and humans[13] have concluded that males catabolized relatively more protein than females during a period of starvation.

Evidence from a number of studies has indicated that the menstrual phase also may influence protein kinetics. Lamont et al.[53] reported that females who completed 60 minutes of cycle ergometry at 70% of their VO_{2peak} had a greater urinary and total (urine plus sweat) urea excretion during the midluteal phase of their menstrual cycle, when compared to the follicular phase. A similar observation was made by Lariviere et al.,[54] who noted that leucine flux, an indicator of protein breakdown, was elevated ~13% in the midluteal compared with the midfollicular phase of the menstrual cycle. Furthermore, it appeared that the extra leucine being released due to increased protein breakdown was directed toward increased oxidation, which also increased ~23% in the midluteal compared to the midfollicular phase of the menstrual cycle.[54] The disproportionate increase in progesterone during the midluteal compared to the midfollicular phase of the menstrual cycle may indicate that an

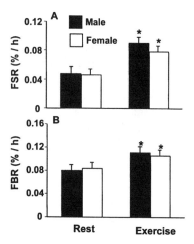

Figure 7.4 A. Mixed muscle protein fractional synthetic rate (FSR in % · h⁻¹) following single-leg knee flexion eccentric exercise (see text for details) and in a control resting leg, in males (N = 8) and females (N = 8). **B.** Mixed muscle protein fractional breakdown rate (FBR in % · h⁻¹). *, significantly different from resting value. Values are means ± SE.

elevated progesterone/estrogen ratio could exert a catabolic effect on body proteins.[53,54] This hypothesis awaits further evaluation.

III. MUSCLE AND WHOLE BODY PROTEIN TURNOVER DURING AND AFTER EXERCISE

A. Protein Degradation

The breakdown or proteolysis of muscle protein is controlled by multiple proteolytic pathways that are constantly active in skeletal muscle, but the activity of which can be increased by a variety of stressors, including exercise.[59-61] The primary protein-degrading systems include the lysosomal pathway,[59,60,62] the ATP-dependent-ubiquitin-pathway (AUP),[63] and the calcium activated neutral protease (CANP) or calpain pathway.[61,64]

The acid hydrolases of the lysosomal system degrade endocytosed proteins, some cell membrane proteins, and some cytosolic proteins. Originally, the lysosomal system was suspected of playing a significant physiological role in muscle proteolysis.[59,60,62] However, the significance of this pathway in muscle proteolysis is not considered quantitatively important.[63] Nonetheless, the importance of lysosomal proteases from extracellular sources such as monocytes and macrophages may play a delayed role in severe exercise stress to muscle.[65] (See muscle damage, Chapter 10.)

Calpain exists as two isoforms, μ and m, which require micromolar and millimolar calcium (Ca⁺) ion concentrations respectively for activation. An elevation in intramuscular [Ca²⁺] secondary to damage to the sarcoplasmic reticulum (SR),[66] failure of the SR to take up Ca^+ following activation,[67] or diffusion of extracellular Ca^{2+} through an exercise-damaged sarcolemma[68] could activate the proteolytic activity of calpain.[61] If an elevation in sarcoplasmic $[Ca^{2+}]$ is linked to an increase in skeletal muscle protein degradation, it is possible that calpain activation might be an initial mechanism whereby muscle protein degradation[69] and loss[70] occur following muscle damage. Calpain has been shown to degrade primarily Z-line proteins such as α-actinin and vimentin.[61] This high degree of specificity has led to the suggestion that the sarcomeric disruption and Z band streaming that are seen following exercise[71,72] (see Chapter 3) are due to activation of calpain.[61] To date, the contribution of Ca^{2+}-activated, calpain-mediated proteolysis as a result of exercise and muscular contraction has not been quantified yet.

The mechanism behind the ATP-dependent-ubiquitin proteolytic pathway involves the covalent conjugation of activated ubiquitin molecules to the protein targeted for degradation.[63] Formation of a polyubiquinated protein substrate appears to be a requirement for degradation by the 20S core proteasome, part of the 26S proteasome complex.[63] Within the central core of the 20S proteasome, the protein substrate is cleaved by multiple catalytic sites to small peptides, which are released and rapidly degraded to free amino acids by oligopeptidases and exopeptidases.[63]

Only a paucity of data is available showing how the activities of any of these three proteolytic pathways are activated with exercise.[73-75] It also has been shown recently that these proteolytic pathways are responsive to amino acid concentrations for increasing concentrations of exogenous amino acids reduce muscle protein breakdown.[76,77] What little evidence does exist on the pathways responsible for muscle proteolysis has shown that the lysosomal pathway is responsible for only a small portion of the exercise-induced proteolysis that occurs in muscle.[73,75] This means that either the CANP or AUP pathway is responsible for the remainder of the muscle proteolysis. Evidence from other catabolic states seems to favor the involvement of the AUP pathway[63] although the activity of CANP proteolytic pathway appears to be elevated by exercise.[61] Further investigation needs to address which proteolytic pathways are activated by exercise and to what extent the various pathways are responsible for total muscle proteolysis.

At the same time that synthesis is elevated following resistance exercise,[69,84-86] protein breakdown is also elevated.[69] Prior to the development of a technique to measure mixed muscle protein breakdown,[69,88] there were only surrogate measures of muscle proteolysis using 3-methylhistidine (3-MH) excretion.[69,86,89-91] However, there have been disparate results with some studies showing an increase[90,94] and others showing no change[69,86,91] in 3-MH excretion following exercise. It may be that only after repeated bouts of exercise, 3-MH excretion is increased.[94] It has been postulated that the pattern of the increase may be due to accumulated damage or a delay before myofibrillar protein degradation occurs following exercise. In support of the latter hypothesis, Fielding et al.[36] showed that urinary 3-MH excretion remained unchanged until ten days following an intense bout of eccentric exercise. Earlier concerns regarding the contribution of gut protein to myofibrillar protein turnover and its effects on urinary 3-MH excretion[95] may not be relevant because other studies have shown that 3-MH balance across limbs (indicating muscle release) can account for almost all urinary 3-MH excretion.[96] Regardless of the results of the studies that have examined 3-MH excretion, two investigations, using two different methods to assess muscle protein turnover, have shown that resistance exercise also stimulates muscle protein breakdown.[69,84] However, muscle protein balance in the previous studies[69,84] was persistently negative, despite an initial large increase in mixed muscle protein FSR and smaller increases in mixed muscle protein fractional breakdown rate (FBR). This finding was expected because the studies were both conducted in the fasted state.[69,84] In a subsequent investigation, when exogenous amino acids were supplied, the net balance in muscle was positive due to a marked stimulation of muscle protein synthesis.[77]

B. Muscle Protein Synthesis

During endurance exercise, it appears that the rate of muscle protein synthesis is reduced.[35,55] However, at moderate exercise intensities it may be that protein synthesis is able to proceed at a rate that is somewhat lower than that at rest.[56] Whole body protein synthesis also appears to be reduced[6,28] or to remain unchanged[3] during endurance exercise. The finding of a reduction in whole body protein synthesis during exercise[6,28] is intriguing, yet it is unknown in what tissue this is occurring. Furthermore, the signal for a reduction in muscle protein synthesis during endurance is unknown although it may be related to intracellular energy status.[57] In the only study examining the effect of an isolated bout of resistance exercise on protein kinetics, whole body protein synthesis was shown to be unaffected.[58]

Adaptations to resistance exercise are fundamentally different from those of endurance exercise because the result is an increase in muscle fiber diameter.[80-82] For an increase in fiber diameter to occur, there has to be synthesis of new muscle proteins of which ~60% are myofibrillar in nature.[83] For muscle fiber hypertrophy to occur, there must be net positive muscle protein balance such that muscle protein synthesis exceeds muscle protein breakdown. A variety of investigations have shown that resistance exercise stimulates mixed muscle protein synthesis[69,84-86] in both trained and untrained subjects. The time course of protein synthesis following an isolated bout of resistance exercise appears to be somewhat different in untrained subjects, for whom changes in mixed muscle protein fractional synthetic rate (FSR) persist for up to 48 h postexercise,[69] whereas mixed muscle protein FSR in trained persons is back to resting levels by this time.[87] It appears that resistance training attenuates the acute immediate response of muscle protein synthesis to an isolated bout of resistance exercise (S.M. Phillips and R.R. Wolfe, unpublished observations).

It may be that myofibrillar protein turnover is relatively insensitive to the effects of exercise and other interventions. The authors have argued previously that the large (~112%) increase in mixed muscle FSR seen following a single bout of resistance exercise must have been due to a change, to some degree, in the synthesis rate of myofibrillar proteins because they comprise ~60% of total muscle protein by weight.[84,85] At the same time, however, it appears that myofibrillar protein degradation is unchanged.[69,86,91] The effect of both endurance and resistance exercise on the turnover of specific proteins has yet to be investigated.

C. Sex-Specific Responses in Protein Synthesis and Degradation

Interestingly, it may be that there is sex-based difference in the susceptibility to the damaging effects of exercise, particularly eccentric exercise, evidenced by a lower efflux of muscle enzymes in female rats. The mechanism of this lower muscle enzyme efflux is theorized to be due to the higher levels of circulating estrogen in females[78] and is discussed in other chapters (by P.M. Tiidus and P.M. Clarkson) in this volume. However, a recent study has shown exercise-induced muscle enzyme release bore no correlation to measurements of muscle injury, muscle protein breakdown, and force decrement.[79] These findings provided some of the strongest evidence to support that muscle enzyme release and creatine phosphokinase activity, in particular, is an unreliable quantitative indicator of muscle damage and likely of protein degradation.

Several studies now have been published in which the adaptations in muscle cross-sectional areas and muscle fiber characteristics following resistance-training programs were reported for females.[81,97-100] These investigations have shown that in spite of a markedly (~10-fold) lower serum testosterone concentration, females undergo skeletal muscle hypertrophy.[81] Similarly, resistance exercise in females resulted in similar changes in strength and muscle fiber characteristics as seen in males.[98] Recently, the authors observed that a group of males (N = 8, 79 ± 3 kg, 25 ± 3 yr) and females (N = 8, 62 ± 4 kg, 26 ± 4 yr) who had completed ten sets (eight repetitions per set) of unilateral eccentric knee flexion (weight lowering) at 120% of their predetermined single repetition maximum with their nondominant leg (the nonexercised leg was used as a control) showed no gender differences in mixed muscle FSR, FBR, or net muscle balance (synthesis minus breakdown; Figure 7.4). Muscle protein turnover was determined using muscle biopsies from the lateral vastus and a primed constant infusion of $^2H_5$-phenylalanine to determine muscle FSR, by tracer incorporation into muscle protein. In addition, a recently developed technique using a primed constant infusion of ^{15}N-phenylalanine was used to determine mixed muscle protein FBR.[88] Hence, it appears that there are no sex-based differences in the acute and early responses to resistance exercise. However, the results from Alway et al.[81] show that highly trained males have greater muscle cross-sectional area (~76%) and muscle fiber diameter (~100%) than highly trained female bodybuilders. These findings indicate that longer-term training may result in differences that favor greater muscle hypertrophy in male athletes possibly related to the training-induced increase in serum testosterone in males.[98] Longer-term resistance training studies examining the adaptations in muscle protein turnover and serum hormone concentrations will have to be conducted to resolve the observation of sex-based differences in muscle hypertrophy and muscle fiber size.

IV. ENDURANCE TRAINING AND AMINO ACID AND PROTEIN METABOLISM

To date, no study of humans has examined the effects of endurance training on amino acid metabolism during exercise. In rats, Henderson et al.[21] observed that training increased whole-body leucine turnover and oxidation during exercise at a given VO_2. This could be due to a training-induced increase in total muscle BCKAD activity, a mitochondrial enzyme. In contrast, Hood and Terjung[39] found that training reduced the relative contribution of leucine oxidation to VO_2 in electrically stimulated, perfused rat hindquarters. It is possible that the previous results[39] were due to a reduced activation of muscle BCKAD during exercise due to smaller perturbations of energy homeostasis (i.e., lower ADP, Pi), as pointed out by the authors and/or due to higher muscle glycogen concentration.[31] Hood and Terjung[39] therefore suggested that the training-induced increase in whole-body leucine oxidation observed previously[21] must have occurred in the liver, which is plausible because rats have a relatively high liver BCKAD activity that is not found in humans.[39]

The subcellular location of BCKAD has been shown to be on the inner mitochondrial membrane.[22] Given that the number of mitochondria increases following endurance training,[101] it is possible that there would be an increased absolute number of BCKAD enzymes post-training. However, it is known that training results in an attenuation of muscle glycogen utilization, resulting in a relatively greater muscle glycogen concentration post-training.[101,102] The higher relative glycogen concentration, combined with the improved cellular energy status post-training, indicates that although there may be a greater maximal BCKAD activity the active portion (dephosphorylated) of the enzyme would be reduced following training.[32]

Exercise increases leucine oxidation.[3,6,20,21,33-35] In addition, exercise increases the overall rate of appearance (Ra) of alanine.[103] Moreover, oxidation of leucine during exercise is increased in proportion to exercise intensity,[33,104] presumably due to a greater activation of BCKAD.[31,32] The increased Ra of alanine during exercise however, is far greater than its concentration in muscle;[19] hence, it must be due to *de novo* alanine production.[103] The release of alanine from muscle during exercise arises due to the transamination of pyruvate with a variety of amino acids, but is predominantly due to BCAA transamination.[103] This is not the case at rest where an increase in BCAA concentration results in increased glutamine release.[38] One might expect that following training, because glycolytic flux is reduced and pyruvate is directed toward oxidation,[105] there would be a reduction in the amount of carbon precursors available to form alanine. In addition, as argued above, one would expect that BCAA transamination and oxidation also would be reduced following training, hence there would be a reduced flux of α-amino nitrogen to form alanine from pyruvate. However, in contrast to what one might expect, alanine release from trained rat muscle was found to be greater.[106] Future research needs to address the hypothesis that glutamate could act as the nitrogen donor to form alanine because training apparently results in an increase in the activity of glutamine dehydrogenase, and there was no change in the release of glutamine from skeletal muscle of trained rats.[106] No study to date has examined the effect of endurance training on alanine or glutamine flux in humans. Similarly, no studies have been conducted to examine the potential for a sexual-dimorphic amino acid oxidation response to endurance training.

V. NON-MUSCLE AMINO ACID AND PROTEIN
METABOLISM DURING EXERCISE

The alanine and glutamine released from skeletal muscle during exercise can serve as precursors for gluconeogenesis after the nitrogen is incorporated into urea.[17,19] In addition, the uptake of other amino acids (serine, proline, and glycine) is also increased by the liver during prolonged exercise.[17] This occurs at the same time, as there is a marked increase in the hepatic-free amino acid concentration following exhaustive exercise.[108] The implication of these findings is not only that liver increases the uptake of amino acids during exercise but that the rate of proteolysis in the liver is increased markedly by exercise, potentially to provide gluconeogenic precursors. Some support for this idea comes from the findings of Kasperek et al.,[74] who showed that exercise resulted in a ~10 to 12% decrease in liver protein content following 2 to 3 h of exhaustive exercise. Given the large increase in hepatic uptake of amino acids and hepatic proteolysis, the findings of no increase in urinary urea production[42,43,48] during exercise are difficult to reconcile.

Recently, Williams et al.[109] showed that proteolysis of both gut and liver tissue contributed essential amino acids to the circulation during exercise. These results showed that exercise resulted in an increase in whole body leucine Ra and rate of disappearance (Rd), and yet splanchnic bed amino acid uptake did not change.[109] These authors speculated that muscle was the most likely consumer of the leucine released from both gut and liver.[109] These findings are supported by an earlier study of Wasserman,[47] who showed that dogs have an enhanced release of α-amino nitrogen from the gut during exercise. Interestingly, measurements of the synthetic rate of gut mucosa in humans recently have been made and have shown it to be a very active tissue in terms of its contribution to overall whole body protein synthesis.[110] This could mean that suppression in the gut protein synthetic rate, even without a concomitant change in mucosal tissue breakdown, could result in the provision of extra amino acids for other tissues. The idea that the gut could act as a labile pool of amino acids for other tissues, including liver and muscle, is interesting.[111] The signal for increased degradation of gut proteins during exercise is likely the reduced amino acid delivery to the tissue along with the increased glucagon to insulin ratio that occurs during exercise.[112]

An interesting observation made by Wasserman et al.[47] was that the total of the hepatic nitrogen uptake (the sum of amino acid and ammonia) was almost complete (i.e., uptake-matched delivery). Calculation revealed that amino acids can account for almost 20% of total gluconeogenic substrates.[17] At the same time, however, release of urea from the liver did not match nitrogen uptake, suggesting either that the urea pool in the liver had expanded or that there was another route of disposal of the α-amino nitrogen. One possibility is that the α-amino nitrogen could have been incorporated into proteins via increased synthesis. Support for such a hypothesis comes from the work of Carraro et al.,[48] who showed that the FSR of fibronectin was elevated at the end of exercise and that the FSR of fibrinogen was increased during recovery. However, this study did not find an effect of exercise upon the FSR of albumin. It remains to be seen whether similar increases in the FSR of plasma proteins can be observed at higher exercise intensities.

In this relatively new area of investigation there has been no studies looking at a sex-specific response. Examination of the glucagon to insulin ratios in the study by Tarnopolsky et al.[4] showed that they were much higher in males. This observation may indicate that gut proteolysis enhancement may be a partial explanation for the increased urea excretion observed in that study[4] and the increased leucine oxidation in males and females in a subsequent study.[3]

VI. EXERCISE AND REQUIREMENTS FOR DIETARY PROTEIN

A variety of studies examining protein requirements in athletes have concluded that protein requirements of habitually exercising individuals are elevated compared to those of sedentary persons.[3,5,8,9,113] It is obvious that the role of any extra dietary protein required by exercising persons would depend on the nature of the exercise because endurance exercise presumably would increase protein requirements through increased indispensable amino acid oxidation and resistance exercise by increasing protein requirements to support growth of muscle. Protein requirements established by the Food and Agricultural Organization of the World Health Organization of the United Nations (FAO/WHO/UNU)[114] are found by utilizing the nitrogen balance approach. Hence, using this same approach, several studies have attempted to determine protein requirements by conducting nitrogen balance studies.[5,7,9]

A. Resistance Exercise

Tarnopolsky and co-workers[9] conducted a study using the nitrogen balance approach to examine the protein requirements of a group of endurance-trained and resistance-trained athletes and a group of sedentary controls. As pointed out earlier, Tarnopolsky et al.[58] demonstrated that an isolated bout of resistance exercise did not increase leucine oxidation or perturb whole body protein turnover, perhaps due to the relatively low intensity of a resistance workout versus an endurance workout. Hence, it would appear that any extra protein required by strength-trained individuals is directed, for the most part, toward muscular hypertrophy. Protein requirements of trained bodybuilders were found to be 12% greater than those of sedentary controls, who had a protein requirement of 0.84 g protein $\cdot$ kg^{-1} $\cdot$ day^{-1}. The study by Tarnopolsky et al.,[9] examining the nitrogen balance of the resistance-training athletes, does highlight some bewildering results, however. For example, on a protein intake (actually equivalent to the habitual protein requirement of the bodybuilders) of ~2.8 g protein $\cdot$ kg^{-1} $\cdot$ day^{-1}, all bodybuilders were in highly positive nitrogen balance (~12–20 g N $\cdot$ day^{-1}). When extrapolated back to protein, this would have meant that the bodybuilders should have gained ~200 g of lean mass $\cdot$ day^{-1}.[9] Such shortcomings of nitrogen balance long have been recognized and have led to the recommendation of combining tracer and nitrogen balance approaches to determining protein requirements. Using such an approach, this same group later showed that strength-training athletes, who were also performing some endurance exercise,

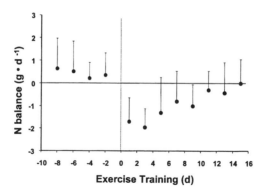

Figure 7.5 Nitrogen (N) balance in males (all subjects were consuming ~1 g protein · kg⁻¹ · day⁻¹) prior to and at the onset of a program of physical activity. Adapted from data in reference 117. Values are means ± SD.

had protein requirements almost 100% greater than those of sedentary controls.[7] In fact, consumption of the low protein diet (0.86 g protein · kg^{-1} · day^{-1}) by the strength-trained group resulted in an accommodated state where whole body protein synthesis was reduced compared to the medium (1.4 g protein · kg^{-1} · day^{-1}) and high protein (2.4 g protein · kg^{-1} · day^{-1}) diets.

In contrast to the results of Tarnopolsky et al.,[7,9] nitrogen balance studies conducted in the elderly initiating a moderate program of strength-training in the elderly have shown that protein requirements were reduced due to the anabolic stimulus of the resistance exercise.[115] Support for such a possibility can be seen in the results of Phillips et al.,[69] who showed that in the fasted state an isolated bout of resistance exercise resulted in increased muscle net protein balance, implying an improved intracellular recycling of amino acids. Butterfield and Calloway[116] also found a similar effect in persons beginning moderate exercise programs. Moreover, in an early study by Gontzea,[117] nitrogen balance became transiently negative at the onset of an exercise-training program, but the subjects were able to achieve nitrogen balance after ten days of training consuming 1 g protein · kg^{-1} · day^{-1} (Figure 7.5). It is possible that these latter results indicate a more efficient utilization of protein or an accommodation mechanism[118,119] that has resulted in the suboptimal functioning of some protein synthetic pathway. The discrepancy between the studies is explained almost certainly by the differences in the training status of the subjects as well as the different intensity, frequency, and duration of the exercise bout.

B. Endurance Exercise

Studies also have examined the adequacy of recommended protein intakes in persons engaged in vigorous endurance exercise. A study by Phillips et al.[3] examined the adequacy of the Canadian RNI for protein of (0.86 g protein · kg^{-1} · day^{-1})[120] in individuals engaged in habitual endurance exercise. Males and females were adapted to an isoenergetic diet for a period of ten days prior to conducting a three-day nitrogen balance experiment.[3] Endurance athletes consuming adequate energy and protein at the Canadian RNI were unable to maintain positive nitrogen balance.[3]

There was a trend for the males to be in a more negative nitrogen balance as compared to the females.[3] Friedman and Lemon[8] studied habitually exercising male athletes and conducted nitrogen balance experiments at two levels of protein intake. On the low protein intake (~0.86 g protein $\cdot$ kg^{-1} $\cdot$ day^{-1}) the athletes were also in negative nitrogen balance.[8] Both of these studies indicate that the Canadian RNI and the U.S. RDA for protein (both ~0.86 g protein $\cdot$ kg^{-1} $\cdot$ day^{-1}) were inadequate for habitually exercising male and female athletes. Meredith et al.[5] also conducted nitrogen balance experiments in habitually training endurance athletes. The mean protein intake to maintain zero nitrogen balance was 0.94 g protein $\cdot$ kg^{-1} $\cdot$ day^{-1} (~109% of the protein RNI[5,120]), which translated into an actual protein requirement of 1.26 g protein $\cdot$ kg^{-1} $\cdot$ day^{-1}. A weakness of the previous studies, however, was the failure to include any sedentary controls.[3,5,8] When a sedentary control group was included, Tarnopolsky et al.[9] found that the protein requirement of a group of endurance athletes was 1.67 times that of the control group. This finding translated into a daily protein requirement of 1.6 g protein $\cdot$ kg^{-1} $\cdot$ day^{-1} (~186% of the RNI for protein). It should be pointed out that in all the studies mentioned[3,5,7-9] the adaptation periods to the altered protein intakes were at least ten days in duration, which appears to be adequate for adaptation of specific urea cycle and other protein metabolic enzymes.[121]

Recently, a well-controlled study examined 24 h continuous leucine oxidation and urea kinetics in subjects who completed a total of 3 h (two exercise bouts lasting 1.5 h in duration in the fasted and fed state) of mild exercise.[34] These investigators concluded that the two exercise bouts did not result in negative leucine balance while consuming 1 g protein $\cdot$ kg^{-1} $\cdot$ day^{-1} (~100 mg leucine $\cdot$ kg^{-1} $\cdot$ day^{-1}). In addition, they found that the estimates of protein turnover from leucine oxidation, was only moderately increased during exercise. (A minimal estimate of the increase in leucine oxidation was 27% above resting, whereas a maximal estimate was closer to 45%, depending on which bicarbonate retention factor was employed.) These data compared quite well with protein turnover data from urea nitrogen kinetics, which showed very little change throughout rest, exercise, and recovery.[34] Furthermore, the modest exercise-induced increase in leucine oxidation during the two exercise bouts amounted to only ~4 to 7% of daily leucine oxidation. At the moderate level of exercise used by El-Khoury and co-workers;[34] however, it is perhaps not surprising that their subjects were in leucine balance because leucine oxidation increases in direct proportion to exercise intensity.[35] Further support for this contention comes from the exercise-induced increase in leucine oxidation observed by Phillips et al.[3] of 84% (from ~28 to ~51 μmol $\cdot$ kg^{-1} $\cdot$ min^{-1}) in males exercising at (65% VO$_{2peak}$, compared to the smaller increase reported by El-Koury[34] in males exercising at between 45 and 50% VO$_{2peak}$ (from ~27 to ~39 μmol $\cdot$ kg^{-1} $\cdot$ min^{-1}). Critical to the interpretations of the results of leucine oxidation studies, corrections were made for shifts in background[13] CO$_2$ enrichment and bicarbonate retention in both studies.[3,34] It would be very informative if the same elegant techniques used in the study by El-Koury[34] were employed in a study where more rigorous exercise was performed. Given the opposing points of view regarding protein requirements,[3,7,9,10,34] future research needs to examine protein requirements and perhaps amino acid requirements during endurance exercise.

C. Sex-Specific Protein Requirements

As mentioned above, both male and female endurance athletes habitually performing vigorous endurance exercises were in negative nitrogen balance while
consuming a weight-maintaining energy intake with a protein intake equivalent to
the Canadian RNI (close to the U.S. RDA).[3] Although the habitual dietary intake of
protein is usually in excess of the Canadian RNI (see Tarnopolsky Chapter 1, Table
1.2), it is important that leucine, and possibly oxidation of other amino acid may
increase in proportion to exercise intensity. Thus, dietary protein requirements could
be increased in a proportional relationship to exercise intensity. In addition, because
exercise and dietary restriction frequently are used in combination for weight loss
by certain female athletes (i.e., gymnastics, ballerinas), they may be more likely to
have an inadequate protein intake. Furthermore, an increasing number of females
are participating in sports during pregnancy and lactation, which may pose a further
stress upon dietary protein requirements.

VII. OVERALL SUMMARY

Amino acid oxidation contributes between three and six percent of the total energy
cost of endurance exercise. At lower exercise intensities, there is likely no negative
impact upon dietary protein requirements. In well-trained endurance athletes exercising on a daily basis, the amino acid contribution to energy expenditure may result in
a increased dietary protein requirement. For the well trained athlete who is exercising
more than 5 times per week, both the Canadian and United States recommended
protein intakes may be inadequate. Fortunately, both male and female athletes habitually consume enough protein to cover even a modest increase in requirements.
Although there is some evidence that females catabolize less protein than males
during endurance exercise, they may be the group at greatest risk for a suboptimal
dietary intake. For example, the following confounding variables are unique or more
frequent with females: dietary energy restriction, anorexia, pregnancy, and lactation.

Studies need to address the issues of the longitudinal adaptive responses of
BCKAD activity and amino acid oxidation to endurance exercise training in both
males and females. Potential gender differences in alanine and glutamine flux as
well as hepatic amino acid oxidation during exercise need to be examined further.
The effect of estrogen and the progesterone/estrogen ratio on both protein synthesis
and degradation needs further clarification.

Research into sex differences in protein metabolism remains an embryonic, yet
fruitful, area to explore.

REFERENCES

1. Romijn J. A., Coyle E. F., Sidossis S., Gastaldelli A., Horowitz J. F., Endert E., and
    Wolfe R. R., Regulation of endogenous fat and carbohydrate metabolism in relation
    to exercise intensity and duration, *American Journal of Physiology,* 265, E380, 1993.

2. Tarnopolsky M. A., Atkinson S. A., Phillips S. M., and MacDougall J. D., Carbohydrate loading and metabolism during exercise in men and women, *Journal of Applied Physiology,* 78, 1360, 1995.

3. Phillips S. M., Atkinson S. A., Tarnopolsky M. A., and MacDougall J. D., Gender differences in leucine kinetics and nitrogen balance in endurance athletes, *Journal of Applied Physiology,* 75, 2134, 1994.

4. Tarnopolsky L. J., MacDougall J. D., Atkinson, S. A., Tarnopolsky M. A., and Sutton J. R., Gender differences in substrate for endurance exercise, *Journal of Applied Physiology,* 68, 302, 1990.

5. Meredith C. N., Zackin M. J., Frontera W. R., and Evans W. J., Dietary protein requirements and body protein metabolism in endurance-trained men, *Journal of Applied Physiology,* 66, 2850, 1989.

6. Knapik J., Meredith C. N., Jones B., Fielding R., Young V., and Evans W. J., Leucine metabolism during fasting and exercise, *Journal of Applied Physiology,* 70, 43, 1991.

7. Tarnopolsky M. A., Atkinson S. A., MacDougall J. D., Chesley A., Phillips S., and Schwarcz H. P., Evaluation of protein requirements for trained strength athletes, *Journal of Applied Physiology,* 73, 1986, 1992.

8. Friedman J. E. and Lemon P. W., Effect of chronic endurance exercise on retention of dietary protein, *International Journal of Sports Medicine,* 10, 118, 1989.

9. Tarnopolsky M. A., MacDougall J. D., and Atkinson S. A., Influence of protein intake and training status on nitrogen balance and lean body mass, *Journal of Applied Physiology,* 64, 187, 1988.

10. Millward D. J., Bowtell J. L., Pacy P., and Rennie M. J., Physical activity, protein metabolism and protein requirements. *Proceedings of the Nutrition Society,* 53, 223, 1994.

11. Bier D. M., Intrinsically difficult problems: the kinetics of body proteins and amino acid in man, *Diabetes and Metabolism Reviews,* 5, 111, 1989.

12. Millward D. J., The endocrine response to dietary protein: the anabolic drive on growth, in *Milk Proteins,* Barth, C.A. and Schlimme, E. Eds., Steinkoppf Verlag, Darmstadt, 1989.

13. Runcie J. and Hilditch T. E., Energy provision, tissue utilization, and weight loss in prolonged starvation, *British Medical Journal,* 2, 352, 1974.

14. Goldberg A. L. and Chang T. W., Regulation and significance of amino acid metabolism in skeletal muscle, *Federation Proceedings,* 37, 2301, 1978.

15. Biolo G., Gastaldelli A., Zhang X., and Wolfe R. R., Protein synthesis and breakdown in skin and muscle: a leg model of amino acid kinetics, *American Journal of Physiology,* 267, E467, 1996.

16. Biolo G., Fleming D., Maggi S. P., and Wolfe R. R., Transmembrane transport and intracellular kinetics of amino acids in human skeletal muscle, *American Journal of Physiology,* 268, E75, 1995.

17. Ahlborg G., Felig P., Hagenfeldt L., Hendler R., and Wahren J., Substrate turnover during prolonged exercise in man, *Journal Clinical Investigation,* 53, 1080, 1974.

18. Graham T. E., Turcotte L. P., Kiens B., and Richter E. A., Training and muscle ammonia and amino acid metabolism in humans during prolonged exercise, *Journal of Applied Physiology,* 78, 725, 1995.

19. Felig P., Amino acid metabolism in man, *Annual Review of Biochemistry,* 44, 933, 1975.

20. Wolfe R. R., Goodenough R. D., Wolfe M. H., Royle G. T., and Nadel E. R., Isotopic analysis of leucine and urea metabolism in exercising humans, *Journal of Applied Physiology,* 52, 458, 1982.

21. Henderson S. C., Black A. L., and Brooks G. A., Leucine turnover and oxidation in trained rats during exercise, *American Journal of Physiology*, 249, E137, 1985.

22. Boyer B. and Odessey R., Kinetic characterization of branched chain ketoacid dehydrogenase, *Archives of Biochemistry and Biophysics*, 285, 1, 1991.

23. Khatra B. S., Chawla R. K., Sewell C. W., and Rudman D., Distribution of branched-chain α-keto acid dehydrogenases in primate tissues, *Journal Clinical Investigation*, 59, 558, 1977.

24. King P. A., Goldstein L., and Newsholme E. A., Glutamine synthetase activity of muscle in acidosis, *Biochemical Journal*, 216, 523, 1983.

25. MacLean D. A., Graham T. E., and Saltin B., Branched-chain amino acids augment ammonia metabolism while attenuating protein breakdown during exercise, *American Journal of Physiology*, 276, E1010, 1994.

26. MacLean D. A. and Graham T. E., Branched-chain amino acid supplementation augments plasma ammonia responses during exercise in humans, *Journal of Applied Physiology*, 74, 2711, 1993.

27. Hutson S. M. and Hall T. R., Identification of the mitochondrial branched chain amino transferase as a branched chain alpha-keto acid transporter protein, *The Journal of Biological Chemistry*, 268, 3084, 1993.

28. Rennie M. J., Edwards R. H. T., Davies C. T. M., Krywawych S., Halliday D., Waterlow J. C., and Millward D. J., Protein and amino acid turnover during and after exercise, *Biochemical Society Transactions*, 8, 499, 1980.

29. Fielding R. A., Evans W. J., Hughes V. A., and Moldawer L. L., and Bistrian, B. R., The effects of high intensity exercise on muscle and plasma levels of alpha-ketoisocaproic acid, *European Journal of Applied Physiology*, 55, 482, 1986.

30. May R. C., Hara Y., Kelly R. A., Block K. P., Buse M. G., and Mitch W. E., Branched-chain amino acid metabolism in rat muscle: abnormal regulation in acidosis, *American Journal of Physiology*, 252, E712, 1987.

31. Wagenmakers A. J., Beckers E. J., Brouns F., Kuipers H., Soeters P. B., van der, Vusse G. J., and Saris W. H., Carbohydrate supplementation, glycogen depletion, and amino acid metabolism during exercise, *American Journal of Physiology*, 260, E883, 1991.

32. Wagenmakers A. J., Brookes J. H., Coakley J. H., Reilly T., and Edwards R. H., Exercise-induced activation of the branched-chain 2-oxo acid dehydrogenase in human muscle, *European Journal of Applied Physiology*, 59, 159, 1989.

33. Lemon P. W., Nagle F. J., Mullin J. P., and Benevenga N. J., *In vivo* leucine oxidation at rest and during two intensities of exercise, *Journal of Applied Physiology*, 53, 947, 1982.

34. El-Khoury A. E., Forslund A., Olsson R., Branth S., Sjödin A., Andersson A., Atkinson A., Selvaraj A., Hambraeus L., and Young V. R., Moderate exercise at energy balance does not affect 24-h leucine oxidation or nitrogen retention in healthy men, *American Journal of Physiology*, 273, E394, 1997.

35. Rennie M. J., Edwards R. H. T., Krywawych S., Davies C. T. M., Halliday D., Waterlow J. C., and Millward D. J., Effect of exercise on protein turnover in man, *Clinical Science*, 61, 627, 1981.

36. Fielding R. A., Meredith C. N., O'Reilly K. P., Frontera W. R., Cannon J. G., and Evans W. J., Enhanced protein breakdown after eccentric exercise in young and older men, *Journal of Applied Physiology*, 71, 674, 1991.

37. Katz A., Broberg S., Sahlin K., and Wahren J., Muscle ammonia metabolism and amino acid metabolism during dynamic exercise in man, *Clinical Physiology*, 6, 365, 1986.

38. Elia M. and Livesey G., Effects of ingested steak and infused leucine on forelimb metabolism in man and the fate of carbon skeletons and amino groups of branched chain amino acids, *Clinical Science,* 64, 517, 1983.

39. Hood D. A. and Terjung R. L., Effect of endurance training on leucine metabolism in perfused rat skeletal muscle, *American Journal of Physiology,* 253, E648, 1987.

40. Eriksson L. S., Broberg S., Björkman O., and Wahren J., Ammonia metabolism during exercise in man, *Clinical Physiology,* 5, 325, 1985.

41. Graham T. E., Kiens B., Hargreaves M., and Richter E. A., Influence of fatty acids on ammonia and amino acid flux from active human muscle, *American Journal of Physiology,* 261, E168, 1991.

42. Wolfe R. R., Wolfe M. H., Nadel E. R., and Shaw J. H., Isotopic determination of amino acid-urea interactions in exercise in humans, *Journal of Applied Physiology,* 56, 221, 1984.

43. Carraro F., Kimbrough T. D., and Wolfe R. R., Urea kinetics in humans at two levels of exercise intensity, *Journal of Applied Physiology,* 75, 1180, 1993.

44. Lemon P. W. and Nagle F. J., Effects of exercise on protein and amino acid metabolism, *Medicine and Science in Sports and Exercise,* 13, 141, 1981.

45. Lemon P. W., Dolny D. G., and Yarasheski K. E., Effect of intensity on protein utilization during prolonged exercise, *Medicine and Science in Sports and Exercise,* 16, 151, 1984.

46. Haralambie G. and Berg A., Serum urea and amino nitrogen changes with exercise duration, *European Journal of Applied Physiology,* 36, 39, 1976.

47. Wasserman D. H., Geer R. J., Williams P. E., Becker T. A., Lacy D. B., and Abumrad N. N., Interaction of gut and liver on nitrogen metabolism during exercise, *Metabolism: Clinical and Experimental,* 40, 168, 1991.

48. Carraro F., Hartl W. H., Stuart C. A., Layman D. K., Jahoor F., and Wolfe R. R., Whole body and plasma protein synthesis in exercise and recovery in human subjects, *American Journal of Physiology,* 258, E821, 1990.

49. Wagenmakers A. J., Coakley J. H., and Edwards R. H., Metabolism of branched-chain amino acids and ammonia during exercise: clues from McArdles disease, *International Journal of Sports Medicine,* 11, S101, 1990.

50. Lemon P. W., Yarasheski K. E., and Dolny D. G., Validity/reliability of sweat analysis by whole-body washdown vs. regional collections, *Journal of Applied Physiology,* 61, 1967, 1986.

51. Dohm G. L. and Louis T. M., Changes in androstenedione, testosterone and protein metabolism as a result of exercise, *Proceedings of the Society for Experimental Biology and Medicine,* 158, 622, 1978.

52. Widdowson E. M. and McCance R. A., The effects of chronic undernutrition and of total starvation in growing and adult rats, *British Journal of Nutrition,* 10, 363, 1956.

53. Lamont L. S., Lemon P. W., and Bruot B. C., Menstrual cycle and exercise effects on protein catabolism, *Medicine and Science in Sports and Exercise,* 19, 106, 1987.

54. Lariviere F., Moussalli R., and Garrel D. R., Increased leucine flux and leucine oxidation during the luteal phase of the menstrual cycle in women, *American Journal of Physiology,* 267, E422, 1994.

55. Dohm G. L., Tapscott E. B., Barakat H. A., and Kasperek G. J., Measurement of *in vivo* protein synthesis in rats during an exercise bout, *Biochemical Medicine,* 27, 367, 1982.

56. Carraro F., Stuart C. A., Hartl W. H., Rosenblatt J., and Wolfe R. R., Effect of exercise and recovery on muscle protein synthesis in human subjects, *American Journal of Physiology,* 259, E470, 1990.

57. Bylund-Fellenius A.-C., Ojamaa K. M., Flaim K. E., Li J. B., Wassner S. J., and Jefferson L. S., Protein synthesis versus energy state in contracting muscle of perfused rat hindlimb, *American Journal of Physiology*, 246, E297, 1984.

58. Tarnopolsky M. A., Atkinson S. A., MacDougall J. D., Senor B. B., Lemon P. W. R., and Schwarcz H., Whole body leucine metabolism during and after resistance exercise in fed humans, *Medicine and Science in Sports and Exercise*, 23, 326, 1991.

59. Vihko V., Salminen A., and Rantamaki J., Exhaustive exercise, endurance training, and acid hydrolase activity in skeletal muscle, *Journal of Applied Physiology*, 47, 43, 1979.

60. Salminen A. and Vihko V., Effects of age and prolonged running on proteolytic capacity in mouse cardiac and skeletal muscles, *Acta Physiologica Scandanavica*, 112, 89, 1981.

61. Belcastro A. N., Skeletal muscle calcium-activated neutral protease (calpain) with exercise, *Journal of Applied Physiology*, 74, 1381, 1993.

62. Salminen A., Kainulainen H., and Vihko V., Lysosomal changes related to ageing and physical exercise in mouse cadiac and skeletal muscles, *Experientia*, 38, 781, 1982.

63. Mitch W. E. and Goldberg A. L., Mechanisms of muscle wasting, *New England Journal of Medicine*, 335, 1897, 1996.

64. Belcastro A. N., Parkhouse W. S., Dobson G., and Gilchrist J. S., Influence of exercise on cardiac and skeletal muscle myofibrillar proteins, *Molecular and Cellular Biochemistry*, 83, 27, 1988.

65. Tidball J. G., Inflammatory cell response to acute muscle injury, *Medicine and Science in Sports and Exercise*, 27, 1022, 1995.

66. Byrd S. K., Alterations in the sacoplasmic reticulum: a possible link to exercise-induced muscle damage, *Medicine and Science in Sports and Exercise*, 24, 531, 1992.

67. Byrd S. K., McCutcheon L. J., Hodgson D. R., and Gollnick P. D., Altered sarcoplasmic reticulum function after high-intensity exercise, *Journal of Applied Physiology*, 67, 2072, 1989.

68. Evans W. J. and Cannon J .G., The metabolic effects of exercise-induced muscle damage, in *Exercise and Sport Sciences Reviews*, Holloszy, J.O. Ed., Williams and Wilkins, Baltimore, MD, 1991.

69. Phillips S. M., Tipton K. D., Aarsland A., Wolf S. E., and Wolfe R. R., Mixed muscle protein synthesis and breakdown following resistance exercise in humans, *American Journal of Physiology*, 273, E99, 1997.

70. Lieber R. L., Schmitz M. C., Mishra D. K., and Friden J., Contractile and cellular remodelling in rabbit skeletal muscle after cyclic eccentric contractions, *Journal of Applied Physiology*, 77, 1926, 1994.

71. Friden J., Sjöstrom M., and Ekblom B., Myofibrillar damage following intense eccentric exercise in man, *International Journal of Sports Medicine*, 4, 170, 1983.

72. Friden J., Kjorell U., and Thornell L.-E., Delayed muscle soreness and cytoskeletal alterations: an immunocytological study in man, *International Journal of Sports Medicine*, 5, 15, 1984.

73. Kasperek G. J. and Snider R. D., Total and myofibrillar protein degradation in isolated soleus muscles after exercise, *American Journal of Physiology*, 257, E1, 1989.

74. Kasperek G. J., Dohm G. L., Barakat H. A., Strausbauch D. W., Barnes D. W., and Snider R. D., The role of lysosomes in exercise-induced hepatic protein loss, *Biochemical Journal*, 202, 281, 1982.

75. Kasperek G. J., Conway G. R., Krayeski D. S., and Lohne J. J., A reexamination of the effect of exercise on rate of muscle protein degradation, *American Journal of Physiology,* 263, E1144, 1992.

76. Svanberg E., Möller-Loswick A.-C., Matthews D. E., Körner U., Andersson M., and Lundholm K., Effects of amino acids on synthesis and degradation of skeletal muscle proteins in humans, *American Journal of Physiology,* 271, E718, 1996.

77. Biolo G., Tipton K. D., Klein S., and Wolfe R. R., An abundant supply of amino acids enhances the metabolic effect of exercise on muscle protein, *American Journal of Physiology,* 273, E122, 1997.

78. Tiidus P. M., Can estrogens diminish exercise induced muscle damage? *Canadian Journal of Applied Physiology,* 20, 26, 1995.

79. Van der Meulen J. H., McArdle A., Jackson M. J., and Faulkner J. A., Contraction-induced injury to the extensor digitorum longus muscle of rats: the role of vitamin E, *Journal of Applied Physiology,* 83, 817, 1997.

80. Roman W. J., Fleckenstein J., Stray-Gundersen J., Alway S. E., Peshock R., and Gonyea W. J., Adaptations in the elbow flexors of elderly males after heavy-resistance training, *Journal of Applied Physiology,* 74, 750, 1993.

81. Alway S. E., Grumbt W. H., Stray-Gundersen J., and Gonyea W. J., Effects of resistance training on elbow flexors of highly competitive bodybuilders, *Journal of Applied Physiology,* 72, 1512, 1992.

82. Housch T. J., Housch D. J., Weir J. P., and Weir L. L., Effects of eccentric-only resistance training and detraining, *International Journal of Sports Medicine,* 17, 145, 1996.

83. Welle S., Thornton C., Jozefowicz R., and Statt M., Myofibrillar protein synthesis in young and old men, *American Journal of Physiology,* 264, E693, 1993.

84. Biolo G., Maggi S. P., Williams B. D., Tipton K. D., and Wolfe R. R., Increased rates of muscle protein turnover and amino acid transport after resistance exercise in humans, *American Journal of Physiology,* 268, E514, 1995.

85. Chesley A., MacDougall J. D., Tarnopolsky M. A., Atkinson S. A., and Smith K., Changes in human muscle protein synthesis after resistance exercise, *Journal of Applied Physiology,* 73, 1383, 1992.

86. Yarasheski K. E., Zachwieja J. F., and Bier D. M., Acute effects of resistance exercise on muscle protein synthesis rate in young and elderly men and women, *American Journal of Physiology,* 265, E210, 1993.

87. MacDougall J. D., Gibala M. J., Tarnopolsky M. A., MacDonald J. R., Interisano S. A., and Yarasheski K. E., The time course for elevated muscle protein synthesis following heavy resistance exercise, *Canadian Journal of Applied Physiology,* 20, 480, 1995.

88. Zhang X., Chinkes D. L., Sakurai Y., and Wolfe R. R., An isotopic method for measurement of muscle protein fractional breakdown rate *in vivo, American Journal of Physiology,* 270, E759, 1996.

89. Dohm G. L., Israel R. G., Breedlove R. L., Williams R. T., and Askew E. W., Biphasic changes in 3-methylhistdine excretion in humans after exercise, *American Journal of Physiology,* 248, E588, 1985.

90. Dohm G. L., Williams R. T., Kasperek G. J., and van Rij A. M., Increased excretion of urea and N^{τ}-methylhistidine by rats and humans after a bout of exercise, *Journal of Applied Physiology,* 52, 27, 1982.

91. Hickson J. F., Wolinsky I., Rodriguez G. P., Pivarnick J. M., Kent M. C., and Shier N. W., Failure of weight training to affect urinary indices of protein metabolism in men, *Medicine and Science in Sports and Exercise,* 18, 563, 1986.

92. Young V. R. and Munro H. N., N$^{\tau}$-Methylhistidine (3-methylhistidine) and muscle protein turnover: an overview, *Federation Proceedings,* 37, 2291, 1978.

93. Bonen A., Malcolm S. A., Kilgour R. D., MacIntyre K. P., and Belcastro A. N., Glucose ingestion before and during intense exercise, *Journal of Applied Physiology,* 50, 766, 1981.

94. Pivarnick J. M., Hickson J. F., and Wolinsky I., Urinary 3-methylhistidine excretion increases with repeated weight training exercise, *Medicine and Science in Sports and Exercise,* 21, 283, 1989.

95. Rennie M. J. and Millward D. J., 3-Methylhistidine excretion and the urinary 3-methylhistidine/creatinine ratio are poor indicators of skeletal muscle protein breakdown, *Clinical Science,* 65, 217, 1983.

96. Sjölin J., Stjernström H., Henneberg S., Andersson E., Martensson J., Friman G., and Larsson J., Splanchnic and peripheral release of 3-methylhistidine in relation to its urinary excretion in human infection, *Metabolism: Clinical and Experimental,* 38, 23, 1989.

97. Staron R. S., Leonardi M. J., Karapondo D. L., Malicky E. S., Falkel, J. E., Hagerman F. C., and Hikida R. S., Strength and skeletal muscle adaptations in heavy-resistance-trained women after detraining and retraining, *Journal of Applied Physiology,* 70, 631, 1991.

98. Staron R. S., Karapondo D. L., Kraemer W. J., Fry A. C., Gordon S. E., Falkel J. E., Hagerman F. C., and Hikida R. S., Skeletal muscle adaptations during early phase of heavy-resistance training in men and women, *Journal of Applied Physiology,* 76, 1247, 1994.

99. Hisaeda H., Miyagawa K., Kuno S., and Fukunaga T., and Muraoka I., Influence of two different modes of resistance training in female subjects, *Ergonomics,* 39, 842, 1996.

100. Wang N., Hikida R. S., Staron R. S., and Simoneau J. A., Muscle fiber types of women after resistance training — quantitative ultrastructure and enzyme activity, *European Journal of Applied Physiology,* 424, 494, 1993.

101. Holloszy J. O. and Coyle E. F., Adaptations of skeletal muscle to endurance exercise and their metabolic consequences, *Journal of Applied Physiology,* 56, 831, 1984.

102. Jansson E. and Kaijser L. Substrate utilization and enzymes in skeletal muscle of extremely endurance-trained men, *Journal of Applied Physiology,* 62, 999, 1987.

103. Carraro F., Naldini A., Weber J. M., and Wolfe R. R., Alanine kinetics in humans during low-intensity exercise, *Medicine and Science in Sports and Exercise,* 26, 348, 1994.

104. Evans W. J., Exercise and protein metabolism, *World Review of Nutrition and Dietetics,* 71, 21, 1993.

105. Phillips S. M., Green H. J., Tarnopolsky M. A., and Grant S. M., Increased clearance of lactate following short-term training in men, *Journal of Applied Physiology,* 79, 1862, 1995.

106. Hood D. A. and Terjung R. L., Endurance training alters alanine and glutamine release from muscle during contractions, *FEBS Letters,* 340, 287, 1997.

107. Wibom R. and Hultman E., ATP production rate in mitochondria isolated from microsamples of human muscle, *American Journal of Physiology,* 259, E204, 1990.

108. Dohm G. L., Beecher G. R., Warren R. Q., and Williams R. T., The influence of exercise on free amino acid concentrations in rat tissues, *Journal of Applied Physiology,* 50, 41, 1982.

109. Williams B. D., Wolfe R. R., Bracy D. P., and Wasserman D. H., Gut proteolysis contributes essential amino acids during exercise, *American Journal of Physiology,* 270, E85, 1996.

110. Nakshabendi I. M., Obeidat W., Russel R. I., Downie S., Smith K., and Rennie M. J., Gut mucosal protein synthesis measured using intravenous and intragastric delivery of stable tracer amino acids, *American Journal of Physiology,* 269, E996, 1995.

111. Biolo G., Zhang X., and Wolfe R. R., Role of membrane transport in interorgan amino acid flow between muscle and small intestine, *Metabolism: Clinical and Experimental,* 44, 719, 1995.

112. Wolfe R. R., Nadel E. R., Shaw J. H. F., Stephenson L. A., and Wolfe M. H., Role of changes in insulin and glucagon in glucose homeostasis in exercise, *Journal Clinical Investigation,* 77, 900, 1986.

113. Lemon P. W., Do athletes need more dietary protein and amino acids? *International Journal of Sport Nutrition,* 5, S39, 1995.

114. FAO/WHO/UNU, Energy and Protein Requirements, in *Report of a Joint FAO/WHO/UNU Expert Consultation.* (Tech. Rep. No. 724), Geneva, Switzerland, 1985.

115. Campbell W. W., Crim M. C., Young V. R., Joseph L. J., and Evans W. J., Effects of resistance training and dietary protein intake on protein metabolism in older adults, *American Journal of Physiology,* 268, E1143, 1995.

116. Butterfield G. E. and Calloway D. H., Physical activity improves protein utilization in young men, *British Journal of Nutrition,* 51, 171, 1984.

117. Gontzea I., Sutzescu P., and Dumitrache S., The influence of adaptation to physical effort on nitrogen balance in man, *Nutrition Reports International,* 22, 231, 1975.

118. Young V. R., Nutritional balance studies: indicators of human requirements or adaptive mechanisms? *Journal of Nutrition,* 116, 70, 1985.

119. Young V. R. and Marchini J. S., Mechanisms and nutritional significance of metabolic responses to altered intakes or protein and amino acids with reference to nutritional adaptation in humans, *American Journal of Clinical Nutrition,* 51, 270, 1990.

120. Department of Health and Welfare, Recommended Nutrient Intakes (Protein), in *Nutrition Recommendations: The Report of the Scientific Review Committee.* Canadian Government Publishing Centre, Ottawa, Canada, 1990.

121. Das T. K. and Waterlow J. C., The rate of adaptation of urea cycle enzymes, amino transferases, and glutamine dehydrogenases to changes in dietary protein intake, *British Journal of Nutrition,* 32, 353, 1974.

CHAPTER 8

Gender Differences in Lipid Metabolism During Exercise and at Rest

M. A. Tarnopolsky, M.D., Ph.D., F.R.C.P.(C)

CONTENTS

I. INTRODUCTION

This chapter will focus primarily upon free fatty acid (FFA) metabolism and the potential for a gender-specific difference. Particular emphasis will be placed upon FFA metabolism during exercise. Free fatty acids are a major source of metabolic energy for humans both at rest and during exercise. Quantitatively, the triacylglyceride (TG) pool in adipocytes provides the largest potential source of energy (Table 8.1).

Table 8.1 Total Body Fuel Stores in Male and Female Athletes

Fuel Store	Gender	Mass (kg)	Mass (% total)	Exercise Duration (min)*
Adipose Tissue	M	8.4	12%	3024
	F	11.6	21%	6000
Carbohydrate				
Muscle glycogen	M	0.5	0.7%	133
	F	0.37	0.7%	140
Liver glycogen	M	0.09	0.09%	24
	F	0.08	0.09%	28
Blood glucose	M	0.0054	0.008%	1
	F	0.0045	0.008%	1
Protein (Muscle)	M	9.4	50%	2506
	F	7.0	40%	2666

* Exercise at 60% VO_{2peak} (male VO_{2peak} = 5.0 L/min; female VO_{2peak} = 3.5 L/min). Estimated weight for male = 70 kg; female = 55 kg. Also assumes that all of the given substrate could be oxidized.

It makes sense that humans have evolved to store energy in the form of TG for they are the most energy-dense of the macronutrients and, unlike proteins, they do not have the same regulatory and structural importance. The oxidation of lipid provides about 9 kilocalories (kcal) of metabolizable energy as compared to 4 kcal for both protein and carbohydrate. Assuming that glycogen is stored in association with water on a 1:3–4 ratio basis, it can be estimated that a 70 kg male with 15% body fat, who stored all of his potential energy as glycogen instead of TG, would weigh 156 kg! Given the metabolic storage efficiency of TG, it may be that the sexual dimorphism in adipose tissue content and potentially the ability to utilize it under periods of metabolic stress (i.e., exercise) could have arisen from selective evolutionary pressures for females to withstand starvation and remain ovulatory.[1]

II. GENERAL OVERVIEW OF FATTY ACID METABOLISM

Fatty acid metabolism is a complex and interesting area. A comprehensive review of this area would require a dedicated chapter. Therefore, the author will only review the major highlights of FFA metabolism with a particular focus upon oxidative pathways in skeletal muscle during exercise.

The FFA are categorized by their number of carbons into short (2–4), medium (6–12), long (14–20), and very long (> 22) chains. Unless otherwise specified, the author primarily will be referring to the long chain FFAs in this chapter as they are quantitatively the major source of fuel to exercising skeletal muscle under normal conditions. The focus of the chapter will be on the FFA oxidation pathways and their regulation, particularly during exercise.

A. Pathways

The source of skeletal muscle FFA in the fasted state comes from plasma FFA bound to albumin (from adipose tissue TG hydrolysis), plasma derived TG hydrolysis by endothelial lipoprotein lipase (LPL) of very low density lipoproteins (VLDL), and the liberation from intramuscular TG (IMTG) sources by hormone-sensitive lipase (HSL). In the postprandial state, much of the fat entering the body is in the form of TG-rich chylomicrons that deliver FFA to adipocytes and skeletal muscle for storage as TG.

For plasma FFA (albumin-FFA + LPL liberated), the transport across the sarcolemma has both saturable and nonsaturable kinetics. Two FFA transport proteins, FFA transport protein (FATP)[2] and FFA translocase (FAT),[3] have been cloned. These proteins are expressed ubiquitously and respond rapidly to metabolic stressors.[4] For example, the cytokine IL-1, results in a reduction of FAT and FATP mRNA in rat skeletal muscle.[4] Given the large differences in circulating IL-1 concentrations between the genders (see Chapter 2), there is the potential for FFA transport to be regulated differentially at the sarcolemmal transport level.

Another factor that may contribute to FFA transport is cytosolic fatty acid binding protein (FABP).[5] FABP represents about 1% of total cytoplasmic proteins.[5] This protein may function to create a metabolic sink for the importation of FFA across the sarcolemma. Considering the fact that FABP content has been correlated positively with palmitate oxidative capacity, it is likely that FABP has some role in determining the tissue capacity for FFA oxidation.[5]

Once inside the cytosol the FFA is condensed with CoA via an ATP-dependent reaction catalyzed by acyl-CoA synthase (outer leaflet of outer mitochondrial membrane). The charged acyl-CoA group then can enter the mitochondria through a pore. Once the acyl-CoA group has entered the intermitochondrial space it is converted into an acyl-carnitine moiety by carnitine acyl transferase I (CAT I) on the inner leaflet of the outer mitochondrial membrane. This moiety then passes into the mitochondrial matrix via carnitine:acylcarnitine translocase. The acyl group finally is available to β-oxidation after the carnitine acyl transferase II (CAT II) reaction, which occurs on the inner leaflet of the inner mitochondrial membrane (Figure 8.1). It should be noted that short and medium chain FFAs can enter the mitochondrial matrix directly without the carnitine carrier process. Thus, medium chain triglyceride supplements have been used in the treatment of patients with CPT II deficiency and also have been tried in athletic supplement drinks.[6]

Beta oxidation is the major final common pathway for the oxidation of most FFA in humans. Essentially, the acyl group with N carbons (i.e., 16 for palmitate) is catabolized sequentially (thiolysis) into two carbon fragments at the b carbon after each passes through the four enzyme cycles. The acetyl-CoA that is produced enters the TCA cycle at the citrate synthase step.

The first step in β-oxidation is catalyzed by acyl CoA dehydrogenase (short-, medium-, long-, and very long-chain length genetically distinct forms) with the release of FADH$_2$. The next step involves enoyl-CoA hydratase (crotonase and long-chain enoyl-CoA hydratase forms). Following this step an oxidation reaction is catalyzed by the FFA oxidation enzyme most frequently measured in exercise physiology studies, namely, β L-3-hydroxyacyl-CoA-dehydrogenase (HAD) short- and long-chain specific forms. The terminal thiolysis step results in the formation of an acetyl-CoA group and an acyl group (N-2 carbons) (acetaoacetyl-CoA thiolase and a generalized 3-ketoacyl-CoA thiolase) (Figure 8.2). In addition to mitochondrial β-

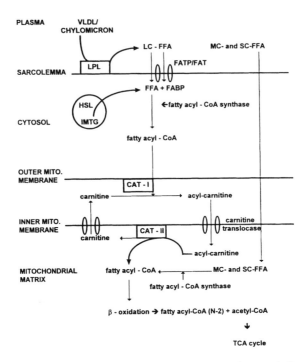

Figure 8.1 Pathways of fat oxidation in skeletal muscle. LPL = lipoprotein lipase, SC, MC, LC = short, medium, and long chain FFA; FATP = fatty acid transport protein; FAT = fatty acid translocase; HSL = hormone sensitive lipase; IMTG = intramuscular triglyceride; CAT — I and II = carnitine acyl transferase I and II; TCA = tricarboxylic acid cycle; MITO = mitochondria.

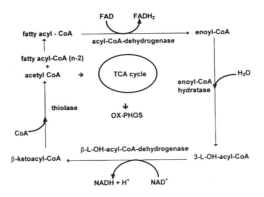

Figure 8.2 β-oxidation pathway in skeletal muscle. FAD = flavin adenine dinucleotide (FADH$_2$ = reduced form); NAD$^+$ = nicotine adenine nucleotide (NADH + H$^+$ = reduced form); CoA = coenzyme A; n-2 = acyl group less 2 carbons after each cycle.

oxidation, there exists a peroxisomal β-oxidation pathway and ω-oxidation in microsomes. To this author's knowledge, the contribution of these latter pathways to energy production during exercise has not been explored.

In skeletal muscle and adipocytes, FFA are stored along with glycerol as TG. Indirect evidence for FFA synthesis pathways comes from the observation of malonyl-CoA in both human[7] and rodent[8] skeletal muscle. This process is energy-dependent (requires NADPH) and occurs in the cytosol (both opposite to β-oxidation). The process also requires a protein scaffold called acyl-carrier protein (ACP). The first committed step in FFA synthesis is catalyzed by a biotin-dependent enzyme, acetyl-CoA carboxylase (ACC) (acetyl-CoA + $CO_2 \rightarrow$ malonyl-CoA). ACC is regulated by phosphorylation (+Pi = decreased activity; –Pi = increased activity). In essence, FFA synthesis is the reverse of β-oxidation, with two carbon fragments being added sequentially to an acyl group. Propionyl CoA is important in the formation of odd chain fatty acids; there are specific desaturase enzymes that insert double bonds at specific loci in mammals.

B. Regulation

The regulation of skeletal muscle β-oxidation is multifaceted. One of the first levels of regulation is the delivery of FFA to the muscle. This glucose-fatty acid cycle was demonstrated either by direct FFA infusion[9] or by the infusion of Intralipid (chemically similar to chylomicrons) and heparin (activates LPL).[10,11,12] It has been proposed that an increased FFA delivery to skeletal muscle will result in a mass action increase in FFA uptake and oxidation and a subsequent decrease in glucose uptake[9] and glycogenolysis.[9,13] The decrease in glycogenolysis and glycolysis was thought to be due to an increased glucose-6-phosphate and citrate that inhibited phosphorylase and phosphofructokinase (PFK), respectively.[9] A glycogen sparing effect consequent to FFA elevation has been shown during exercise in humans.[10] Contrary to these results, a nearly identical study found no effect of Intralipid infusion on glycogenolysis during exercise, yet glucose uptake was inhibited.[12]

An excellent study explored this concept in great detail and found that Intralipid infusion resulted in glycogen sparing as early as 15 minutes of exercise.[11] Citrate was elevated at rest in this latter study; however, there were no differences in citrate at 1 and 15 minutes of exercise for Intralipid vs. placebo infusion.[11]

This group suggested that the locus of glycogenolytic control with elevated FFA was at the level of phosphorylase.[11] The well-known increase in FFA oxidation and glycogen sparing that occurs with endurance training also is felt to be related to a step proximal to PFK (Phosphorylase) and not to citrate-mediated PFK inhibition.[14] On the opposite side of the metabolic coin, glucose and insulin *per se* can inhibit lipolysis.[15] It is clear that there are interactions between glucose and FFA that influence the choice of substrate selection during exercise. These interactions are complex, and the regulation at rest and during exercise may be quantitatively and qualitatively different.

Malonyl-CoA is the most important inhibitory regulator or CPT I activity and, as such, can influence significantly FFA oxidation rates.[16] When the insulin:glucogon ratio is high, such as in the fed state, there is an increase in the activation of acetyl-

CoA carboxylase (ACC) (dephosphorylate) with an increase in malonyl-CoA and resultant FFA synthesis. In the fasted state or during exercise, there is a decrease in the insulin:glucagon ratio, a decrease in ACC activity (phosphorylation), a decrease in malonyl-CoA, a removal of CPT I inhibition, and an increase in β-oxidation. Although ACC can be phosphorylated by either 3'- or 5'-cyclic monophosphate-dependent protein kinase (PKA) and AMP-activated protein kinase (AMPK), in rat skeletal muscle it appears that AMPK phosphorylation of ACC is the most important.[8] The result of AMPK-mediated ACC phosphorylation is an increase in the K_m for ATP, bicarbonate, and acetyl CoA, as well as an increase in the activation constant for citrate.[8] Thus, at the onset of exercise, an increase in AMP triggers a reduction in ACC activity → decreased malonyl-CoA, and an increase in β-oxidation. One study has reported that ACC and FFA synthase activity increases in the liver of OVX rats given estradiol.[17] Whether ACC activity or AMPK-dependent ACC phosphorylation differs between the genders is unclear; however, this would be a fruitful area for future investigation.

From a hormonal standpoint, the catecholamines appear to be the most important in stimulating FFA oxidation in skeletal muscle.[18] Epinephrine increases lipolysis[19] independent of plasma glucose concentrations[20] and stimulates adipocyte lipolysis.[21] Norepinephrine increases the TG-FFA cycle rate nearly four-fold.[22] Repeated epinephrine infusion results in an attenuation of epinephrine-stimulated lipolysis, suggesting a receptor or post-receptor mechanism.[19] Furthermore, the major regulator of HSL is epinephrine (hence its name).[23] Plasma epinephrine and norepinephrine concentrations are lower during exercise at the same absolute intensity of exercise following endurance training.[24]

When this latter observation is interpreted in light of greater fat oxidation attenuated glycogen degradation following endurance exercise training,[24] it is likely that catecholamine-stimulated glycogenolysis and lipolysis respond in opposite ways to endurance exercise training (implying a postreceptor effect). One further piece of evidence to support that glycogenolysis and lipolysis can be attenuated and enhanced simultaneously, respectively, in the presence of an elevated epinephrine comes from studies with caffeine ingestion[25] (see Chapter 13).

C. Acute Effects of Endurance Exercise

The proportion of FFA oxidized during endurance exercise is critically dependent upon the intensity of exercise. Essentially, as the intensity of exercise increases, there is a progressive decrease in the proportion of energy derived from FFA and an increase in the contribution from carbohydrate. As exercise intensity approaches VO_{2max}, FFA cannot supply energy fast enough to keep up with energy demand, and muscle glycogen and blood glucose provide a proportionately greater amount of energy.[26] This well-known phenomenon has been referred to as the cross-over concept by George Brooks[27] (Figure 8.3).

In addition to intensity-dependent alterations in the ratio of FFA:carbohydrate, there are also intensity-dependent differences in the proportional ratio of plasma-derived FFA (peripheral lipolysis):IMTG lipolysis. At an exercise intensity of about 25% VO_{2max}, peipheral lipolysis provides the largest proportion of energy, but at 60

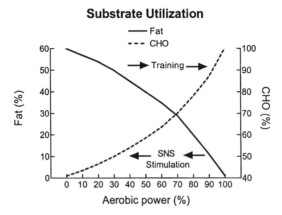

Figure 8.3 Proportion of fat and carbohydrate utilized during endurance exercise as a function of intensity. Aerobic power refers to percentage of VO_{2max}. Training and SNS (sympathetic nervous system) stimulation refer to the effect of these major regulators on the proportion of fat and carbohydrate oxidized. Redrawn and adapted from References 24 and 27.

to 65% VO_{2max}, IMTG lipolysis becomes more predominant.[26] In addition to lipolysis *per se,* some of the FFA available for oxidation comes from a decrease in fatty acid re-esterification.[28] For example, at rest, 70% of released FFA are re-esterified, but at the onset of exercise, this decreases to 25 to 30% until recovery when the percent increases to over 90%.[28] This mechanism may provide a rapid FFA delivery at the onset of exercise and a rapid repletion following completion and may also be a locus for metabolic control.

As the duration of endurance exercise progresses, there is a proportionate increase in the contribution from fat to the total energy expenditure.[18,24,29]

D. Effects of Endurance Exercise Training

In response to endurance exercise training, there is a definite sparing of glycogen utilization and a proportionate increase in FFA oxidation.[30,31,32,33] It is interesting to note that the increased FFA oxidation is primarily in the IMTG pool[24,31,32] (Table 8.2). As one would expect, there is an increase in both the substrate (IMTG)[32] and capacity (HAD[31,34]; CPT[35,36] activity) for intra-muscular β-oxidation in response to endurance training. Even at the ultrastructural level there is an increase in lipid droplets seen following endurance training.[37] Recent evidence also has found that FABP content is increased with endurance training,[38] suggesting that the diffusive flux for FFA may be enhanced with endurance training.

In addition to increases in enzymatic and substrate capacity in response to endurance training, it also appears that the lipolytic sensitivity to catecholamines is increased.[39,24] This may be due to an increase in catecholamine-stimulated adipocyte lipolysis as demonstrated by Despres and colleagues.[21] However, peripheral lipolysis and catecholamine concentrations are significantly lower at the same absolute exercise intensity following endurance training.[24] At the same time, the contribution from IMTG to total energy expenditure is increased two- to three-fold.[24,31] Thus, following

Table 8.2 **Adaptations in Fat Oxidation Consequent to**
             Endurance Training

Variable	Adaptation
Muscle Transport/Storage	↑ FABP, ↑ IMTG, ↑ mitochondria
Muscle Enzyme Capacity	↑ HAD and CPT activity
Whole Body Oxidation	↑ IMTG oxidation, ↑ TG/FFA flux
	↓ peripheral lipolysis
	↑ lipolytic sensitivity to catecholamines

Note: For definition of short forms see text (refs. 18, 24, 26, 31, 32,
         40, 41, 42, and 46).

endurance training, the capacity for adipocyte lipolysis is increased; however, its relative contribution to energy delivery is reduced relative to IMTG oxidation.

Interestingly, LPL gene expression is increased in skeletal muscle and not adipocytes following endurance exercise training, suggesting an enhancement of FFA delivery to skeletal muscle.[40] This observation is consistent with the observation that IMTG concentration is increased following endurance training.[32]

Metabolic tracer studies have demonstrated a greater glycerol and FFA rate of appearance (Ra) at rest in both longitudinal[24] and cross-sectional studies.[26] Glycerol Ra is felt to be an indicator of whole body lipolysis.[18] There are several tissues of origin for glycerol, and it has been estimated that about 15% come from skeletal muscle in untrained dogs.[41] Furthermore, human muscle may take up and release glycerol simultaneously.[42] Contrary to established concepts (namely that liver and kidney are the main sites of glycerol Rd and re-esterification due to their high glycerol kinase activity), it now appears that extra-hepatic and extra-renal tissues contribute significantly to glycerol release and uptake in spite of low glycerol kinase activity.[41,43] There is at least one report of glycerol kinase activity in skeletal muscle.[44] Whether this indicates that triglyceride-FFA cycling can occur directly within skeletal muscle is unclear. However, the combination of unexpectedly high glycerol concentrations in microdialysed human skeletal muscle[45] and the finding that FFA re-esterification can occur in extra-hepatic tissues,[41,43] raises this interesting possibility.

Clearly, endurance training increases TG-FFA cycling at rest by approximately four-fold.[26] This could alter significantly FFA delivery to skeletal muscle during the rest-to-exercise transition, particularly if this occurs to any extent directly within the skeletal muscle.

During endurance exercise at the same relative intensity, there is a greater total and peak glycerol Ra.[18] When tested at the same absolute intensity following endurance training, total glycerol Ra during exercise is similar,[46,24] yet the calculated[24] IMTG oxidation is increased. It would be interesting to calculate the contribution of skeletal muscle to total glycerol Ra before and after endurance training at both the absolute and relative exercise intensities.

III. GENDER DIFFERENCES IN FATTY ACID METABOLISM

From a morphological standpoint, one of the most consistent observations is the greater amount of subcutaneous adipose tissue in females as compared to males. As discussed in Chapter 1, there is some evidence that females may derive a greater proportion of energy from lipids during endurance exercise. The focus of the following section is on an exploration of this possibility.

A. Capacity for Fatty Acid Oxidation

1. Storage of Substrate

It is clear from Table 8.1 that the total amount of adipose tissue available to the average female athlete is much greater than that available to the male. Other than perhaps providing buoyancy for a female endurance swimmer, it is not conceivable under usual circumstances that either a male or female would be limited by the availability of adipose tissue *per se*. From a phylogenetic standpoint, the larger depot in females may provide for starvation resistance. As discussed in more detail in Chapters 9 and 10, females seem to be able to maintain subcutaneous adipose tissue in the face of energy deficit imposed by exercise or energy restriction (see also "lipolytic differences between the genders").

There has been very little research into potential gender differences in IMTG content. It is interesting to speculate whether there may be gender differences in IMTG that would mirror those seen in the peripheral adipose tissue. In one study of males and females aged 19 to 85, it was reported that the total fat content of female muscle was 58 g/kg and of male muscle was 23 g/kg.[47] In untrained females, there appears to be an increase in interfascicular fat that was not seen in trained females nor in males (no IMTG measurements were made).[48] The authors measured the IMTG content of skeletal muscle in six male and six female well-trained endurance athletes from a carbohydrate loading study[49] and found that females had a higher IMTG content (female = 38 mmol/kgdm; male = 32 mmol/kgdm; P < 0.05).[50] Whether this gender difference represents true IMTG or whether it is from adipocytes in the endo- and peri-mysial space around fibers and fasicles remains to be seen. It will be important to look at male and female muscle with light (Oil-red-O) and electron microscopy (see Chapter 3) to determine whether the observed gender difference is truly in the IMTG fraction. It is not likely that the slight increase in type I/II fiber proportions for females compared to males (Chapter 3) could account totally for the IMTG difference. Again, Oil-red-O and ATPase on serial histological sections in males and females will help to answer this question.

It is possible that IMTG content *per se* could influence FFA oxidation directly for its hydrolysis bypasses peripheral lipolysis, plasma transport, and sarcolemmal uptake, which are required for peripheral FFA utilization. Furthermore, endurance training increases IMTG content[32] and proportional oxidation,[24] which indirectly implies that IMTG oxidation is a preferred fuel source under periods of metabolic stress (i.e., exercise). There does not appear to be a gender difference in muscle glycogen concentration under basal conditions; however, females may spare glycogen during endurance exercise in human[51] and animal models[52] (Table 8.2).

2. Enzymatic and Transport Capacity

Probably most of the gender-difference literature in fat metabolism has focused on lipoprotein lipase activity. Several studies in the rodent model have found that estradiol treatment decreased adipocyte LPL activity.[53,54,55,56,57] In contrast, progesterone has little,[55,58] or modest stimulatory[59,60] effects upon adipocyte LPL activity. In contrast, muscle LPL activity either decreases later than adipocyte LPL activity[53] or significantly increases[56,57] in response to estradiol treatment. Ellis and colleagues showed that five days of 17-β-estradiol administration to male rats increased both basal and postexercise LPL activity in red and white vastus and heart.[57] Taken together, these data suggest that estradiol treatment in rodent models induces a greater propensity for the flux of plasma-borne TG-derived FFA toward skeletal muscle and heart. Whether the available FFA is shunted into oxidative or synthetic pathways is likely dependent upon the prevailing hormonal mileau and acute and chronic exercise status. It may be that estrogen induces much greater oscillations in the balance between synthesis and oxidation.[61] Female rat adipocytes have greater insulin binding as compared to male adipocytes, and fatty acid synthase is four times greater.[62] This enhanced insulin sensitivity for females also has been demonstrated in human skeletal muscle.[63] Whether this is related to the observed increase in IMTG is not clear at this point.

It is interesting to speculate that in the postprandial phase (high insulin) females may shunt more FFA into storage due to an increased insulin sensitivity whereas, during exercise, fat oxidation is enhanced. In studying the lipolytic potential of human adipocytes, it is important to note that both LPL activity and lipolysis are influenced by the site of fat depositon.[58,64] For example, females have a greater number of α2 receptors (decreased lipolysis) in the gluteal region as compared to males and as compared to their abdominal region.[64] Furthermore, adipocyte LPL activity is greater in the femoral/gluteal region as compared to the abdominal region.[58] This likely explains the propensity for females to accumulate adipose tissue in the femoral-gluteal region and also is an important factor to consider in gender-comparative work, for the site of fat biopsy could alter the results of a study designed to look at LPL activity or lipolysis.

In humans there has been some discrepancy in results from lipolytic rates obtained from biopsied adipocytes.[21,65] Despres and colleagues[21] found that males had a higher basal and epinephrine-stimulated lipolytic rate as compared to females. On the other hand, Crampes et al.[65] found that females had a greater lipolytic response to elevated concentrations of both epinephrine and isoproterenol as compared to males, and this was accentuated in the trained vs. untrained state. The differences may relate to sampling site as the former study (males greater than females) is sampled from the supra-iliac region (? More α_2 receptors) and the latter from the peri-umbilical region (where female and male β receptor numbers are similar). Furthermore, the sexual dimorphism seen by Crampes et al.[65] was demonstrated predominantly in the endurance-trained subjects, which may indicate that female adipocyte lipolysis is more inducable in response to exercise training. It should be noted that for adipocytes, LPL activity and lipolytic rates trend in opposite directions.[58] To date, the author is not aware of any studies that have reported gender

Table 8.3   Gender Differences in Metabolic Capacity for FFA Oxidation During Exercise

A. Substrate	Gender Difference
1. IMTG	♀ > ♂
2. Adipose Tissue	♀ > ♂
3. Glycogen (Basal)	♀ = ♂

B. Enzyme	Gender Difference
1. Muscle LPL	♀ > ♂
2. Adipocyte LPL	♀ < ♂
3. CPT	♂ = ♀
4. HAD	? ♀ > ♂
5. HSL	No Data
6. Other β-Oxidation	No Data

C. Transporter	Gender Difference
1. FAT/FATP	No Data
2. FABP	? ♀ > ♂
3. Carnitine Translocase	No Data

Note: For definitions, please see text. ♀ = female; ♂ = male.

differences in HSL activity. Clearly these studies must be completed to gain insight into potential gender differences in fat metabolism (Table 8.3).

To date the author is not aware of any gender-specific examinations of FAT nor FATP transporter capacity. There have been two reports that have demonstrated that females have a higher FABP concentration in liver as compared to males.[66,67] Estradiol itself was the likely factor that accounted for the observed gender difference.[66] In rat skeletal muscle there is indirect evidence that estradiol increases FABP content in skeletal muscle.[68] Whether this gender difference is present in human skeletal muscle remains to be seen; however, if it does, then the diffusive flux for FFA may be enhanced in females (Table 8.3).

The next major factor in FFA transport is the malonyl-CoA-regulated step catalyzed by CPT I. An earlier study by Costill and colleagues found no significant gender difference in CPT activity in whole muscle homogenates from male and female athletes.[35] Furthermore, a recent study by Spriet and colleagues isolated mitochondria from male and female athletes using malonyl-CoA inhibition to confirm the CPT I specific fraction and found no gender difference in CPT I activity (L. Spriet, personal communication, 1998). Furthermore, there does not appear to be a gender difference in muscle total carnitine content.[69] In summary, there does not appear to be a gender difference in muscle CPT I activity nor total carnitine (Table 8.3).

Once in the mitochondrial matrix, the FFA-CoA enters the β-oxidation pathway. The author is not aware of any studies of potential gender differences in acyl-CoA dehydrogenase, crotonase, nor thiolase enzyme activities. However, there have been several studies that have examined HAD activity between the genders.[70,71,72] Green and colleagues[71] reported the activity of several key marker enzymes important in substrate metabolism in 16 males and 17 females who were active, but not endurance-trained. This group found that females had a greater ratio of HAD/SDH (an indicator of aerobic fat oxidation capacity to total aerobic potential) as compared to males.[71] Furthermore, they showed that the PFK/HAD ratio was higher in males as compared to females (indicating a higher glycolytic/fat oxidation potential).[71] There has been only one longitudinal study that examined potential gender differences in HAD activity with altered contractile function (electrical stimulation).[70] Although they did not find a gender difference in HAD activity, the activity increased to a greater extent for the females (+30%; $P < 0.01$) as compared to the males (+12%; $P < 0.05$).[70] Taken together, these data indicate that females may have a greater induction of HAD as compared to males and that the activity of HAD relative to the TCA cycle capacity may be slightly greater. Future studies should examine the activity of the thiolysis step, as it is a non-equilibrium step that is thought to be rate-limiting (Table 8.3).

In summary, there are greater subcutaneous adipose stores and probably IMTG stores for females as compared to males. This may be related to a greater insulin sensitivity in females mediating an increase in FFA synthase. LPL activity in adipocytes appears to be higher in males as compared to females and this is correlated with estrogen concentrations. Epinephrine and isoproterenol-stimulated lipolysis seems to be higher in trained females as compared to males. Data exists to suggest that FABP should be greater in female muscle; however, no direct studies have been conducted in humans. There are no gender differences in CAT I nor in total muscle carnitine. Finally, the HAD/TCA potential may be slightly greater in females and more responsive to exercise-induction.

B. Studies of Lipid Metabolism at Rest

In a very large study of 720 healthy Caucasian males (N = 427) and females (N = 293), it was reported that basal fat oxidation was lower for females as compared to males.[73] This may be related to the effects of estradiol for it has been shown that E_2 replacement to postmenopausal females decreased FFA availability (FFA Ra).[74] An interesting case report found that with increasing doses of ethinyl estradiol, there was a progressive decrease in fat oxidation in both the basal and postprandial states.[75] It may be that the lesser oxidation of FFA at rest is due to lower delivery from adipocyte stores. Jensen and colleagues[76] found that in abdominal adipose tissue there was similar FFA release for males and females, whereas in lower body adipose tissue only the males showed an increase in FFA release in response to epinephrine. This same group also showed that males had a substantially greater TG-derived FFA uptake in the splanchnic region as compared to females.[77]

In summary, it appears that basal fat oxidation is lower in untrained females as compared to males. It could be that under nonstressed or well-fed physiological conditions (i.e., relatively high insulin:glucagon ratio), females direct FFA into storage and not into oxidation. The increased insulin sensitivity towards FFA synthesis is also consistent with this notion. Furthermore, the well-known greater subcutaneous adipose tissue stores in females is also consistent with this hypothesis. The situation is the opposite during endurance exercise.

C. Studies of Lipid Metabolism During Exercise

As seen in Chapter 1, there is a lower RER during endurance exercise in females as compared to males (Tables 8.4 and 8.5). These studies have indicated a greater reliance on lipid for energy under these circumstances for the female. If one calculates the RER values for the studies listed in Table 8.5 (N = 52 males; N = 52 females), there is a lower RER for females by about 5% [males = 0.91 (0.06); females = 0.87 (0.05)]. From a metabolic standpoint this amounts to about a 70% higher fat oxidation for females [~22% of total energy expenditure (males) to ~39% of total energy (females)] during endurance exercise at about 65% VO_{2max} (Table 8.4). Others have not found a gender difference in fat oxidation during endurance exercise.[35,78] In one of these studies the RER values were not reported and the untrained subjects were exercised at 75% VO_{2peak} although the trained subjects were exercised at 80% VO_{2peak}.[78] Clearly, some of the subjects would have been close to or over their anaerobic thresholds. Furthermore, it is likely that females only will show enhanced fat oxidation at intensities about 65% VO_{2peak} for the reasons stated previously (namely, that females may have a greater propensity for IMTG oxidation, and its greatest contribution to energy production is about 50 to 65% VO_{2peak}). In the other study reporting no gender differences in fat oxidation during endurance exercise there were interesting matching issues that may have confounded the interpretation.[35] First, the female athletes were much younger than the males (23 vs. 35 y, respectively), and more importantly, there is no mention of menstrual status, nor of the phase of the menstrual cycle.[35] It is unlikely that many of the females were eumenorrheic when running 80 to 115 km/wk. In any case, the bulk of the data in humans shows that the RER is lower for females as compared to males during submaximal endurance exercise. There has been only a single study that has used metabolic tracers to examine the question of potential gender differences in the metabolic response to exercise.[79] They reported no differences in palmitate Ra between the genders in response to endurance exercise; unfortunately, there were only four subjects per group and glycerol Ra was not determined.[79]

In humans there has been a recent paper using an estradiol and stable isotope of glucose and glycerol to explore further the metabolic effects of estradiol during exercise.[80] This group studied six amenorrhiec females following each of three treatments (C72 = 72 h placebo patch; E_2 72 = 72 h of 17-β-estradiol patch; and E_2 144 = 144 h of E_2 patch).[80] They found that plasma FFA was greater for both E_2 trials vs. placebo and reported a trend toward slightly lower RER values later in exercise (data not shown).[80] There was no effect of treatment upon glycerol Ra, and glucose Ra was attenuated for both E_2 treatments.[80] Furthermore, there was a significant attenuation in the postexercise catecholamine concentration for the E_2 treatment trials.[80] Our group also has used an estrogen patch protocol in males (Chapter 2) and found no effect on the RER during endurance exercise and no attenuation of muscle glycogen utilization.[81] Unfortunately, although the estrogen patch allows for a within group design, it does not mimic all of the differences between males and

Table 8.4 Energy and Substrate Utilization from 4 Studies in the Same Laboratory

		kcal/hr	kcal/kg/hr	kcal/kg LBM/hr	CHO (%)	FAT (%)	PRO (%)
Tranopolsky, L. et al., 1991	6 ♂	797	11.9	14	81	10	9
	6 ♀	620	10.1	13.5	61	41	0
Phillips, S. M. et al., 1993	6 ♂	729	11.4	12.7	47	49	3
	6 ♀	590	10.2	12.5	35	61	2
Tarnopolsky, M. A. et al., 1995	7 ♂	1019	13.6	15.9	83	8	6
	8 ♀	666	11.6	14.2	72	24	1
Tarnopolsky, M. A. et al., 1997	8 ♂	806	11.1	12.5	75	23	2
	8 ♀	616	10.1	13.0	68	29	3
Total mean (±S.D.)	28 ♂	838 (126)**	12 (1)*	13.7 (1.6)+	72 (17)**	22 (19)**	5 (3)**
	27 ♀	623 (32)	10.5 (0.7)	13.3 (0.7)	59 (17)	39 (16)	2 (1)

Note: ** $p \leq 0.001$; * $p \leq 0.05$; + NS.

Table 8.5 Respiratory Exchange Ratios from Several Gender Comparative Studies

			RER	
Study	Subjects	Exercise	Males	Females
Phillips, S. M. et al., 1993	6 ♂ 6 ♀	90 min. treadmill run @ 65% VO_{2peak}	0.86	0.83 $p \leq 0.001$
Tarnopolsky, L. et al., 1991	6 ♂ 6 ♀	97 min. ♀ & 93 min ♂ treadmill run @ 63% VO_{2peak}	0.94	0.87 $p \leq 0.0001$
Tarnopolsky, M. A. et al., 1995	7 ♂ 8 ♀	90 min. cycle ergometry @ 65% VO_{2peak}	0.92	0.89 $p \leq 0.05$
Tarnopolsky, M. A. et al., 1997	8 ♂ 8 ♀	60 min. cycle ergometry @ 72% VO_{2peak}	0.99	0.93 $p \leq 0.001$
Blatchford, F. K. et al., 1985	6 ♂ 6 ♀	90 min. treadmill walk @ 35% VO_{2max}	0.85	0.81 $p \leq 0.05$
Froberg, K. et al., 1984	6 ♂ 6 ♀	53.8 min. ♀ & 36.8 min. ♂ cycle ergometry @ 80% VO_{2max}	0.97	0.93 $p \leq 0.01$
Costill, D. et al., 1979	13 ♂ 12 ♀	60 min. treadmill run @ 70% VO_{2max}	0.84	0.83 NS

Note: ♀ = females; ♂ = males; NS = non-significant.

females, but rather changes only one parameter (i.e., estradiol). For example, in both of these studies the plasma estradiol concentration only was increased by approximately 100%, whereas a eumenorrhiec female has peak estradiol concentrations (luteal phase) that are about 700% greater than basal levels. The model also does not consider the other female sex hormone, progesterone, that may also be an important factor in determining male from female metabolic responses to endurance exercise.

There are clearly difficult matching issues to consider; however, true gender comparative studies will require very labor-intensive, large between-gender longitudinal training studies with sensitive biochemical indices (i.e., muscle biopsies, molecular genetic techniques, and metabolic tracers) and tight control for extraneous confounding variables.

In the rodent model there is convincing evidence for an effect of 17-β-estradiol to influence metabolism during endurance exercise.[57,82,83] An early study found that eight days of E_2 injection into OVX rats resulted in a significantly lower $^{14}CO_2$ evolution from labeled glucose and a significantly greater $^{14}CO_2$ evolution from labeled palmitate.[83] This suggested that fat oxidation was enhanced and glucose oxidation inhibited by E_2. Similar results also were found with a five-day E_2 treatment protocol in male rats where both pre- and postexercise FFA concentrations were elevated as compared to placebo oil injected rats.[82] In this latter study, there was a significant attenuation of muscle and liver glycogen utilization, and it was suggested that this was secondary to the increase in fat availability.[82] This same group went on to further explore the effect of E_2 on fat oxidation by administering E_2 to male rats for five days and measuring plasma FFA, glycerol, and TG as well as muscle, heart, and adipose LPL activity.[82] They found that E_2 treatment resulted in an increased resting glycerol and FFA and a lower TG, which corresponded to a decrease in adipocyte- and an increase in muscle and heart-LPL activity.[57] The ratio of muscle/adipocyte-LPL activity was 4.65 for the E_2 group and 1.15 for the placebo group, and they suggested that this indicated an E_2 mediated distribution of plasma TG-FFA toward heart and skeletal muscle.[57]

IV. CONCLUSIONS

There appear to be significant gender differences in both the storage and utilization of fats. Females have more subcutaneous adipose tissue and probably IMTG as compared to males. During submaximal endurance exercise there is a greater fat oxidation for females as compared to males, and this may lead to glycogen and protein sparing (see Chapters 6 and 7). Estradiol appears to be a major mediator of the aforementioned metabolic effects, particularly when one considers work from the rodent model.

There still remains a huge amount of work to do in the area of gender differences in fat metabolism including

1. Longitudinal training study of males and females using metabolic tracers and muscle measurements,
2. Determination of FABP content of skeletal muscle,
3. Determination of FAT and FATP content in skeletal muscle,
4. Quantitation of intracellular lipid content,
5. Examination of glucose-FFA cycle, and
6. Examination of effect of caffeine upon FFA oxidation.

The author expects that over the next few years the answers to some or all of these questions will be found, creating a better position to make some definitive conclusions about gender differences in fat metabolism. The question as to why gender differences in fat metabolism have been selected may never be answered and will remain speculative. Perhaps selective pressures have favored the survival of females, who under periods of stress (i.e., exercise and starvation), could utilize the efficient fat stores and thus survive and reproduce.[1]

REFERENCES

1. Widdowson, E. M., The response to the sexes to nutritional stress, *Proc. Nutr. Soc.,* 35, 175, 1976.
2. Abumrad, N. A., Raafat El-Maghrabi, M., Amri, E-Z., Lopez, E., and Grimaldi, P. A., Cloning of a rat adipocyte membrane protein implicated in binding or transport of long-chain fatty acids that is induced during preadipocyte differentiation, *The Journal of Biological Chemistry,* 268(24), 17665, 1993.
3. Schaffer, J. E. and Lodish, H. F., Expression cloning and characterization of a novel adipocyte long chain fatty acid transport protein, *Cell,* 79, 427, 1994.
4. Memon, R. A., Feingold, K. R., Moser, A. H., Fuller, J., and Grunfeld, C., Regulation of fatty acid transport protein and fatty acid translocase mRNA levels by endotoxin and cytokines, *Am. J. Physiol.,* 274 (*Endocrinol. Metab.,* 37), E210, 1998.

5. Peeters, R. A., in't Groen, M. A., and Veerkanp, J. H., The fatty acid-binding protein from human skeletal muscle, *Arch. Biochem. Biophys.*, 274(2), 556, 1989.

6. Jeukendrup, A. E., Saris, W. H. M., Schrauwen, P., Brouns, F., and Wagenmakers, A. J. M., Metabolic availability of medium-chain triglycerides coingested with carbohydrates during prolonged exercise, *J. Appl. Physiol.*, 79(3), 756, 1995.

7. Odland, L. M., Heigenhauser, J. F., Lopaschuk, G. D., and Spriet, L. L., Human skeletal muscle malonyl-CoA at rest and during prolonged submaximal exercise, *Am. J. Physiol.*, 270 (*Endocrinol. Metab.*, 33), E541, 1996.

8. Winder, W. W., Wilson, H. A., Hardie, D. G., Rasmussen, B. B., Hutber, C. A., Call, G. B., Clayton, R. D., Conley, L. M., Yoon, S., and Zhou, B., Phosphorylation of rat muscle acetyl-CoA carboxylase by AMP-activated protein kinase and protein kinase A, *J. Appl. Physiol.*, 82(1), 219, 1997.

9. Rennie, M. J. and Holloszy, J. O., Inhibition of glucose uptake and glycogenolysis by availability of oleate in well-oxygenated perfused skeletal muscle, *Biochem. J.*, 168, 161, 1977.

10. Costill, D. L., Coyle, E., Dalsky, G., Evans, W., Fink, W., and Hoopes, D., Effects of elevated plasma FFA and insulin on muscle glycogen usage during exercise, *J. Appl. Physiol.*, 43(4), 695, 1977.

11. Dyck, D. J., Putman, C. T., Heigenhauser, G. J. F., Hultman, E., and Spriet, L. L., Regulation of fat-carbohydrate interaction in skeletal muscle during intense aerobic cycling, *Am. J. Physiol.*, 265 (*Endocrinol. Metab.*, 28), E852, 1993.

12. Hargreaves, M., Kiens, B., and Richter, E. A., Effect of increased plasma free fatty acid concentrations on muscle metabolism in exercising men, *J. Appl. Physiol.*, 70(1), 194, 1991.

13. Rennie, M. J., Winder, W. W., and Holloszy, J. O., A sparing effect of increased plasma fatty acids on muscle and liver glycogen content in the exercising rat, *Biochem. J.*, 156, 647, 1976.

14. Coggan, A. R., Spina, R. J., Kohrt, W. M., and Holloszy, J. O., Effect of prolonged exercise on muscle citrate concentration before and after endurance training in men, *Am. J. Physiol.*, 264 (*Endocrinol. Metab.*, 27), E215, 1993.

15. Klein, S., Holland, O. B., and Wolfe, R. R., Importance of blood glucose concentration in regulating lipolysis during fasting in humans, *Am. J. Physiol.*, 258 (*Endocrinol. Metab.*, 21), E32, 1990.

16. McGarry, J.D., Mills, S.E. Long, C.S., and Foster, D.W., Observations on the affinity for carnitine, and malonyl-CoA sensitivity, of carnitine, palmitoyltransferase-I in animal and human tissues, *Biochem. J.*, 214, 21, 1983.

17. Mandour, T., Kissebah, A. H., and Wynn, V., Mechanism of oestrogen and progesterone effects on lipid and carbohydrate metabolism: alteration in the insulin: glucagon molar ratio and hepatic enzyme activity, *Eur. J. Clin. Invest.*, 7, 181, 1977.

18. Klein, S., Weber, J-M., Coyle, E. F., and Wolfe, R. R., Effect of endurance training on glycerol kinetics during strenuous exercise in humans, *Metabolism*, 45(3), 357, 1996.

19. Townsend, R. R., Klein, S., and Wolfe, R. R., Changes in lipolytic sensitivity following repeated epinephrine infusion in humans, *Am. J. Physiol.*. 266 (*Endocrinol. Metab.* 29), E155, 1994.

20. Klein, S., Holland, O. B., and Wolfe, R. R., Importance of blood glucose concentration in regulating lipolysis during fasting in humans, *Am. J. Physiol.*, 258 (*Endocrinol. Metab.*. 21), E32, 1990.

21. Depres, J. P., Bouchard, C., Savard, R., Tremblay, A., Marcotte, M., and Theriault, G., The effect of a 20-week endurance training program on adipose-tissue morphology and lipolysis in men and women, *Metabolism*, 33(3), 235, 1984.

22. Kurpad, A. V., Calder, K. A. G., and Elia, M., Muscle and whole body metabolism after norepinephrine, *Am. J. Physiol.,* 266 (*Endocrinol. Metab.,* 29), E877, 1994.

23. Oscai, L. B., Essig, D. A., and Palmer, W. K., Lipase regulation of muscle triglyceride hydrolysis, *J. Appl. Physiol.,* 69(5), 1571, 1990.

24. Phillips, S. M., Green, H. J., Tarnopolsky, M. A., Heigenhauser, G. J. R., Hill, R. E., and Grant, S. M., Effects of training duration on substrate turnover and oxidation during exercise, *J. Appl. Physiol.,* 81(5), 2182, 1996.

25. Spriet, L. L., MacLean, D. A., Dyck, D. J., Hultman, E., Cederblad, G., and Graham, T.E., Caffeine ingestion and muscle metabolism during prolonged exercise in humans, *Am. J. Physiol.,* 262 (*Endocrinol. Metab.,* 25), E391, 1992.

26. Romjin, J. A., Klein, S., Coyle, E. F., Sidossis, S., and Wolfe, R. R., Strenuous endurance training increases lipolysis and triglyceride-fatty acid cycling at rest, *J. Appl. Physiol.,* 75(1), 108, 1993.

27. Brooks, F.A., Fahey, T.D., and White, T.P., *Exercise Physiology: Human Bioenergetics and its Applications,* Mayfield Publishing Co., Mountainview, CA, 1996.

28. Wolfe, R. R., Klein, S., Carraro, F., and Weber, J-M., Role of triglyceride-fatty acid cycle in controlling fat metabolism in humans during and after exercise, *Am. J. Physiol.,* 258 (*Endocrinol. Metab.,* 21), E382, 1990.

29. Sial, S., Coggan, A. R., Carroll, R., Goodwin, J., and Klein, S., Fat and carbohydrate metabolism during exercise in elderly and young subjects, *Am. J. Physiol.,* 271 (*Endocrinol. Metab.,* 34), E983, 1996.

30. Holloszy, J. O., Dalsky, G. P., Nemeth, P. M., Hurley, B. F., Martin, W. H. III, Hagberg, J. M., Utilization of fat as substrate during exercise: effect of training, in *Biochem. of Exercise VI,* Vol. 16, Saltin, B., (Ed.), Human Genetics, Champaign, IL, 1986.

31. Jansson, E. and Kaijser, L., Substrate utilization and enzymes in skeletal muscle of extremely endurance-trained men, *J. Appl. Physiol.,* 62, 999, 1987.

32. Hurley, B. F., Nemeth, P. M., Martin, W. H. III, Hagberg, J. M., Dalsky, G. P., and Holloszy, J. O., Muscle triglyceride utilization during exercise: effect of training, *J. Appl. Physiol.,* 60(2), 562, 1986.

33. Poehlman, E. T., Gardner, A. W., Ariciero, P. J., Goran, M. I., and Calles-Escandon, J., Effects of endurance training on total fat oxidation in elderly persons, *J. Appl. Physiol.,* 76(6), 2281, 1994.

34. Tremblay, A., Simoneau, J-A., and Bouchard, C., Impact of exercise intensity on body fatness and skeletal muscle metabolism, *Metabolism,* 43(7), 814, 1994.

35. Costill, D. L., Fink, W. J., Getchell, L. H., et al., Lipid metabolism in skeletal muscle of endurance-trained males and females, *J. Appl. Physiol.,* 47(4), 787, 1979.

36. Mole, P. A., Osgai, L. B., and Holloszy, J. O., Increase in levels of palmityl CoA synthetase, carnitine palmityltransferase, and palmityl CoA dehydrogenase, and in the capacity to oxidize fatty acids, *J. Clin. Inves.,* 50, 2323, 1971.

37. Howald, H., Hoppeler, H., Claassen, H., Mathieu, O., and Straub, R., Influences of endurance training on the ultrastructural composition of the different muscle fiber types in humans, *Pflügers Arch.,* 403, 369, 1985.

38. Veerkamp, J. H. and van Moerkerk, H. T. B., Fatty acid-binding protein and its relation to fatty acid oxidation, *Mol. Cell Biochem.,* 123, 101, 1993.

39. Poehlman, E. T., Gardner, A. W., Ariciero, P. J., Goran, M. I., and Calles-Escandon, J., Effects of endurance training on total fat oxidation in elderly persons, *J. Appl. Physiol.,* 76(6), 2281, 1994.

40. Seip, R. L., Angelopoulos, T. J., and Semenkovich, C. F., Exercise induces human lipoprotein lipase gene expression in skeletal muscle but not adipose tissue, *Am. J. Physiol.,* 268 (*Endocrinol. Metab.,* 31), E229, 1995.

41. Previs, S. F., Martin, S. K., Hazey, J. W., Soloviev, M. V., Keating, A. P., Lucas, D., David, F., Koshy, J., Kirschenbaum, D. W., Tserng, K-Y., and Brunengraber, H., Contributions of liver and kidneys to glycerol production and utilization in the dog, *Am. J. Physiol.*, 271 (*Endocrinol. Metab.*, 34), E118, 1996.

42. Elia, M., Khan, K., Calder, G., and Kurpad, A., Glycerol exchange across the human forearm assessed by a combination of tracer and arteriovenous exchange techniques, *Clinical Science*, 84, 99, 1993.

43. Landau, B. R., Wahren, J., Previs, S. F., Ekberg, K., Chandramouli, V., and Brunengraber, H., Glycerol production and utilization in humans: sites and quantitation, *Am. J. Physiol.*, 271 (*Endocrinol. Metab.*, 34), E110, 1996.

44. Newsholme, E. A. and Taylor, K., Glycerol kinase activities in muscles from vertebrates and invertebrates, *Biochem. J.*, 112, 465, 1969.

45. Maggs, D. G., Jacob, R., Rife, F., Lange, R., Leone, P., Durling, M. J., Tamborlane, W. V., and Sherwin, R. S., Interstitial fluid concentrations of glycerol, glucose, and amino acids in human quadricep muscle and adipose tissue, *J. Clin. Invest.*, 96, 370, 1995.

46. Martin, W. H. III, Dalsky, G. P., Hurley, B. F., Matthews, D. E., Bier, D. M., Hagberg, J. M., Rodgers, M. A., King, D. S., and Holloszy, J. O., Effect of endurance training on free fatty acid turnover and oxidation during exercise, *Am. J. Physiol.*, 265 (*Endocrinol. Metab.*, 28), E708, 1994.

47. Forsberg, A. M., Nilsson, E., Werneman, J., Bergström, J., and Hultman, E., Muscle composition in relation to age and sex, *Clin. Sci.*, 81, 249, 1991.

48. Prince, F. P., Hikida, R. S., and Hagerman, F. C., Muscle fiber types in women athletes and non-athletes, *Pflügers Arch.*, 371, 161, 1977.

49. Tarnopolsky, M. A., Atkinson, S. A., Phillips, S. M., and MacDougall, J. D., Carbohydrate loading and metabolism during exercise in men and women, *J. Appl. Physiol.*, 78(4), 1360, 1995.

50. Tarnopolsky, M. A. and Phillips, S. M., Gender Differences in intra-muscular triglyceride and β-3-hydroxyacl-CoA dehydrogenase activity, *Can. J. Appl. Phys.*, 20, 51P, 1995.

51. Tarnopolsky, L. J., MacDougall, J. D., Atkinson, S. A., Tarnopolsky, M. A., and Sutton, J. R., Gender differences in substrate for endurance exercise, *J. Appl. Physiol.*, 68, 302, 1990.

52. Kendrick, Z. V. and Ellis, G. S., Effect of estradiol on tissue glycogen metabolism and lipid availability in exercised male rats, *J. Appl. Physiol.*, 71(5), 1694, 1991.

53. Ramirez, I., Estradiol-induced changes in lipoprotein lipase, eating, and body weight in rats, *Am. J. Physiol.*, 240 (*Endocrinol. Metab.*, 3), E533, 1981.

54. Hamosh, M. and Hamosh, P., The effect of estrogen on the lipoprotein lipase activity of rat adipose tissue, *J. Clin. Invest.*, 55, 1132, 1975.

55. Gray, J. M. and Wade, G. N., Food intake, body weight, and adiposity in female rats: actions and interactions of progestins and antiestrogens, *Am. J. Physiol.*, 240 (*Endocrinol. Metab.*, 3), E474, 1981.

56. Wilson, D. E., Flowers, C. M., Carlile, S. I., and Udall, K. S., Estrogen treatment and gonadal function in the regulation of lipoprotein lipase, *Atherosclerosis*, 24, 491, 1976.

57. Ellis, G. S., Lanza-Jacoby, S., Gow, A., and Kendrick, Z. V., Effects of estradiol on lipoprotein lipase activity and lipid availability in exercised male rats, *J. Appl. Physiol.*, 77(1), 209, 1994.

58. Rebuffe-Scrive, M., Sex steroid hormones and adipose tissue metabolism in ovariectomized and adrenalectomized rats, *Acta Physiol. Scand.*, 129, 471, 1987.

59. Steingrimsdottir, L., Brasel, J., and Greenwood, M. R. C., *Am. J. Physiol.*, 239 (*Endocrinol. Metab.*), E162, 1980.

60. Shirling, D., Ashby, J. P., and Baird, J. D., Effect of progesterone on lipid metabolism in the intact rat, *J. Endocr.,* 90, 285, 1981.

61. Hansen, F. M., Fahmy, N., and Nielsen, J. H., The influence of sexual hormones on lipogenesis and lipolysis in rat fat cells, *Acta Endocrinologica,* 95, 566, 1980.

62. Guerre-Millo, M., Leturque, A., Girard, J., and Lavau, M., Increased insulin sensitivity and responsiveness of glucose metabolism in adipocytes from female versus male rats, *J. Clin. Invest.,* 76, 109, 1985.

63. Nuutila, P., Knuuti, M. J., Mäki, M., Laine, H., Ruotsalainen, U., Teräs, M., Haaparanta, M, Solin, O., and Yki-Järvinen, H., Gender and insulin sensitivity in the heart and in skeletal muscles, *Diabetes,* 44, 31, 1995.

64. Richelsen, B., Increased α_2- but similar β-adrenergic receptor activities in subcutaneous gluteal adipocytes from females compared with males, *European Journal of Clinical Investigation,* 16, 302, 1986.

65. Crampes, F., Riviere, D., Beauville, M., Marceron, M., and Garrigues, M., Lipolytic response of adipocytes to epinephrine in sedentary and exercise-trained subjects: sex-related differences, *Eur. J. Appl. Physiol.,* 59, 249, 1989.

66. Ockner, R. K., Lysenko, N., Manning, J. A., and Monroe, S. E., Sex steroid modulation of fatty acid utilization and fatty acid binding protein concentration in rat liver, *J. Clin. Invest.,* 65, 1013, 1980.

67. Luxon, B. A. and Weisiger, R. A., Sex differences in intracellular fatty acid transport: role of cytoplasmic binding proteins, *Am. J. Physiol.,* 265 (*Gastrointest. Liver Physiol.,* 28), G831, 1993.

68. van Breda, E., Keizer, H. A., York, M. M., Surtel, D. A. M., de Jong, Y., van derVusse, G. J., and Glatz, J. F. C., Modulation of fatty-acid-binding protein content of rat heart and skeletal muscle by endurance training and testosterone treatment, *Pflügers Arch.,* 421 (*European Journal of Physiology*), 274, 1992.

69. Jansson, G. M. E., Degenaar, P. P., Menheere, C. A., et al., Plasma urea, creatinine, uric acid, albumin, and total protein concentrations before and after 15-, 25-, and 42-km contests, *Int. J. Sports Med.,* S132, 1989.

70. Gauthier, J. M., Thériault, R., Thériault, G., Gélinas, Y., and Simoneau, J-A., Electrical stimulation-induced changes in skeletal muscle enzymes of men and women, *Med. Sci. Sports Exerc.,* 24(11), 1252, 1992.

71. Green, H. J., Fraser, I. G., and Ranney, D. A., Male and female differences in enzyme activities of energy metabolism in vastus lateralis muscle, *Journal of Neurological Sciences,* 65, 323, 1984.

72. Simoneau, J-A. and Bouchard, C., Human variation in skeletal muscle fiber-type proportion and enzyme activities, *Am. J. Physiol.,* 257 (*Endocrinol. Metab.,* 20), E567, 1989.

73. Nagy, T. R., Goran, M. I., Weinsier, R. L., Toth, M. J., Schutz, Y., and Poehlman, E. T., Determinants of basal fat oxidation in healthy caucasians, *J. Appl. Physiol.,* 80(5), 1743, 1996.

74. Jensen, M. D., Martin, M. L., Cryer, P. E., and Roust, L. R., Effects of estrogen on free fatty acid metabolism in humans, *Am. J. Physiol.,* 266, E914, 1994.

75. O'Sullivan, A.J., Hoffman, D.M., and Ho, K.Y., Estrogen, lipid oxidation, and body fat, *New Eng. J. Med.,* 333(10), 669, 1995.

76. Jensen, M. D., Cryer, P. E., Johnson, C. M., and Murray, M. J., Effects of epinephrine on regional free fatty acid and energy metabolism in men and women, *Am. J. Physiol.,* 270 (*Endocrinol. Metab.,* 33), E259, 1996.

77. Nguyen, T. T., Mijares, A. H., Johnson, C. M., and Jensen, M. D., Postprandial leg and splanchnic fatty acid metabolism in nonobese men and women, *Am. J. Physiol.,* 271 (*Endocrinol. Metab.,* 34), E965, 1996.

78. Friedmann, B. and Kindermann, W., Energy metabolism and regulatory hormones in women and men during endurance exercise, *Eur. J. Appl. Physiol.,* 59, 1, 1989.

79. Mendenhall, L. A., Sial, S., Coggan, A. R., and Klein, S., Gender differences in substrate metabolism during moderate intensity cycling, *Med. Sci. Sport. Exerc.,* 27, S213, 1995.

80. Ruby, B. C., Robergs, R. A., Waters, D. L., Bruge, M., Mermier, C., and Stolarczyk, L., Effects of estradiol on substrate turnover during exercise in amenorrheic females, *Med. Sci. Sports Exerc.,* 29(9), 1160, 1997.

81. Tarnopolsky, M. A., Bosman, M., MacDonald, J. R., Vandeputte, D., Martin, J., and Roy, B. D., Postexercise protein-carbohydrate and carbohydrate supplements increase muscle glycogen in men and women, *J. Appl. Physiol.,* 83(6), 1877, 1997.

82. Kendrick, Z. V. and Ellis, G. S., Effect of estradiol on tissue glycogen metabolism and lipid availability in exercised male rats, *J. Appl. Physiol.,* 71(5), 1694, 1991.

83. Hatta, H., Atomi, Y., Shinohara, S., Yamamoto, Y., and Yamada, S., The effects of ovarian hormones on glucose and fatty acid oxidation during exercise in female ovariectomized rats, *Horm. Metabol. Res.,* 20, 609, 1988.

CHAPTER 9

Sex Differences on Regulation of Energy Homeostasis, Growth, and Body Composition During Periods of Energy Imbalance: Animal Studies

Ronald N. Cortright

CONTENTS

I. OVERVIEW

Growth, body composition, and survival are affected by both environmental and genetic variables. The food supply is the most important extrinsic factor affecting these variables. A diet insufficient in energy and/or protein adversely will effect the rate of growth in the young and reduce protein and fat mass in adults.[1,2] In addition, chronic physical activity will elevate energy requirements over those needed to support basal energy needs. If the increased energy expenditure due to physical activity is not compensated for by increased dietary energy intake, the resulting energy imbalance will lead to a loss of body tissue.[3] Although this may be favorable in the obese state,[4] a negative energy balance will result in losses in body tissue that will compromise physiological function in adults or growth in the young.[5,6] More recently, studies with very active people[7-9] or exercise-trained animals[10,11] have reported elevations in nitrogen excretion and amino acid oxidation. As a result, exercise scientists have suggested that protein requirements (originally devised for sedentary adults) may be greater for physically active individuals.[12] However, these earlier studies only have been done in either male rats or humans. It is only recently that studies investigating potential gender differences in substrate utilization during acute endurance exercise or whole body tissue changes following chronic exercise have emerged. For example, it has been suggested that as a consequence of endurance exercise, females selectively oxidize fat for fuel,[13,14] implying a greater capacity to spare protein mass during periods of energy deficit. This area requires further study because of the potential for reduction in protein mass, growth, and exercise capacity in males but not females.[15]

The hormonal milieu orchestrates the orderly sequence of maturational events during growth. The growth process is a complex phenomenon that is affected not only by growth hormone and somatomedins, but also by gonadal hormones. To illustrate, males are typically larger than females in terms of body mass and height/length. In addition, the lean to fat ratio is typically greater in the male. These differences generally are attributed to the influence of male androgens.[16] In contrast, differences in fat mass and fat patterning observed in the female[17] have been attributed to ovarian hormones.[18] Progesterone increases adiposity[19] whereas estrogens have been shown to reduce body mass in the rat.[20] Physical activity has been shown to lower plasma testosterone[21,22] and estrogen.[23,24] The effect of physical activity on gonadal hormones also suggests that the growth process is more likely to be affected negatively by chronic exercise in males than in females.

It appears that females are more resistant to food restriction and/or starvation than males.[25] Widdowson[26] suggested that because females are responsible for the survival (gestation and caretaking) of the young, they have been affected more favorably by natural selection pressures to resist the loss of body energy stores during times of food scarcity. Ovarian hormones have been proposed as a mechanism by which females enhance fat storage and energy conservation to increase survivability.[25,26] This hypothesis may have important implications with respect to disease. In terms of substrate availability diabetes is similar to starvation (inability to utilize blood glucose). As a result, it may be that the deleterious effects of this disease on growth and body composition are less pronounced in the female than in the male.

Recently, several discoveries in the area of endocrinology and metabolism have provided new insights into the control of food intake and energy conservation. Namely, the product of the newly cloned obesity gene named leptin (Greek for leptos, which means thin) has been demonstrated to control appetite[27] and more recently to be involved in energy substrate partitioning[28] and thermogenesis[29] in animals. In addition, the cloning of two new uncoupling proteins, one expressed predominately in white adipose tissue (UCP2), the other in skeletal muscle (UCP3), offer potential explanations for the observed gender differences in growth, body composition and survival in response to energy imbalance (over or under eating, starvation, and energy imbalance due to elevated activity).

In summary, food availability, exercise, and metabolic diseases such as diabetes represent physiological perturbations to the energy and protein status of an animal. These conditions require metabolic and dietary adjustments to support growth and maintain existing body tissues. Females, perhaps due to the presence of ovarian hormones and variable differences in other factors (perhaps leptin and uncoupling proteins) that regulate food intake and energy efficiency, appear to respond more favorably than males to periods of energy deficit or starvation. Consequently, a consistently greater and more permanent affect on physical growth, body composition, and survival should occur in males in response to perturbations in energy and protein homeostasis.

II. FACTORS THAT AFFECT GROWTH AND BODY COMPOSITION

To facilitate the discussion on the sexual dimorphism of growth, body composition, and survival in animals, this section will describe those physiological factors that affect the variables of concern. The entire review will focus mainly on studies from rodents (rat and mouse) because the majority of the current literature centers on these models; however, parallels in the human will be mentioned for the sake of comparison. For a comprehensive discussion of the factors that contribute to the sexual dimorphism of growth, body composition, and energy balance in the human, the reader is directed to the chapter in this book by Westerterp. In addition, the author does not intend to diminish the importance of other experimental models in defining this topic and therefore further readings are suggested.[25,30-35]

A. Energy Status

The energy requirement of an animal is defined as that amount of energy needed to maintain health, growth, and physical activity.[1] In the adult, maintenance of normal body weight results from achieving a state of energy balance (energy stored = energy$_{in}$ − energy$_{out}$) in which total energy intake from food is matched to total energy expenditure. The balance between energy intake and energy expenditure is controlled precisely and is the result of many neural and hormonal influences. An imbalance between energy intake and expenditure leads to either weight gain or weight loss and concomitant changes in body composition in the adult or tissue accretion and linear growth in the young. (See Figure 9.1 for a summary of this section.)

1. Control of Feeding and Metabolism of Energy Nutrients

Energy or food intake is under the control of the central nervous system (CNS). In the brain, the hypothalamus is a focal point that accounts for and regulates the perception of when nutrients are needed, when they are consumed, and how they are utilized.[6,36] Quantitative and qualitative adjustments in food intake (e.g., appetite for specific nutrients) are derived from sensory and metabolic inputs to the hypothalamus.[37] Two areas of the hypothalamus have been regarded as important in the control of food intake:[38] the ventro-medial hypothalamic area (VMHA) and the lateral hypothalamic area (LHA). The VMHA has been labeled the satiety center. (electrical stimulation of the VMHA leads to cessation of eating.) The LHA has been labeled the feeding center. (electrical stimulation of the LHA causes animals to begin eating.) In addition, the paraventricular nuclei are believed to act as integrators of satiety, although laterally, the perifornical region of the hypothalamus integrates the influences of feeding.[39] Centrally, four classes of compounds (monoamines, amino acids, prostaglandins, and peptides) have been identified in the modulation of feeding behavior.[40,41] The majority of these compounds inhibit food intake [e.g., cholecystokinin, thyroid releasing hormone, serotonin, amphetamines, most neuro-peptides/calcitonin, corticotrophin-releasing factor (CRF), bombesin, neurotensin]. Only a few stimulate food ingestion (e.g., norepinephrine, neuropeptide Y, several opioid peptides). Therefore, the system may be described as one that primarily seeks food that is held in check by inhibitory inputs.[40] Peripheral factors that are believed to provide information to the central control modulating food intake include 1) gastrointestinal factors (physical and chemical changes transmitted via the vagus nerve), 2) liver metabolism (sensing of substrate availability), 3) adipose tissue status (sensing the size of adipose tissue stores), and 4) endocrine factors. Furthermore, α-agonists (norepinephrine) promote feeding and β-agonists (epinephrine) inhibit feeding. These control mechanisms are obviously complex and not well understood.[6] The importance of the newly discovered satiety factor leptin in the control of feeding and peripheral energy metabolism will be discussed in detail below.

Control of nutrient metabolism is exerted directly by innervation of hepatic, muscle, and adipose tissues and by control over the release of adrenal and pancreatic hormones that regulate the metabolism of the cells of a given tissue. Glycogenolysis in the liver is enhanced by VMHA-mediated norepinephrine stimulation of the VMHA by increasing glycogen phosphorylase activity, and glycogenesis is enhanced by vagal stimulation of the LHA by increasing the rate of glycogen synthase activity.[42] In adipose tissue, sympathetic arousal by β-adrenergic systems in the VMHA increases lipolysis, whereas the opposite effect is observed following activation of the parasympathetic system.[43] Stimulation of the LHA increases vagal tone and raises insulin concentrations.[44] In muscle and fat and a variety of other tissues, insulin facilitates the entry of glucose into the cells. Anabolic effects include stimulation of protein synthesis, inhibition of protein degradation, and promotion of lipogenesis

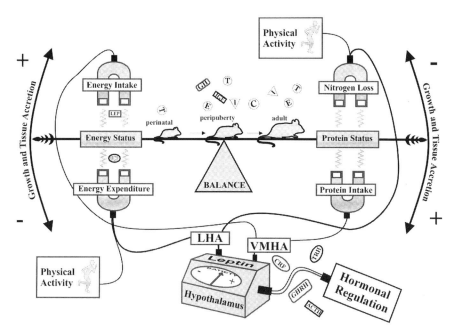

Figure 9.1 Factors that affect growth and body composition. Growth in animals occurs as an orderly sequence of events. When energy/protein intake exceeds losses, linear growth and tissue accretion occurs. There are two periods of rapid growth, the first in infancy and the second at the time of puberty due to an interaction between sex steroids [estrogens (E) and androgens (T)] and growth factors (e.g., GH, IGF-1). Unlike humans, rats continue to grow, although at a declining rate, over most of their life span. In males, the peak in mass velocity is greater and its duration is longer such that by adulthood male rats weigh approximately 40 to 50% more than the females. During periods of undernutrition, the body is capable of conserving existing energy/protein to continue the growth process, but inevitably compromised physiological function or death occur. Consequently, the mammalian body has evolved an intricate and integrative neuronal and hormonal system to maintain energy and protein balance. Energy intake is controlled centrally by the hypothalamus, which receives input about the state of the body's energy reserves. In this respect, the satiety hormone leptin (Lep) dictates to the brain the status of energy stored in adipose tissue via its influence on feeding behavior. Energy expenditure also is regulated by the hypothalamus, which functions by neural (sympathetic/parasympathetic) and hormonal (hypothalmic releasing factors; e.g., GHRH, CRF, TRH) mechanisms to adjust the endocrine (e.g., catecholamines, C; insulin, I; thyroid hormone, T) control of nutrient metabolism. Energy expenditure also can be regulated in the periphery by uncoupling proteins (UCP), which are important for thermoregulation but also may play a significant role in energy homeostasis. Accordingly, it has been suggested that not only may leptin act as a regulator of substrate metabolism in skeletal muscle but levels of fat and lean mass may be related to leptin's regulation of UCPs. Finally, other factors such as chronic physical activity can elevate energy/protein needs which, if not compensated by increased dietary intake, will result in energy/protein imbalance reducing the rate of growth in the young or causing a loss of body tissue in the adult. (See text for details.)

by favoring glucose metabolism to two carbon fragments. Stimulation of the VMHA depresses insulin secretion and raises glucagon concentrations.[45] In the liver, pancreatic release of glucagon increases the breakdown of glycogen and increases gluconeogenesis using available amino acids derived from muscle. Glucagon is also lipolytic, which leads in turn to increased ketogenesis. Another area centrally controlled is the sympathoadrenal system, which is comprised of the sympathetic nervous system and the adrenal medulla. In response to norepinephrine by sympathetic nerve endings, catecholamines are released into the general circulation, which serves to regulate both glucose and fatty acid concentrations in the blood.[46] Epinephrine, through β-receptor action, stimulates glycogenolysis in muscle and liver. Epinephrine also stimulates hormone-sensitive lipase, which acts to raise arterial fatty acid concentrations. Catecholamines increase the secretion of insulin and glucagon via β-adrenergic mechanisms and inhibit the secretion of these hormones via α-adrenergic mechanisms.

The hypothalamus also contains peptide neurosecretory-releasing factors that regulate the secretion of pituitary hormones.[47,48] Growth hormone releasing hormone (GHRH) acts on the somatotrophs of the anterior pituitary to release growth hormone (GH). GH promotes the accumulation of lean body mass directly by increasing the uptake of amino acids from the blood, decreasing glucose uptake, and stimulating lipolysis. GH also stimulates the production of a group of peptides from the liver known as insulin-like growth factors (somatomedins; e.g., IGF-I and IGF-II). IGF-I is primarily responsible for the stimulation of the events leading to linear growth of the skeleton, although IGF-II is involved in the stimulation of tissue growth (increased protein and RNA synthesis) and repair.[49] Hypothalamic secretion of corticotropin-releasing factor (CRF) leads to a release of adrenocorticotropic hormone (ACTH), which regulates the synthesis and secretion of glucocorticoids from the adrenal cortex. Glucocorticoids decrease protein synthesis and promote protein catabolism in muscle and transfer amino acids to the liver for gluconeogenesis. In addition, corticosteroids increase glucagon secretion, thereby assisting (hepatic uptake of amino acids) in this function.[50] Another hypothalamic trophic factor, thyroid releasing hormone (TRH), causes the release of thyroid stimulating hormone (TSH) by thyrotroph cells in the anterior pituitary and stimulates the release of the thyroid hormones (thyroxine and triiodo-thyronine) from the thyroid gland. Thyroid hormones stimulate calorigenesis (heat production) in most tissues (brain, spleen, and testes are exceptions) of the body. In addition, they increase glycogen formation in the liver (in the presence of insulin), facilitate the uptake of glucose from the blood into adipose and muscle tissue, and stimulate the synthesis, mobilization, and oxidation of lipids. The oxidation of lipids is affected more than their synthesis, so the net effect is a decrease in the size of most fat stores. Thyroid hormones also promote the overall accumulation of protein (increase protein synthesis) and bone growth through stimulation of GH.[51]

2. The Role of Leptin in the Control of Feeding

In 1958, G.R. Hervey first demonstrated the presence of a hormone that regulated body weight through an interaction with the hypothalamus.[52] G.C. Kennedy had suggested five years earlier that the site of this hormone was the adipose tissue, which developed later into a lipostatic theory of body weight control.[53] Hervey's experimental destruction of the VMH in one member of a parabiotic rat pair led to death by starvation in the unlesioned animal. Hervey proposed that a circulating satiety factor was produced in excess by the lesioned parabiont as body fat accumulated. The unlesioned parabiont thus became hypophagic and died. Similarly, Coleman and Hummel,[54] using parabiotic mice, suggested that obese (ob/ob) mice lacked the lipostatic factor, and diabetic (db/db) mice became obese because they were resistant to the satiety factor although they over-produced it (lean mice in parabiosis with obese db/db mice died of starvation). In 1994, Zhang, Friedman, and co-workers[55] reported the identification and cloning of the gene responsible for obesity in the ob/ob mouse as well as the human homolog. In subsequent studies, this group of investigators was able to demonstrate that injections of the ob-protein reduced the body weight and fat mass of obese mice.

Currently it is hypothesized that leptin, which is secreted by adipose tissue into the blood, dictates to the animal how much adipose tissue it harbors via control of feeding behavior. In this regard, leptin is a centrally acting satiety factor that acts at the level of the hypothalamus to reduce food intake.[56] In humans and animals, caloric restriction reduces serum leptin concentrations and mRNA levels in adipose tissue, and refeeding increases these levels.[57] The effect of fasting can be mimicked by norepinephrine and the effect of feeding by either insulin or glucocorticoids.[58-61] Accordingly, during times of substrate availability, insulin and glucocorticoid concentrations are elevated and act to increase lipogenesis, resulting in leptin secretion causing subsequent cessation of feeding behavior. Reductions in insulin/glucocorticoids, as in the acutely fasted state, or reductions in fat mass as with prolonged underfeeding or starvation would promote a diminished leptin secretion favoring activity to increase food intake.

A potential link between adiposity, leptin secretion, and feeding behavior is through the appetite-stimulating hypothalamic peptide neuropeptide Y (NPY). An emerging hypothesis is that the decreased food intake caused by leptin secretion is due to a reduction in NPY gene expression via receptors in the arcuate nucleus (located just below the ventromedial nucleus) of the hypothalamus.[61,62] High hypothalamic concentrations of NPY elicit food intake, whereas low concentrations have opposite effects.[63] Interestingly, in most animal models of obesity, hypothalamic concentrations of NPY are high, and intracerebroventricular infusions of NPY cause obesity in normal rats.[63] When leptin is administered for long periods to ob/ob mice, their food intake is reduced as is their body weight, and their overall metabolic rate is raised (indicated by elevated oxygen consumption). These beneficial effects on whole body and fat mass are accompanied by marked decreases in hypothalamic NPY.[64]

The ob-gene and its protein product leptin have important implications for obesity, diabetes, and cardiovascular disease. In the ob/ob mouse, it is apparent that the observed obesity was due to a mutated gene, and hence a nonfunctional protein. In contrast, obese humans do not possess a mutated form of the protein and in fact overproduce leptin.[65] However, the db/db mouse (also obese) was found to encode a mutated receptor for the ob protein and consequently overproduced leptin in an attempt to overcompensate for the genetic defect.[66,67] Currently, it is under intense investigation as to whether humans are insensitive to leptin due to mutations of the gene for leptin receptors in the brain or at the level of the cerebral spinal fluid where leptin must cross the blood brain barrier to reach its putative effect site in the hypothalamus. Regardless, the recent identification of additional mechanisms regulating feeding behavior by the brain, which are independent and additive to the effects of the putative leptin pathway, indicate that the control of feeding is very complex and made even more so by potential gender differences in their regulation.[68]

3. Regulation of Energy Expenditure

Control of energy expenditure is divided into several components: 1) the basal metabolic rate, 2) the thermic effect of feeding, 3) adaptive thermogenesis, and 4) the thermic effect of physical activity.[3,69,70] Basal metabolic rate (BMR) refers to the minimum amount of energy needed by the body at rest in the postabsorptive state (10 to 12 h after last meal). In comparison, resting metabolic rate (RMR) is the energy expenditure under similar conditions except the measurement may be made several hours (3 to 4) after the last meal. In the great majority of the cases BMR is the largest component of energy requirements (60 to 75% of the daily energy expenditure). Several factors can affect basal metabolism: 1) body surface area (metabolic rate increases with surface area), 2) body composition (a large proportion of adipose tissue lowers the BMR), 3) gender [basal metabolic rate is generally lower in females (5 to 10%)], and 4) age (metabolic rate is increased during periods of rapid growth and at the onset of puberty and lower in the elderly). In the human, the energy cost for growth is low compared to basal requirements because growth is a slow process.[1] However, in the rat, which accumulates body tissue more rapidly, the energy cost of growth is much greater.[2] Thyroid hormones are believed to carry a major responsibility for the regulation of the basal metabolic rate.[69]

The thermic effect of feeding (TEF) is the energy expended in excess of resting metabolic rate for digestion, absorption, transport, metabolism, and storage of food. It accounts for approximately 10% of daily energy expenditure.[69] Although the TEF represents a smaller fraction of 24 h energy expenditure than the RMR, variations in TEF may have consequences for long-term body fat regulation.

Adaptive thermogenesis may be considered a change in the normal status of daily energy expenditure, primarily by altering the resting metabolic rate and the thermic effect of feeding. These alterations are the result of environmental and physiological stresses. Nonshivering thermogenesis and alterations in the thermic effect of feeding as a result of physical activity may be considered examples of adaptive thermogenesis.[71]

Next to basal needs, the thermic effect (energy expenditure) due to physical activity is the single most important factor influencing the energy needs of an animal. Physical activity raises the metabolic rate both during and after the event. Due to the elevated energy demand, the utilization of stored energy substrate (carbohydrate and fat) will increase.[70] This increased utilization of substrate must be returned to the body from the diet, or body tissues will be affected. In humans, the thermic effect of exercise may be as little as 10% or as high as 50% in very active individuals.[72]

Weight (mass) gain in the adult occurs when energy intake is greater than expenditure. This is necessary in the young to promote growth, but leads to obesity in adults. Acutely, the body responds to carbohydrate and protein overfeeding by increasing oxidation of both substrates. However, this metabolic response and the storage capacity of these nutrients is limited. The eventual result of overeating is the conversion of both substrates to fat with the inevitable outcome being the development of obesity.[72] In a growing animal, energy must be provided above that required for basal metabolism, physical activity, and diet-induced thermogenesis. During this time, a higher nutrient demand for tissue deposition requires food intake to increase.[36] This additional energy is necessary to cover the cost of increasing body mass and height. As the young mature, the rate of growth diminishes and the energy requirement for growth is reduced.

Body mass loss occurs when energy intake is less than expenditure. In the short term, undernutrition can result in a decrease in resting metabolic rate in both animals and humans beyond that accounted for by mass loss.[3,73-75] This metabolic adaptation may serve as a protective mechanism to prevent excessive loss of energy stored in vital tissues during periods of starvation.[76] The decrease in resting metabolic rate during periods of undernutrition is most likely a result of decreased sympathetic nervous activity[46] and thyroid function.[77] However, in the long term, growth or body mass and body composition are compromised.

Starvation represents an extreme energy imbalance that leads to losses in body mass. The metabolic events of starvation occur in two phases.[78] The initial response to starvation is concerned with the maintenance of glucose production to meet the needs of the CNS. An absence of metabolic fuel from the diet leads to lower insulin and elevated glucagon concentrations. This results in increased lipolysis, reflected by increased circulation of free fatty acids and glycerol. In addition, increased protein catabolism and release of amino acids result from the action of cortisol and glucagon. The liver takes up these fatty acids and amino acids (primarily alanine) for ketogenesis and gluconeogenesis (glucose-alanine cycle). The glucose-alanine cycle[79] is complimented by the Cori cycle whereby lactate is resynthesized back to glucose in the liver and the kidney. The CNS utilizes the glucose formed, and the rest of the body's tissues rely on fatty acids and ketones. The second phase of starvation is directed at minimizing the rate of protein breakdown. This adaptation occurs as a result of a reduction of glucose utilization by the brain. In addition, lower circulating alanine concentration is observed, signaling a reduction in protein catabolism with prolonged starvation. Ketones are the substrates that provide the protein-sparing signal to muscle tissue during this phase of starvation. In this regard, the physiologic increments of ketones can inhibit the oxidation of branched-chain amino acids in muscle, which is the major source of nitrogen for alanine synthesis. In the final stages of starvation, however, fat stores are used up, and the entire energy requirement must be met by visceral organ and plasma proteins. Depletion of these proteins is apparent by edema and finally death results.[76,78,80]

4. The Role of Leptin and Uncoupling Proteins in Energy Homeostasis

The biochemical mechanisms regulating the efficiency of energy usage still elude scientists. However, recent data concerning the metabolic role(s) that leptin and uncoupling proteins (UCP) have in energy homeostasis offer intriguing possibilities for better understanding how mammals regulate energy balance, adiposity, and hence growth and body composition.

The potential for a role of leptin in the control of metabolism has been heightened by the discovery and characterization of the leptin receptor (OB-R) from mouse choriod plexus.[66,81] OB-R is homologous to members of the cytokine receptor super-family and is a single membrane-spanning receptor most related to the gp130 signal-transducing component of the IL-6 receptor, the G-CSF receptor, and the LIF receptor.[66] Splice variants of the receptor that differ in their cytoplasmic domain have been identified. Functionally, in the db/db mouse a short form of the OB-R lacking a cytoplasmic domain is expressed predominantly, indicating that these animals are unable to transduce the leptin signal into the cell interior to exert its metabolic effects.[81] In contrast, the ob/ob mouse, which secretes a mutated form of leptin, has normal OB-R function. More recently, it has been reported that binding of ligand to the receptor activates the JAK kinase and leads to phosphorylation of cytoplasmic target proteins including STAT (signal transducers and activators of transcription) cytoplasmic transcription factors. Phosphorylation of STAT proteins induces dimerization and translocation into the nucleus and results in specific acti-vation of gene transcription.[82] The short form of the receptor is unable to activate STAT proteins and thus provides evidence that reduced expression of the long form is sufficient to cause the db/db phenotype.[81]

When leptin is administered to ob/ob mice, in addition to reductions in food intake, energy expenditure is increased. Both lean and obese animals treated with leptin lose fat mass but retain lean body mass.[64,83] In ob/ob mice, leptin also nor-malizes serum concentrations of glucose, insulin, and lipids.[64] The latter effects are observed at low leptin doses that do not affect body weight, suggesting that leptin's metabolic effects precede its effects on food intake and weight. In pair-feeding studies, leptin-injected mice lose 30 to 50% more weight and 50 to 100% more fat mass than pair-fed controls.[84] In contrast, food restriction (with associated decreased leptin levels) is associated with decreased energy expenditure.[84,85]

Skeletal muscle accounts for the major portion of postprandial insulin-stimulated glucose uptake[86] and whole-body lipid oxidation[87] and is the major tissue contrib-uting to resting metabolic rate. Furthermore, skeletal muscle has been demonstrated to express both the long and short form of the leptin receptor isoforms.[81] Conse-quently, it has been hypothesized that leptin might influence directly skeletal muscle substrate metabolism. Muoio[28] studied leptin's effects on glucose and fatty acid (FA) metabolism in isolated mouse soleus and extensor digitorum longus (EDL) muscles. Leptin increased soleus muscle FA oxidation by 42% and decreased FA incorporation in triacylglycerol (TAG) by 35% in a dose-dependent manner. In contrast, insulin decreased soleus muscle FA oxidation by 40% and increased incorporation of TAG by 70%. When both hormones were present, leptin attenuated both the antioxidative and the lipogenic effects of insulin by 50%. Less pronounced hormone effects were observed in EDL muscle. Leptin did not alter insulin-stimulated muscle glucose metabolism. According to Muoio,[28] leptin modulates energy homeostasis, in part, through mechanisms that are independent of food intake, and it directs metabolic fuels toward oxidation and away from storage. This has two important implications. First, it is possible that post-receptor abnormalities exist in the signal transduction pathway(s) under pathological conditions such as obesity or diabetes. Second, leptin may be an important regulator of whole-body energy metabolism, having a catabolic role in times of substrate availability (e.g., in the fed state), with an attenuated secretion response being important during periods of underfeeding, starvation, or physiological perturbations that mimic these situations (e.g., chronic endurance exercise; see below). Similar results have been demonstrated by Shimabukuro[88] who found that in rats with normal leptin receptors, *in vivo* hyperleptinemia induces a depletion of TAG content in liver, skeletal muscle, and pancreas without increasing plasma free fatty acids (FFA) or ketones or altering insulin sensitivity. This study also suggests that leptin increases intracellular oxidation of lipids and may be useful therapeutically as an antiadipogenic agent in diabetes.

Body fat stores and energy balance also are controlled largely by the adrenergic system. Thus, catecholamines stimulate lipolysis in adipose cells and thermogenesis in skeletal muscles and brown adipose tissue through adrenergic receptors coupled to guanine nucleotide-binding proteins, adenylate cyclase, and cAMP. Until recently, only β_1- and β_2-adrenergic receptors (βAR) were recognized as functionally active receptors in humans.[89,90] In rodents, it appears that β_3AR are the predominant mediators of catecholamine-stimulated thermogenesis in brown adipose (enriched with UCP), and lipolysis in white adipose tissue (β_3AR in white adipose tissue function to stimulate lipolysis). Thus, $\beta_3$3AR are important regulators of energy balance and adiposity in rodents.[29] In support of this hypothesis, impaired expression and functional activity of β_3AR in adipose tissue of congenitally obese C57BL/6J (ob/ob) mice have been demonstrated. Adipose tissue of ob/ob mice contains 300 times fewer β_3 adrenergic receptors than their lean counterparts,[91] and the receptors are less responsive to β_3 agonists. A similar phenomenon may occur in humans as evidence indicates that point mutations exist in gene encoding the β_3-adrenergic receptor in the obese, insulin-resistant Pima Indian tribe, as well as in other groups of obese persons studied.[89,90] In the groups studied, a mutation in the gene that results in the substitution at position 64 of the amino acid arginine for tryptophan in the first intracellular loop of the receptor was associated with slower metabolism and a propensity to gain weight. In turn, sex differences in adiposity and the response to altered states of energy balance may be explained someday by alterations of the β_3AR. For example, a mutated (Trp64Arg) form of the β_3-adrenergic receptor (β_3AR) may be expressed according to sex. The Trp64Arg-β_3AR has been associated with obesity and increased visceral fat in women but not in men.[92]

Leptin has been speculated to be associated with elevated sympathetic activity, which subsequently, through the release of norepinephrine, stimulates β_3 adrenergic receptors in brown (and perhaps white) fat cells.[62] The nerves are part of neuronal circuit that leads from the VMH to the spinal cord. Stimulation of β_3 receptors causes an increase in transcription and translation of a gene encoding for metabolic uncoupling protein (UCP). Therefore, leptin may act to regulate body weight and body composition by regulating overall energy expenditure in the periphery through β_3-activated UCP activity. Indeed, a role for leptin in the regulation of thermogenesis has been established.[64,83,93] Consequences of increased leptin secretion would be increased utilization of excess stored energy as whenever fat mass begins to over-accumulate due to a positive energy balance. Leptin production then would be expected to mirror the energy status of the animal in a reciprocal manner (i.e., reduced leptin production during periods of compromised tissue energy stores). In support, Pelleymounter et al.[64] have demonstrated that C57BL/6J obese/diabetic mice with a mutation in the ob gene, when injected with recombinant leptin protein, increase their metabolic rate, body temperature, and activity levels. Ten mg/kg of injected leptin increased oxygen consumption 25% and raised core body temperature from 35 to 37°C. As expected, leptin also lowered body weight, percent fat, food intake, and serum concentrations glucose and insulin.

There is no precedence established for sex differences in circulating leptin concentrations under conditions that alter energy intake or expenditure in animals. However, in the human, Hickey et al.[94] reported gender differences under exercise-training conditions. Nine male and nine females were compared before and after 12 weeks of aerobic training. It was shown that the women had higher circulating leptin concentrations despite lower fat mass and that training lowered systemic leptin levels in females but not in males. Given the thermogenic effect described for leptin, an attenuated leptin response to exercise may facilitate energy conservation in the females vs. males.

Regulation of body mass maintenance and/or thermoregulation occurs, in part, by the dissipation of energy solely as heat by futile metabolic cycles. In animals, thermogenesis is the major function of brown adipose tissue (BAT)[29,95] that contains uncoupling protein (termed UCP1) found on the mitochondrial membrane. It is thought that UCPs transport fatty acid anions from the inner to the outer surface of the inner mitochondrial membrane and become protonated. Then the neutral molecules return inside. The net result is the exothermic movement of protons from outside to inside the inner mitochondrial membrane, down the concentration gradient resulting in uncoupled ATP synthesis.[29] UCP1 is found exclusively in brown adipose tissue (BAT). Recently, however, two new uncoupling proteins, UCP2 and UCP3, have been discovered.[96-99] Although their metabolic and physiological roles have not been elucidated, UCP2 has been shown to be widely distributed among body tissues, although UCP3 is expressed predominantly in skeletal muscle.

Skeletal muscle is the major determinant of both resting and activity-related metabolic rate. Therefore, it is logical to speculate that factors that would regulate UCP gene expression in muscle, such as hormones that are associated with the control of metabolic rate (e.g., thyroid hormone), would also effect UCP levels and thus could provide a mechanism for the regulation of energy homeostasis and thermogenesis. Experiments investigating these possibilities are ongoing. Recently, Gong[29] reported that muscle UCP3 levels are increased six-fold in hyperthyroid but decreased three-fold in hypothyroid rats. However, although thyroid hormone (T3) stimulates UCP1 gene expression, BAT apparently becomes less active under this condition. Therefore, a compensatory mechanism by BAT may be set in place to adjust for the extra heat production from the muscle and perhaps other tissues.[29] Interestingly, leptin, which elevates metabolic rate in rodents, also increases muscle and BAT UCP mRNA levels in the ob/ob mouse. The induction of UCP by leptin in muscle and BAT presumably explains some of leptin's thermogenic effect in rodents.

Starvation (48 h) in rats results in an eight-fold increase in UCP3 mRNA (with no change in UCP2) in skeletal muscle whereas refeeding is associated with a marked reduction in UCP3 below basal.[29] As suggested by Gong,[29] the starving animal, despite loss of body tissue and compromised energy substrate supply, is still required to maintain body core temperature for survival. Thus, UCP3 may serve this function, suggesting a shift in the predominant role of thermogenic regulation from BAT to skeletal muscle in the rodent during a compromised state of nutrition.

In summary, the mammalian body has evolved an intricate and integrative neuronal and hormonal system to maintain energy balance. Energy intake is controlled centrally by the hypothalamus, which receives input about the state of the body's energy reserves. In this respect, the discovery of the hormone leptin has done much to further the understanding of the control of feeding behavior. Energy expenditure also is regulated by the hypothalamus, which functions to control expenditure by peripheral adjustments in nutrient metabolism. During periods of undernutrition, the body is capable of changing its normal status of energy expenditure, primarily via alterations in the metabolism of substrate and reductions in both resting metabolic rate and the thermic effect of feeding. The overall effect of these adaptations is the preservation of organ tissue for maintenance of physiological homeostasis and a high energy flux for continuation of an elevated activity level. Under extreme conditions such as chronic starvation, metabolic adjustments fail and death of the organism ensues. Skeletal muscle-uncoupling proteins (UCP2 and UCP3) may play a significant role in thermoregulation and energy homeostasis. During times of compromised heat production (e.g., starvation), UCP activity may be upregulated despite inadequate energy availability with maintenance of body core temperature taking precedence. Reductions in BAT activity may act to counterbalance this physiological response. In contrast, during physiological conditions of excess heat production, down regulation of uncoupling proteins in muscle may serve to protect against excessive heat build-up and to conserve energy. Finally, the identification of leptin as a regulator of substrate metabolism in skeletal muscle offers exciting opportunities to further the understanding of the mechanisms by which energy homeostasis is maintained. Furthermore, because the maintenance of body mass and body composition depend on establishing an energy balance between energy intake and energy expenditure, the levels of fat and lean mass may be related to leptin's regulation of UCPs. Mechanisms that may operate differently in females have not been investigated and represent an exciting new frontier in our understanding of sexual dimorphism in energy metabolism.

5. Effects of Endurance Exercise on Energy Status

Endurance exercise results in alterations in energy expenditure both during and after the event. The obvious effect of exercise is to raise energy expenditure during the course of purposeful activity. The greater the energy output the greater the overall daily energy expenditure. Fine-tuning energy and nutrient intake with expenditure result in maintenance of body mass although a failure to do so results in tissue loss.

An increased metabolic response also occurs following a single bout of exercise [termed excess postexercise oxygen consumption (EPOC)].[100] A major portion of EPOC most likely is related to the energy expended to resynthesize high energy phosphate compounds and to refill muscle glycogen stores. However, any factor that influences mitochondrial oxygen consumption (e.g., metabolic hormones such as catecholamines, thyroxine, and glucocorticoids) will contribute to EPOC.[101] EPOC appears to increase with exercise intensity (> 70% VO_{2max}) and duration (> 60 min).[100] Although at equivalent absolute workloads EPOC seems to be reduced in trained individuals,[102] an important factor to consider is the cumulative EPOC effect. As such, over sufficient time, relatively modest elevations in resting metabolic rate could have large effects on body composition.[3]

The overall effect of endurance exercise training on postexercise thermogenesis is not clear. Poehlman[103] has identified a positive, linear relationship between VO_{2max} and relative resting metabolic rate, whereas other investigators have failed to show a relationship.[104] The mechanism by which exercise might elevate resting metabolic rate is at present unknown although Poehlman[69] has suggested that it may be related to a high energy turnover (increased energy intake and expenditure) in a state of energy balance. As such, a high rate of energy flux through the metabolic system would require elevations in enzyme activity resulting in an increased thermic response due to substrate cycling. It also is debatable whether endurance exercise training results in a change in the thermic effect of feeding. It appears that the response is curvilinear and dependent on exercise intensity. The thermic effect of feeding is highest in moderately trained and lower in highly trained individuals.[105]

An increased sensitivity to thermogenic hormones may increase the thermogenic effect of feeding after an acute exercise bout.[106] In contrast, decreased sympathetic nervous activity as a result of exercise training has been suggested to be a mechanism to account for the decreased thermic effect of feeding in trained individuals. According to Poehlman,[69] there is a large degree of genetic variability in the thermic effect of activity and the thermic effect of feeding with exercise training. This could explain discrepancies in the literature on this topic.

The predicted consequence of a mismatch in energy intake and expenditure due to exercise would be a change in body mass. In humans, significant reductions in body mass often have been reported with chronic exercise programs.[107] However, meta-analysis investigations generally indicate that the effect of exercise is to produce a modest effect on total body mass when a constant energy intake is maintained.[3] Measuring body mass alone does not assess completely the specific thermic effect of activity on mass loss. It also is important to consider the body composition changes induced during mass loss with exercise. In general, the literature indicates that chronic exercise increases fat-free mass and reduces fat mass. However, there appears to be a gender-specific response. (See gender differences in the response to endurance exercise.)

B. Protein Status

1. Protein Requirements and Nitrogen Balance

The growth process and maintenance of body tissues in the adult require adequate dietary intake of protein. The protein requirement of an adult animal is defined as the quantity of dietary protein that will balance the losses of nitrogen from the body when energy balance is maintained.[1,108] Protein requirements are higher when there is rapid growth, the nitrogen for protein being provided for the formation, maturation, and maintenance of new tissue.[1] In humans, the protein content increases from 11% (at birth) to 19% (adult value) by 4 years of age.[1] As the growth rate declines the maintenance requirement represents a gradually increasing proportion of the total protein requirement. Therefore, dietary needs decline with age. In the rat, protein requirements decline from about 28% of the diet at 30 days to 10% at 50 days.[109]

Protein homeostasis is maintained by supplying the body with amino acids from the diet. Amino acids exist as part of various pools including the circulation and various tissues (liver, skeletal muscle, and the gut). The free pool of amino acids is small (containing only a few percent of the body's total amino acids), but central to protein/amino acid metabolism because all amino acids must pass through it.[12] Part of the free amino acid pool is incorporated regularly into tissue proteins (synthesis). However, because of protein breakdown, these amino acids return to the free pool after a variable length of time and thus become available for reutilization (protein synthesis or oxidation). The contribution to and removal from the amino acid pool of constituent amino acids is termed turnover. Part of the pool also undergoes catabolic reactions. This process leads to loss of carbon skeletons as CO_2 (oxidation) or its deposition as glycogen or fat, and the nitrogen is eliminated primarily as urea by the kidney. Other routes of amino acid nitrogen loss are sweat urea, ammonia (representing endogenous nitrogen loss from the kidney, sweat glands, and perhaps the lungs), and feces (after exchanging with the free amino acid pool). Some free amino acids are used for synthesis of new nitrogen-containing compounds (e.g., purine bases and creatine in skeletal muscle). These subsequently are degraded without the return of end products to the free amino acid pool (e.g., purine degraded to uric acid). In addition, the nonessential amino acids are made in the body using amino groups derived from other amino acids and carbon skeletons formed by reactions common to intermediary metabolism.[110]

When the dietary input of nitrogen (grams of nitrogen/day) is equal to that excreted (urinary, sweat, and fecal nitrogen), the individual maintains nitrogen balance. In this situation, the rate of synthesis and degradation of body protein is balanced so that the total pool of amino acids is constant. This constancy is maintained by dietary input of new amino acids into the central pool required to compensate for losses via irreversible oxidation, rearrangement of material within the body, and amino acid conversion to carbohydrate and fat. Without dietary input, the needs of any one amino acid compartment can be met for only a short time via other compartments. Eventually the central pool and allied compartments will be depleted. It is this irrevocable loss of amino acids that determines the protein requirement of mammals.

The efficiency by which the body can retain nitrogen changes with the energy and protein composition of diet. Consequently, an accurate knowledge of the interaction of these variables is important to the understanding of the amino acid requirements for growth or maintenance of body tissues. When protein intake is altered, the body is capable of adapting to the new intake, during which time nitrogen excretion will be unstable despite the new constant intake. The length of time necessary to achieve a new steady state will depend to a large extent on the magnitude of the change in intake and the absolute quantity of nitrogen fed.[111] When nitrogen intake is decreased, a dramatic negative nitrogen balance will be observed on the first day. However, nitrogen balance will increase toward some equilibrium level over the subsequent days.[112,113] As a consequence, the concentration of total nitrogen in the urine can be expected to reflect changes in protein intake. Conversely, when nitrogen intake is increased, there is a large positive balance the first few days, which falls toward the point of balance over time.[114] The possibility of an adaptation period to altered protein intake makes the timing of sample collection for NBAL studies critical for meaningful interpretation of results. Data collected during the adaptation period may suggest an increased need for protein although the data collected after adaptation is complete may suggest that the need is unchanged or decreased. Guidelines for determining protein and amino acid requirements specify a minimum of a 10 d adaptation when nitrogen intake is changed.[1] At a fixed protein intake, a change in energy intake also can influence the status of the amino acid pool. For a given protein intake, even below that needed for nitrogen balance, energy intake will improve nitrogen retention.[115] Conversely, for any protein intake, if energy intake is decreased to less than expended, some tissue protein will be degraded and oxidized for energy, the result evidenced as an increased nitrogen excretion. The negative nitrogen balance in this case would not be indicative of the adequacy of protein intake to meet the amino acid requirements of the individual. Under the condition of a decreased energy intake, amino acid needs would be overestimated. In the circumstance of increased energy intake, amino acid requirements would be underestimated due to decreased nitrogen excretion.

In this regard, the effect of elevated activity on energy balance has been shown to be critical in the utilization of protein and hence maintenance of nitrogen equilibrium.[116] For example, Butterfield and Calloway[112] studied previously untrained males on variable energy intakes and found that increasing energy intake 15% of that amount required to maintain body weight increased nitrogen retention by 0.5 g per day. In contrast, Todd[117] found that individuals in energy deficit due to moderate exercise were in negative NBAL despite consuming the RDA for protein (0.8 g/kg · d^{-1}).

2. Effects of Endurance Exercise on Protein Metabolism

Traditionally, it has been assumed that protein contributes in only a minor way to the energy cost of exercise. However, Felig and Wahren[118] have demonstrated a continual flux of amino acids (e.g., alanine) between muscular and nonmuscular tissue (particularly the liver and kidney) suggesting that protein does play a role in the generation of energy during exercise (glucose-alanine cycle). Earlier, Yoshimura[119] reported an increased catabolism of protein in response to endurance exercise. Increases in serum[120] and urinary urea[121,122] and declines in nitrogen balance[123] with endurance exercise support the contention that protein is catabolized for energy during endurance exercise. Given these findings, several exercise scientists have conducted further studies to determine the role of protein as an energy substrate during endurance exercise.[12,124-127]

The first demonstration of increased amino acid oxidation *in vivo* with exercise in mammals was by White and Brooks.[11] They used pulse injection of ^{14}C tracer to study oxidation of glucose, alanine, and leucine in rats during rest and two intensities of exercise. Results demonstrated that the relative oxidation of leucine was related to the metabolic rate. Significant increases in alanine oxidation also were observed with exercise. A number of other studies since have documented increases in whole-body leucine oxidation with exercise.[11,128-131] Consequently, both White and Brooks[11] and Lemon[129] have suggested a reevaluation of the traditional views of amino acid utilization during exercise.

Elevated protein/amino acid metabolism also has been demonstrated with chronic endurance exercise. Dohm[22] reported a significant increase in whole-body leucine oxidation both at rest and during exercise comparing endurance-trained and untrained rats. Similarly, Henderson[10] demonstrated that the rate of leucine oxidation is 40% greater in trained vs. untrained rats. Comparable results have been obtained in humans.[8] Furthermore, others have demonstrated increased protein catabolism in endurance-trained runners or cyclists.[7,9,132,133] The significance of these findings is that protein requirements may be higher in individuals that chronically exercise. Failure to compensate for the irreversible loss of essential amino acids could result in a reduction of lean tissue or an attenuation of growth in the young.

Despite the evidence of elevated protein catabolism with exercise training, other exercise scientists have argued that the elevation is relatively minor, with no significant physiological consequences. It has been known for some time that the body can adapt to sudden increases in physical activity, whereby the efficiency of nitrogen retention is improved.[111,116] Gontzea[134] showed that the initial decrease in nitrogen balance that occurs in exercising untrained men will return to equilibrium after 12 to 14 days of the training protocol. Furthermore, Yoshimura[135] reported that initial losses of blood proteins (albumin and hemoglobin) observed during the first week of endurance training return to pre-exercise concentrations after 2 to 3 weeks of daily exercise. Some tracer data support these findings. Using ^{15}N-glycine and monitoring urinary ammonia, Stein[5] found no differences in protein synthesis or breakdown in the trained athletes when compared to the controls. More recently, Stein[136] reported that protracted endurance exercise can result in a decrease in amino acid flux. From blood samples taken on eight elite triathlon athletes exercising for eight hours on a cycle ergometer (3 h) and a treadmill run (5 h), leucine flux was shown to decrease after 4 h of exercise with a new plateau reached about 20% lower than the pre-exercise conditions. The leucine flux data are consistent with the hypothesis of an adaptation (down regulation) in protein metabolism with endurance exercise. These studies suggest that there is a reduction in catabolism with long-term endurance exercise.

Young and colleagues[137,138] have cautioned, however, that a reduction in the protein/amino acid turnover (flux) may place subjects at a disadvantage for coping with potential metabolic stresses. For example, a reduction in turnover of skeletal muscle proteins presumably would compromise the role of skeletal muscle in energy production during exercise (e.g., the glucose-alanine cycle). In addition, a decreased flux of these substrates through the Krebs cycle could compromise the organism's ability to maintain normal energy metabolism during prolonged exertion. In support of this possibility, Newsholme[139,140] suggested a close relationship between the adequacy of dietary leucine, amino acid turnover, and immune function. Glutamine is both essential for and has a high flux in lymphocytes, macrophage, and other rapidly growing and dividing cells. The source of glutamine is either from dietary protein or via amino acid metabolism in muscle where leucine serves as the nitrogen donor for glutamine synthesis. It has been speculated that a high rate of muscle protein turnover would facilitate the continued availability of glutamine and, presumably, the maintenance of a high flux of glutamine for the support of lymphocyte metabolism and function.

In addition to the debate regarding elevations in protein requirements with increased physical activity, it is noteworthy that there is very little information regarding the effects of variable protein intakes on growth, body composition, or exercise performance in the young. This is especially important because protein requirements are greater in the young,[1] and any adverse effects during growth could have long-lasting consequences. Furthermore, theoretical arguments have been made that supplemental protein will enhance exercise performance, yet few studies have investigated this possibility and at least one study has demonstrated that high protein intakes do not improve exercise performance.[141]

To address these issues, Cortright and co-workers[142] determined whether endurance (moderate intensity) training would alter protein metabolism sufficiently to affect growth, body composition, or exercise capacity in young (28 d) male rats. In addition, they assessed whether supplemental dietary protein would minimize any potential adverse effects on performance. Animals were divided into two exercise (E = voluntary wheel running) and two sedentary (S) groups. Animals were fed 14% (NRC's recommendation for optimal growth) of their energy intake as protein or a similar diet with 20% energy as protein for 72 d. In addition, both exercised groups received a carbohydrate supplement to compensate for the exercise energy expenditure, thereby accounting for the known inverse relationship between energy balance and protein need.[116] In addition to daily wheel running, the animals completed an exercise performance test over three consecutive days following nine weeks of training. Nitrogen balance (NBAL) was measured twice prior to the performance test to assess the acute (d 10 to 14) and chronic (d 48 to 52) protein metabolic response to the diet and exercise protocol. NBAL also was measured immediately after the performance test (d 65 to 66) to determine the effects of the protein supplement. Linear growth [tibial bone (TBL); body (ano-nasal, ANL) lengths] and body composition by chemical analysis were assessed at the end of the experiment.

The exercise stimulus was sufficient to produce a training effect (elevated soleus citrate synthase activity). Total energy (72 d) intake among the four groups was similar, and, as expected, total nitrogen intake was greater in the two protein supplemented groups. With respect to growth, although linear growth (Table 9.1) was not affected by exercise training, final body mass was significantly less in trained vs. sedentary animals (Figure 9.2). The trained animals had less absolute protein mass than the sedentary animals although protein content was similar among groups when expressed as a percentage of body mass (Table 9.1). These results agree with

Table 9.1 Body Composition[1] and Measures of Growth of Sedentary and Trained Rats at Two Levels of Protein Intake

	Sedentary		Exercise	
	14% Diet$_{pro}$	20% Diet$_{pro}$	14% Diet$_{pro}$	20% Diet$_{pro}$
BM (g)	504^a ± 18.3	520^a ± 21.9	444^b ± 17.9	430^b ± 23.7
TBW (g)	300^a ± 12.1	307 ± 8.4	276^b ± 4.4	280^b ± 14.9
%	61.4^a ± 1.3	61.3 ± 1.2	63.7^b ± 0.8	65.0^b ± 0.6
FAT (g)	69^a ± 8.6	74^a ± 9.9	48^b ± 7.0	42^b ± 6.0
%	13.9^a ± 1.4	14.3^a ± 1.4	10.9^b ± 1.2	9.6^b ± 1.0
PRO (g)	98^a ± 4.5	102 ± 4.6	89^b ± 3.0	87^b ± 4.9
%	20.0 ± 0.2	20.2 ± 0.4	20.5 ± 0.3	20.2 ± 0.5
ASH (g)	15 ± 0.3	15 ± 0.6	15 ± 0.5	14 ± 0.5
%	3.1^a ± 0.1	3.0^a ± 0.1	3.5^b ± 0.1	3.3^b ± 0.1
TBL (mm)	44 ± 0.6	44 ± 0.6	44 ± 0.5	43 ± 0.6
ANL (cm)	26 ± 0.4	26 ± 0.5	25 ± 0.3	25 ± 0.6

Note: Values are mean ± SE, unlike letters P < 0.05. TBW, total body-water; BM, body mass; PRO, protein; TBL, tibial bone length; ANL, anno-nasal length. [1]Data computed from depilitated carcass, minus feces.

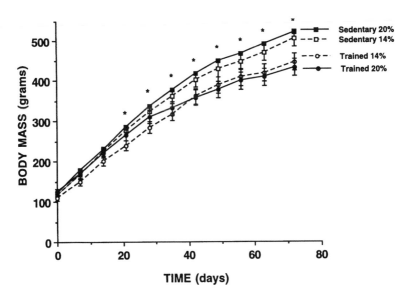

Figure 9.2 Changes in body mass at two levels of protein intake in male rats engaged in daily spontaneous wheel running. Trained animals gained less body mass than sedentary controls regardless of dietary protein intake. Differences in body mass were evident beginning at week four of exercise training. No differences in body weight were evident between the trained animals. Data are mean ± SE; * P <0.05 trained vs. sedentary animals.

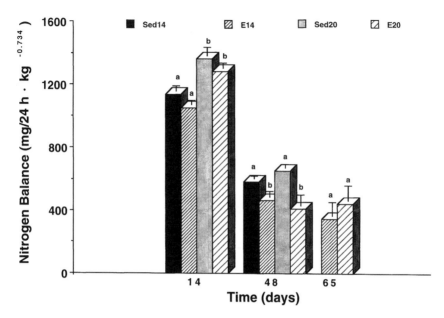

Figure 9.3 Effect of acute, chronic, and intense exercise on nitrogen balance (NBAL). NBAL was significantly less positive in trained vs. the respective sedentary control group following chronic exercise training (d 48 to 52) only. There were no differences evident within either the trained or sedentary groups. Protein supplementation did not alter the effect of three days of intense exercise performance on NBAL. Data are mean ± SE; unlike letters (within time period) P < 0.05.

the findings of Baur[143] who demonstrated that decreased nitrogen deposition can be associated with poor weight gain but does not preclude normal linear growth. The trained animals also had less fat mass than sedentary controls whether expressed as absolute mass or as a percentage of body mass (Table 9.1).

NBAL was positive in both sedentary and running groups following 10 d adaptation to the diet and exercise treatments (Figure 9.3). Following exercise training (d 48 to 52), NBAL remained positive in both activity groups but at a significantly lower level in the trained vs. sedentary groups. NBAL following the exercise performance test was similar between both running groups. Likewise, no difference in the total work accomplished over the 3 d performance test was observed between the running groups. The significantly less positive NBAL observed in the trained vs. sedentary groups suggests that the overall protein synthesis rate was lower in the running groups. Accordingly, the carcass analysis revealed that both the exercising groups contained significantly less absolute protein (E14 = –9%; E20 = –15%) than their respective controls. These data are consistent with the previously observed elevated amino acid oxidation during exercise[10,11,130] and greater nitrogen excretion[123] following endurance exercise. Although these data suggest that protein needs might be greater with this type of exercise, the absence of an effect of supplemental protein on NBAL, body, or protein mass in the E20 group indicates that the protein intake of the E14 animals adequately met their protein needs.

Total testosterone plasma concentration was measured following chronic training and showed trends ($P \leq 0.07$) toward lower values (2.06 ± 0.27 nM) in the exercised vs. sedentary (4.57 ± 1.23 nM) groups. This finding agrees with previous results,[22] suggesting that lower testosterone concentration may contribute to reductions in protein mass observed in exercising animals. Although the differences in plasma testosterone were not statistically different, the 65% reduction in plasma levels may have physiological significance. Furthermore, it has been suggested that reductions in testosterone are exercise intensity-dependent[21] and, if so, the stimulus received by the animals in this study may have been insufficient to statistically lower plasma testosterone concentration.

The study was subject to the limitation that the protein requirements of the growing rat decline with age.[1] Therefore, a diet containing 14% of the total energy consumed as protein may represent a nitrogen intake in excess of the animal's requirement by the end of the experiment. If true, the effect of exercise training on protein status may have been attenuated. Accordingly, if the protein intake had been reduced to a lower yet sufficient level to maintain NBAL in the sedentary groups, the elevated protein catabolism due to exercise may have produced a negative nitrogen balance in the runners. Over time this could result in greater effects on both body and protein mass, which would be expected to adversely affect health and performance.

The data from this experiment have contributed to further knowledge of the effects of exercise on protein requirements. Several studies indicate that protein needs are increased by about 50% with regular endurance exercise.[7,9,133] Some have interpreted this to mean that protein supplementation is necessary for optimal performance. However, this assumes that typical protein intakes are inadequate and that a linear effect exists between protein intake and endurance performance. Neither has been shown to be true. Few studies have attempted to access endurance performance with varying protein intakes. It has been shown in one study that high protein diets can increase body protein stores and muscle mass during intensive endurance training in young men.[141] However, physical work capacity was not improved in the study by Cortright.[142] These results support the contention that supplementation above the recommended intake provides no ergogenic benefit for improving exercise performance. Furthermore, despite being significantly smaller than control, the non-supplemented animals were apparently healthy and capable of performing repeated, high-intensity exercise as well as the protein-supplemented group. Extrapolating to the human, these data suggest that the American diet, which typically provides about 150% of the current RDA for protein, should be sufficient to meet the needs of individuals involved in moderate endurance training.

To summarize this section, growth and maintenance of body tissues depends on an adequate supply of amino acids in the diet. With an adequate protein intake, the amino acid pool remains stable, which is reflected by nitrogen equilibrium in the adult or a positive balance during the growth process. When attempting to evaluate protein requirements in man, it is crucial to take into account 1) the adaptive capacity of the body to change its efficiency of nitrogen retention when protein intake is altered, 2) the effects of altered energy intake or expenditure on nitrogen retention at fixed protein intakes, and 3) alterations in protein status due to exercise training.

Finally, one study suggests that although protein catabolism is elevated due to moderate endurance exercise, the current recommendation for adequate protein intake (provided that additional energy needs are met) is still sufficient to maintain NBAL and performance. This most likely is because the RDA represents that amount of protein needed to maintain NBAL plus a margin of safety to accommodate individual variability in diet, physical activity and metabolism. Recommendations for future studies include experiments comparing chronic, more intense activity at protein intakes near the requirement level for NBAL. These studies need to be performed in the young as well as the adult.

C. Ovarian and Testicular Hormones

In addition to other factors (e.g., growth hormone, IGFs), growth and body composition are regulated by ovarian and testicular hormones. The influence of these sex steroids on the growth process and their effects on body composition are discussed in detail in Chapter 2. Briefly, however, estrogens are thought to increase adiposity, cause an increase in total body protein, and stimulate but eventually cause cessation of linear growth in the human.[18] In contrast, in the rat, estradiol acts to lower adiposity purportedly by lowering lipoprotein lipase activity, and progesterone increases fat storage by increasing the activity of this enzyme.[19,20] Other potential mechanisms that regulate body mass and tissue composition in the female include ovarian action on the hypothalamus, the pituitary, and the liver to alter feeding behavior and substrate availability.[19,20] In humans, male androgens exert important protein-anabolic, growth-promoting effects, in part by increasing GH and hence IGF-1 production.[144] Like estrogens, testosterone stimulates but eventually ceases linear growth by causing the epiphyses of long bones to fuse.[16] In the rat, it appears that testosterone alters body mass and composition in rats by 1) stimulating growth in genital tissues via 5α-reductase metabolite dihydro-testosterone, 2) its anabolic actions on kidney and skeletal muscle, and 3) estrogenic metabolites of testosterone acting directly on adipose tissue to suppress adiposity.[145]

III. GENDER DIFFERENCES IN GROWTH, BODY COMPOSITION, AND SURVIVAL (Figure 9.4)

A. The Growth Process

Growth occurs as an orderly sequence of events that are dependent on an intact endocrine system and adequate nutrition.[146] It involves the accretion of body tissues and an increase in height/length. Patterns of growth vary from species to species. In humans, there are two periods of rapid growth. The first, in infancy, is partly a continuation of fetal growth. Growth hormone is elevated in infants (IGF-1 levels remain constant) but falls until the time of puberty. The second growth spurt, at the time of puberty, is due to an interaction between sex steroids, growth hormone, and IGF-1, and the protein anabolic effects of adrenal androgens. Sex steroids produce

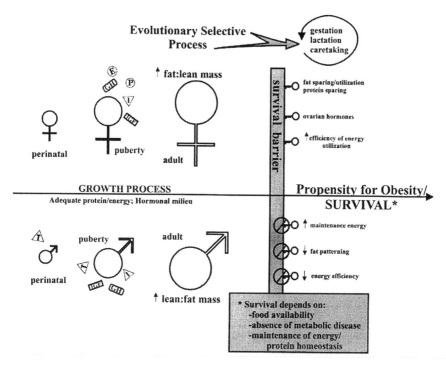

Figure 9.4 Gender differences in factors regulating growth, body composition, and survival. In animals, the growth process is dependent on receiving an adequate supply of energy and protein, whereas maintenance of body tissues in the adult requires that energy/protein intake matches expenditure or nitrogen loss. Accordingly, factors that disrupt energy intake or elevate energy/protein requirements (e.g., food availability, elevated energy expenditure due to activity, and metabolic diseases) will impact negatively growth, alter body composition, and threaten survival. The physiological processes that regulate growth, nutrient utilization, and energy storage are controlled by the neuro-endocrine system. In this regard, males and females differ with respect to the mechanisms available for regulation of growth and metabolism under varying conditions of energy/protein imbalance. It has been suggested that because females are responsible for the survival (gestation and caretaking) of the young, they have been more favorably affected by natural selection pressures to resist the loss of body energy stores. For example, food restriction and/or starvation appear to have a consistently greater and more permanent effect on physical growth in males than females. Females also appear to defend body fat and protein mass during periods of negative energy balance induced by elevated physical activity. The robust mechanisms present in the female to preserve body tissues become more evident in the diabetic state, which simulates starvation due to the inability to utilize glucose. Again, females resist the deleterious effects of this metabolic disease to a greater extent than males. Therefore, perhaps due to the presence of ovarian hormones and variable differences in other factors (leptin and uncoupling proteins) that regulate food intake and energy efficiency, females appear to respond more favorably than males to periods of energy deficit or starvation. (See text for details.)

an increase in the amplitude of spikes in growth hormone, which act to increase IGF-1 secretion; this in turn promotes growth.[147]

The increase in height for boys and girls parallel each other almost exactly until the end of the first decade of life. Between the ages of 11 and 13 years the female estrogens cause a rapid increase in growth, but early uniting of the epiphysis (14th to 16th year of life) causes growth in height to cease. This contrasts with the effect of testosterone in boys, which causes growth at a slightly later age (13th to 17th year). The male, however, undergoes much more prolonged growth so that his final height is considerably greater than that of the female.

Unlike humans, rats continue to grow, although at a declining rate, over most of their life span. Male rats are 5 to 8% heavier at birth than females and this difference increases throughout development. By adulthood (12 weeks old) male rats (Sprague-Dawley) weigh approximately 40 to 50% more than the females. In the intact rat, males and females grow similarly through the first four weeks of life. During the fifth week, the growth rate increases sharply for both sexes. However, in males, the peak in mass velocity is greater and its duration is longer.[148]

Several studies indicate that the neonatal gonad is responsible for the gender dimorphic pattern of growth in the rat.[148-151] Slob[148] and co-workers have demonstrated that if male rats are castrated at birth, they do not achieve as great a body weight or bone length as sham-operated males. Castration at day 21 also reduces growth but not to the same extent. In contrast, castrated females grow to a larger size than intact females. This is because estrogens have an inhibitory effect on body growth.[152,153]

Postnatally, days two to three of age is the period of greatest sensitivity to testosterone. Tarttelin[151] injected female rats with testosterone propionate on any of days two to five and compared the growth response to control animals. Rats injected beyond day three grew substantially less compared to those injected earlier. Apparently, there is a critical period perinataly (d 2 to 3) where testosterone must be present for the male growth pattern to occur.

Castration experiments indicate that the female gonad acts to decelerate the growth pattern found in the male. Tarttelin[151] studied the growth response of neonate female rats under three conditions: 1) injected with testosterone propionate (TP) and ovariectomized on day 21, 2) injected with TP and sham-operated on day 21, and 3) injected with sesame oil and sham-operated. Results demonstrated that although both testosterone-treated groups grew more than controls, the sham-operated, TP-injected group grew less than the ovariectomized, TP-injected animals. Perry[150] corroborated this finding with testosterone-treated ovariectomized neonate females who were shown to grow and utilize food more efficiently than untreated, intact females. Furthermore, Tarttelin[151] have demonstrated that ovariectomized females treated perinataly with estradiol (benzoate) exhibit a depressed growth rate compared to untreated intact litter-mate females.

In summary, male rats grow to a larger size prenatally than females, but their potential for postnatal growth is similar to that of females. In females, the potential for postnatal body growth is sequestered by estrogens throughout adulthood unless the ovaries are removed. In postnatal males, testosterone secretion from the testes during the first few days of life irreversibly elevates the rate of growth to a point greater than that of the female.[154]

B. Response to Undernutrition and Starvation

The response of utilization of ingested energy to long-term underfeeding in male rats has been studied by Hill.[155] Weight reductions were produced in Wistar rats by starvation or by variable degrees of underfeeding. Afterward, body weights were maintained by adjusting daily food intake for 18 days. It was observed that energy conservation in the male rat did occur (i.e., a reduction in the amount of energy required for maintenance of body weight) and developed in proportion to the reduction in body weight. Furthermore, energy conservation increased even while reduced body weights were maintained at lower levels. Suggested mechanisms in the male rat to account for the above observations included the utilization of body fat stores (~30%) and loss of the fat-free body (~9%) although no further changes were observed during the period when the animals were weight-stable despite reduced energy intake. Associated reductions in the resting metabolic rate, the thermic effect of feeding, and reductions in lipoprotein lipase activity during food restriction/ fasting also were reported. However, with males that were more severely food-restricted, a significantly reduced carcass energy content continued throughout the study.

This study aids in elucidating the nature of energy conservation initiated during underfeeding and the metabolic strategies that allow animals to adapt to (and survive) progressive degrees of food restriction. The energy cost of maintenance declines with progressive reductions in energy intake and coincides with loss of body weight (and body energy) until a maximal level is reached. The maximal level can be reached quickly with starvation although it can be reached with less severe energy restriction, which produces a comparable loss of body weight (body energy). With severe underfeeding, the male rat is unable to compensate by further energy conservation, and physiological function is compromised.

Hoyenga and Hoyenga[25] have hypothesized that, due to gender dimorphic evolutionary selection pressures, female mammals have evolved a greater capacity to conserve energy than males. These investigators suggest that because of their extended role as caretakers for the young as well as their obvious role during pregnancy, females have developed mechanisms to better cope with food scarcity. Accordingly, food restriction has been reported to have a greater and more permanent effect on physical growth in males than in females.[25,26,33,156-159] Widdowson[26] cited data from post-WW II Germany, which showed that the majority of people adversely affected by undernutrition were male (60% of those affected). Hall[160] supports this finding with data from seven nineteenth-century northcoast populations in British Columbia, which indicated that the growth process in males is more vulnerable to environmental changes than that in females.

Similar gender differences have been shown in animals that are food-restricted. In one study, Widdowson[26] subjected rats to complete starvation for six days. Although body mass loss was similar after starvation, males lost a greater percentage (16%) of their body mass as protein (especially as catabolism of vital organs such as the liver and heart) than females (8%). The ratio of lipid to protein lost (g) was 1.16 for males vs. 3.26 for females. The greater utilization of fat by females presumably would confer a survival advantage (e.g., less vulnerability to disease or organ failure) during prolonged starvation. Widdowson[26] also subjected ten-day old pigs to a program of undernutrition for one year. At the end of that time, 87% of the females were still alive compared to only 22% of the males. Similarly, McPhee[157] starved five-week old mice for four weeks. Afterward, the difference in mass from *ad libitum* controls was 2.5 times greater in males than in females.

In support of these earlier findings, Hill[161] performed a study examining energy utilization in food-restricted female rats. Female Wistar rats that were food-restricted demonstrated a remarkable ability to reduce maintenance energy costs and to achieve zero-energy balance at food intakes that were 40 to 50% of controls. By contrasting these results with previous results in food-restricted male rats,[155] it appears that female rats can preserve lean mass to a greater degree than male rats by utilizing relatively more fat for energy needs. This preference for fat as a fuel during negative energy balance suggests that females would lose less body weight for a given reduction in carcass energy than males because fat is more energy-dense than lean mass.

The mechanism(s) responsible for the enhanced survivability of the female during times of undernutrition are unknown. In the human, females apparently catabolize more fat and males more protein during starvation. According to Merimee,[162] women have a more rapid rise in blood concentrations of free fatty acids and ketone bodies with starvation, suggesting greater lipid catabolism. A greater ketosis in women could spare protein because ketosis decreases amino acid efflux from muscles. As mentioned, results by Tarnopolsky[14] and Phillips[8] with endurance exercise in humans (acute energy imbalance) support the hypothesis that females utilize stored lipids to a greater extent (lower RER during exercise) and that males rely more on stored glycogen (higher RER during exercise) and body protein (greater leucine oxidation) than females.

Ovarian hormones may be involved, at least in part, in the gender response to undernutrition. In postmenopausal women, there is a gain in central fat mass. Hormone replacement attenuates fat gains in humans, and the decrease in basal metabolic rate associated with postmenopause is attenuated with estrogen replacement.[163] In the rat, estrogens suppress body mass by decreasing food consumption and fat deposition.[164-168] In contrast, progestins have been shown to increase carcass fat content and body mass.[19,20,153,169,170] In the male, androgens either may increase or reduce food intake, fat, and body mass.[171] In the castrated rat, low doses of androgens have been found to increase food intake and body weight, but higher doses (still physiological) reduce body mass and fat (perhaps due to aromatization of testosterone to estrogen).[167,172]

An additional role for estradiol in changing body mass could be via alterations in BAT thermogenesis. Changes in energy expenditure (increased VO_2) already have been linked to estrogen-enhanced thermogenesis,[173,174] but these findings have been inconsistent. McElroy and Wade[175] have reported that at least the dynamic phase of ovariectomy-induced mass gain in rats could not be explained by a reduction in brown adipose tissue. Whether estrogens (or leptin) influence the genetic expression of the new uncoupling proteins (UCP2 and UCP3) mentioned previously remains to be tested. However, these studies may yield important revelations with regard to a link between the hormonal system and the regulation of energy homeostasis.

Finally, although there is substantial evidence to indicate a gender dimorphic response to starvation favoring female survivability, the theory has not gone unchallenged. Harris and colleagues[176,177] have reported that when allowances are made for differences in mass, no differences between undernourished males and females occur either in the gross use of body protein or fat stores or in the relative effects on individual fat depots, muscles, or organs. In addition, no differences were found in the conservation of body nitrogen, whole body protein-synthesis, or metabolic rate. Moreover, because in this study females required more energy to ensure that both genders lost the same proportion of body mass, it was concluded they were less efficient in their utilization of energy and would probably not survive a period of undernutrition as well as males. It should be noted, however, that in the studies by Harris and co-workers,[176,177] recalculation of the data presented leads to the conclusion that females do possess a protein-sparing mechanism not present in males. Males lost 26 grams of fat whereas females lost 16 grams. When the loss of fat or protein mass was expressed as a percentage of total weight loss from control, females lost 79% of their body weight as fat and 17% as protein. In contrast, males lost equal portions of their weight as fat and protein. Moreover, the ratio of lipid to protein loss in grams was only 0.98 for males but was 4.60 for females. This study does indicate, however, that further research is needed in the area of gender dimorphic responses to undernutrition and other factors that alter energy homeostasis.

In summary, after puberty, female and male animals of most species differ in both their body composition and their efficiency of energy utilization. Females generally have higher proportions of body fat than males and appear to be more efficient in energy utilization, primarily as a result of having a lower basal metabolic rate for their body size.[178] During periods of undernutrition, it would be expected that these gender differences would confer on the female an advantage in withstanding a deficiency in energy. Several studies support this reasoning,[25,26,178] but other work has indicated that it may be premature for general acceptance of this theory.[176,177,179] New discoveries in molecular biology may aid our understanding of the control of energy homeostasis (and thus regulation of growth and survivability) in males and females.

C. Response to Exercise: Energy Imbalance Due to Habitual Activity

Adult males typically experience a significant weight loss with endurance exercise despite only mild energy deficits.[4,180] In contrast, females who regularly exercise have been reported to remain weight-stable despite more substantial energy deficits.[181] As a result, it has been shown that when men and women engage in an endurance exercise-training program, men are more sensitive to fat loss.[4,182,183] These studies suggest that females have an improved energy efficiency associated with endurance exercise training and that they protect against fat and protein loss despite an energy deficit.[184]

When female rats are subjected to endurance exercise training (swimming, treadmill) they are able to gain weight at approximately the same rate as sedentary controls.[185,186] In contrast, male rats subjected to regular exercise typically lose weight.[187-189] These studies investigated the gender-specific weight loss response to physical activity in adult rats, using forced exercise (e.g., treadmill running, swimming). However, the weight-loss response of male and female rats with exercise training has seldom been compared with voluntary exercise in very young animals.[190]

To address these questions, Cortright and associates[15] compared the estimated energy balance, linear growth (body and bone lengths), and body composition (all components including body mass, total body water, fat, protein, and ash) in response to chronic, voluntary exercise in very young male and female Sprague-Dawley rats. The energy status of the runners vs. their respective sedentary controls was computed and compared between genders to explain the results. Energy intake was calculated by multiplying the daily food intake by the energy density of the diet (14.65 kJ/g; 3.5 kcal/g), and data were expressed as g/100 g bm · 24 h^{-1}. The energy cost of wheel activity was estimated from the calculation of the average oxygen cost of running in the wheel apparatus.[191] The energy status of the exercising animals was estimated relative to sedentary controls.

Over a nine-week period, females ran significantly greater distances than males, with the difference in running behavior becoming significant at week two and continuing thereafter. On average, females ran 50 to 80% more than males for any given week of the study. Both male and female running rats consumed more food than their sedentary counterparts. Despite this hyperphagia, estimated energy balance for the running animals was negative vs. control. However, the females were in greater energy deficit than the running males over weeks three to seven. Despite running significantly less distance and thus experiencing a lower energy deficit, the effects of daily wheel running on body mass were greater in the males (Figure 9.5). Trained male rats weighed significantly less than sedentary male rats over weeks seven to nine, resulting in a 9.2% reduction in final body mass (Table 9.2). In contrast, the female runners grew at a similar rate as the sedentary female rats and, as a group, were actually heavier (4 g) at the end of the experiment. Even when corrected for the initial mass differences (ANCOVA), fat and protein mass still decreased significantly in males (fat, males = –48%, females = –26%; protein, males = –17%, females = –4.6%). Results were similar when expressed as a percentage of body mass (Table 9.2).

Gender differences in the growth response to exercise have been attributed to differences in appetite between male and female exercising rats.[190] It has been reported that female rats increase food intake in response to endurance exercise and male rats do not.[190,192,193] However, in the study by Cortright[15] both male and female rats consumed more food than their respective sedentary groups. Over the nine-week study, male running rats ate on average 1.6 ± 0.33 g/100 g bm · d^{-1} (mean ± SE) and female running rats ate 1.9 ± 0.26 g/100 g bm · d^{-1} more food than their respective controls. The similarity in feeding behavior indicates that the significant differences in energy status between genders was the result of a greater running activity by the females. This study supports previous literature in that female rats run significantly more than males when allowed access to running wheels.[194] Despite this difference in energy status, the trained female's growth rate was similar to that of her sedentary control. Moreover, females' fat and protein tissue losses were less than trained males.

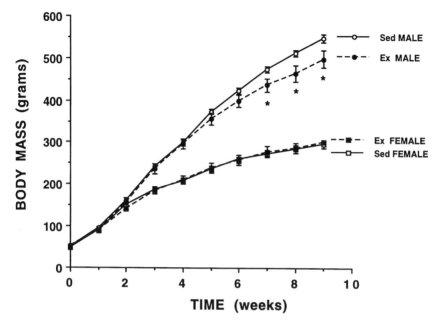

Figure 9.5   Changes in body mass in sedentary (sed) and chronically exercised (Ex) male and female rats. Male but not female rats engaged in chronic wheel-running activity weighed significantly less that their respective sedentary counterparts over weeks 7 to 9. Data are mean ± SE; * P < 0.05 trained vs. sedentary animals.

Table 9.2   Body Composition of Sedentary and Exercised Male and Female Rats

	Male		Female	
	Sedentary	**Exercise**	**Sedentary**	**Exercise**
BM (g)	548.0 ± 9.6	498.0 ± 20.7*	302.0 ± 14.8	297.0 ± 9.9
TBW (g)	336.2 ± 5.3	334.4 ± 9.6#	194.9 ± 6.1	199.6 ± 7.7
%	61.2 ± 0.6	66.6 ± 0.9	64.1 ± 0.8	66.4 ± 0.8
PRO (g)	139.2 ± 2.9	115.0 ± 7.3#	69.7 ± 2.6	64.5 ± 3.5
%	25.3 ± 0.4	22.7 ± 0.6	22.9 ± 0.4	21.7 ± 0.3
FAT (g)	80.4 ± 5.0	41.7 ± 7.3#	33.2 ± 3.4	24.5 ± 4.5
%	14.6 ± 0.8	8.0 ± 1.1	10.8 ± 1.0	7.9 ± 1.0
ASH (g)	15.7 ± 0.6	15.9 ± 0.5	11.1 ± 0.3	11.3 ± 0.4
%	2.9 ± 0.1	3.2 ± 0.1	3.6 ± 0.1	3.8 ± 0.1

Note: Values are means ± SEM; * P < 0.05, diabetic vs. control; BW, body weight; TBW, total body water; PRO, protein; TBL, tibial bone length; ANL, ano-nasal length. ¹Data computed from depilitated carcass, minus feces. Comparisons were made between sedentary and exercised rats within the same gender using ANOVA and ANCOVA. * P < 0.05 differences observed with ANOVA, # P < 0.05 differences observed with ANCOVA.

The mechanism responsible for the gender-dimorphic response in growth with endurance exercise is unknown, but may involve gonadal hormones. It has been demonstrated that endurance exercise lowers plasma testosterone in male rats.[22] The loss of this potent anabolic hormone at puberty could result in an attenuated growth response and account for the significantly lower protein mass observed in the male runners. Evidence to support this hypothesis can be derived from several studies. Dohm and associates[195] demonstrated that the rate of weight gain was lower in treadmill trained vs. sedentary male rats, which resulted in a smaller lean body mass. This occurred even when food consumption of untrained rats was restricted to match the hypophagic response of trained male runners. As a follow-up to this study, Tapscott[196] tested the effects of training on changes in protein synthesis and degradation in male and female rats using a perfused hemicorpus preparation. Results indicated that muscle protein degradation was increased in trained male rats, but training did not alter muscle protein synthesis or degradation in female rats. It was concluded that protein metabolism may contribute to the difference in growth-rate response of male and female rats to endurance training. Support for this conclusion comes from other studies demonstrating that training increases urea nitrogen excretion and decreases nitrogen balance in male rats,[195] but nitrogen excretion is not altered in trained female rats.[22] Finally, although Dohm and Louis[22] have reported an association between treadmill exercise and reduced androgen levels in male rats, a study by Rivest and others[172] demonstrated that testosterone treatment in orchidectomized rats did not eliminate the anorexic effects of exercise, nor did such a treatment promote energy deposition as either fat or lean tissue. Accordingly, further studies are needed to discern the importance of testosterone alterations on body composition changes due to endurance exercise.

In contrast, although estrogens suppress body mass, food consumption, and fat deposition in female rats,[164-168] progesterone has been shown to increase carcass fat content and body mass,[19,153,170] perhaps through alterations in energy balance.[19,170] Collectively, these studies suggest that ovarian hormones may be responsible for the maintenance of body mass in the running female. In support of this concept, Chatterton and colleagues[197] reported that chronic treadmill running resulted in extended periods of progesterone secretion associated with acyclic periods of ovulation. The extended periods of progesterone were associated with significant weight gain. For example, exercising female rats actually gained more weight than sham exercised controls (15.9 ± 3.4 vs. 6.2 ± 1.4 g; P < 0.01). In addition, among the exercising animals, those that were anovulatory (i.e., with extended periods of progesterone secretion) gained more weight (21.0 ± 3.4 vs. 13.0 ± 3.0 g; P = 0.15) than those that remained ovulatory. Collectively, this suggests that progesterone may play a significant role, perhaps through alterations in energy efficiency, to protect the female against the loss of body tissue during the energy imbalance experienced from increased activity behavior.

It should be noted that comparisons between forced exercise (treadmill running), which have been shown to disrupt normal estrous cyclicity[198] and voluntary exercise, which produces more variable results,[199,200] do not always demonstrate consistent results with respect to the exercise effects on the anterior pituitary-gonadal axis (i.e., prolongation of the estrous cycle and concomitant changes in ovarian hormones).

Given that an intensity threshold may exist by which disruption of the hypothalamic-pituitary-gonadal axis occurs, alterations in the estrous cycle and thus estrogen and progesterone levels may not be associated always with volitional endurance exercise. This indicates that further confirmatory studies are needed in the voluntary exercise model to link altered gonadal hormone profiles with changes in growth and body composition in females.

The findings by Cortright[15] agree with those of Pitts[190] who demonstrated that voluntary wheel running is associated with a decrease in body and fat-free mass in male but not female rats. However, both studies disagree with the results by Tokuyama.[194] This group studied the effects of wheel running on food intake, mass gain, and body composition in adult rats. Results indicated that both female and male rats were significantly smaller and had less fat than sedentary controls after 50 days of running. Although food intake increased in both males and females, it was not sufficient to compensate for the increased energy expenditure. The rats used in the study by Tokuyama,[194] however, began running as adults (50 d old) whereas in the studies by Cortright[15] and Pitts,[190] the rats began to exercise as weanlings (21 d old). Therefore, differences in ovarian hormones at puberty may explain the contrasting results of these studies.

It is interesting to observe that despite a reduction in body, fat, and protein mass that occurred in the trained male rats in the study by Cortright,[15] linear growth was not affected. This is in contrast to previous studies that have demonstrated reductions in tibia bone length with endurance exercise.[201,202] However, these studies utilized forced rather than voluntary exercise protocols. Rats in running wheels typically exercise intermittently throughout the dark cycle. This behavior may result in a lower exercise intensity stimulus than would occur with forced exercise, for example, treadmill running. In addition, wheel-running activity changes over the lifespan of the laboratory rat, declining with age.[203] This suggests that over the latter portion of a training protocol (8 to 12 weeks), the intensity of training may be much lower for voluntary vs. forced exercise. If bone growth is dependent on the intensity of the exercise stimulus, then differences are more likely to occur with forced vs. voluntary exercise. It has been mentioned that growth in the male is dependent on the anabolic hormone testosterone. Declines in testosterone concentrations occur with endurance exercise, but these reductions are intensity dependent.[21] The testosterone response to voluntary vs. forced exercise may explain the differences in bone growth observed between the present and previous studies.[202,203]

In conclusion, these studies suggest that female rats are less affected than males in terms of growth and body composition when challenged by the energy deficit due to endurance exercise training. This difference occurs despite a greater energy imbalance incurred by the running female. Further study is needed to determine if a similar gender difference exists in humans.

D. Response to Positive Energy Balance: Overfeeding and Implications for Obesity

The previous discussion has interesting implications with regard to obesity and weight control. For example, the data suggest that in times of energy surfeit, females may be more prone toward obesity and, likewise, it may be more difficult for females to lose body and fat mass.[25] In support, sources report that obesity appears to affect women more often than men, especially after the age of 40 years, and the preponderance of women in the super-obese category is greater at all ages.[179] In contrast, males would appear to have the advantage in an overweight population who attempt to reduce body and fat mass for health purposes.[4,180,184,204,205]

Tremblay[183] reported that males were more sensitive to the effects of exercise on adiposity than females. In addition, Westerterp[204] and Goran examined the existing data using the doubly labeled water method for the measurement of daily metabolic rate combined with a measurement of basal metabolic rate and concluded that a higher level of physical activity was related to a lower % body fat in males. In females, there was not such a relationship between physical activity and body composition. Other studies support this conclusion.[205,206]

These findings often are not reported consistently, however. Horton[105] examined energy balance in endurance-trained female cyclists and untrained controls via a whole room calorimeter on two occasions: a cycling day and a noncycling day. Results were that components of daily energy expenditure (RMR, TEF, and activity) were not significantly different between groups. Horton[105] also found no evidence in males that habitual exercise, at moderate or even high levels, led to a significant prolonged stimulation of metabolic rate per unit of active tissue. However, the increased lean body mass associated with exercise did increase the daily energy expenditure by 8 to 14% in males.

In animals, it has been suggested that the sexes show different responses to dietary changes and to the effect of exercise on feeding. Krook[35] looked at the prevalence of obesity among 10,933 canine necropsies. Among the group diagnosed as being obese without being diabetic were 12% of the males and 21% of the females. Sedentary rats offered a palatable, mixed diet ingest excess energy and became obese.[207,208] However, Pitts and Bull[209] found that male rats did not become obese on a high fat diet when forced to exercise on a treadmill. Selafani and Springer[210] on the other hand found that female rats eating a high energy supermarket diet became obese despite being given free access to a running wheel (although they did not gain as much weight as sedentary females). Furthermore, female rats responded to dietary dilution by adjusting food intake and showed compensation for increased energy expenditure during enforced exercise by hyperphagia. Males were less responsive to dietary dilution and did not show compensation for increased energy expenditure during enforced exercise.

To determine whether males and females differ in their response to the development of dietary obesity with exercise, Rolls and Rowe[211] fed Hooded Listar rats either a palatable, mixed, high energy diet with chow or chow only for 9 to 12 weeks. Furthermore, to determine whether obesity would persist after withdrawal of the fattening diet in both sexes, only chow was provided to all groups for seven weeks following the dietary treatment. Both sedentary males and females on the fattening diet were significantly heavier than sedentary animals on the chow diet. In contrast, females on the chow diet did not lose body weight as the result of exercise but exercising males did.

In summary, the majority of studies suggest that females may be more prone toward obesity under conditions of feast. These findings have implications for the treatment of human obesity and suggest that, unlike males, females require both nutritional as well as activity interventions to regulate whole body and fat mass.

E. Response to Diabetes

Diabetes has deleterious effects on growth and body composition due to a reduced ability to utilize glucose.[212,213] However, the effect of diabetes on growth and body composition has not been compared between genders. Therefore, Cortright and collegues[214] tested the hypothesis that diabetes would reduce growth more in male than female rats because females have mechanisms that enhance fat storage and energy conservation.[25,153,169,178]

Male and female weanling rats were assigned to either a control or diabetic group. Diabetes was induced chemically by injections of streptozotocin with supplementation, if necessary, to equalize the severity of the disease between groups (blood glucose over 13.9 mM; 250 mg/dl). Body mass and blood glucose were measured over the ensuing eight weeks. Subsequently, chemical analysis was performed to measure carcass content of body water, protein, fat, and ash. Linear growth was also assessed by measures of body and bone lengths.

Despite being hyperphagic, growth was retarded severely in males (Figure 9.6). This effect became significant early in the experiment (week three) and resulted in a 45% reduction in the final body mass. In contrast, the female diabetic rats grew at a similar rate as female controls, with diabetes causing a more minor difference in the final body mass (13% less than control). Male diabetic rats showed a greater loss of protein mass vs. control than female diabetic rats when expressed in absolute terms (−40 vs. −5 g) and as a percent of body mass (−4.5% vs. 0%). The effect was not due to the larger body size because ANCOVA (covariate = control body weight) demonstrated similar results. Male diabetic rats also had a greater reduction in fat mass than female diabetic rats when expressed in absolute terms (−39 vs. −23 g fat), and ANCOVA demonstrated similar findings. When expressed as a percent change from control rats, diabetes reduced fat mass more in male than in female rats.

Diabetes resulted in a greater reduction in body length in males vs. females (Table 9.3). Ano-nasal length (ANL), when expressed in absolute terms, demonstrated a greater reduction (−4 vs. −1 cm) in males than females, respectively. When expressed as a percent change from control animals, diabetes reduced ANL more in male rats. Similarly, male diabetic rats had a greater reduction in tibial bone length (TBL) when expressed in absolute terms (−5 vs. 0 mm; male vs. female, respectively) or as a percentage change from control.

Similar effects of diabetes on growth (body mass) and body composition in rats have been reported previously.[212,213] However, these studies did not compare responses between genders. Tepper and colleagues[212] reported that moderately diabetic (fasted bGlc = 11.1 ± 1.5 mM) adult male Sprague-Dawley rats, fed a composite diet *ad libitum,* grew substantially less and demonstrated severe wasting of adipose tissue vs. control. Friedman[213] measured fat and fat-free mass after six weeks in

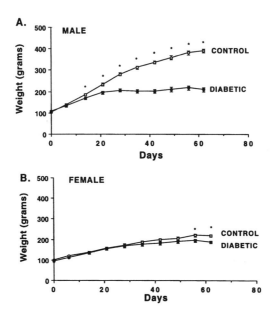

Figure 9.6 Weight of male (Panel A) and female (Panel B) control and diabetic rats. There was a significant disease X time interaction for each gender, which demonstrates that diabetes affected the rate of growth more in male than female rats. Diabetes significantly reduced body weight in male rats beginning at week 2 of the experiment. In contrast, there were not significant differences in body weight between control and diabetic female rats until the eighth week of the experiment. Data are mean ± SE; * P < 0.05 trained vs. sedentary animals.

Table 9.3   Body Composition and Measures of Growth of Control and Diabetic Rats

	Male		Female	
	Control	**Diabetic**	**Control**	**Diabetic**
BM (g)	390 ± 9.3	215 ± 8.4*	221 ± 6.0	192 ± 6.8*
TBW (g)	284 ± 4.9	156 ± 6.0*	132 ± 3.7	130 ± 4.3
%	64 ± 0.5	73 ± 0.2*	60 ± 0.6	68 ± 8.8*
FAT (g)	44 ± 2.7	5 ± 0.3*	35 ± 1.8	12 ± 1.8*
%	11 ± 0.6	2 ± 0.1*	16 ± 0.6	6 ± 0.8*
PRO (g)	84 ± 2.2	44 ± 2.0*	46 ± 1.0	41 ± 1.9*
%	22 ± 0.2	21 ± 0.3*	21 ± 0.5	21 ± 0.4
ASH (g)	12 ± 0.3	7 ± 0.3*	8 ± 0.2	7 ± 0.3*
%	3 ± 0.1	3 ± 0.1	3 ± 0.8	3 ± 0.2
TBL (mm)	40 ± 0.1	35 ± 0.3*	35 ± 0.2	35 ± 0.4
ANL (cm)	23 ± 0.2	19 ± 0.2*	20 ± 0.2	19 ± 0.2*

Note: Values are means ± SEM; * P < 0.05, diabetic vs. control; BW, body weight; TBW, total body water; PRO, protein; TBL, tibial bone length; ANL, ano-nasal length. [1]Data computed from depilitated carcass, minus feces.

severely diabetic adult female Sprague-Dawley rats and also reported a decline in fat mass. An analysis of these two previous studies indicates that, due to diabetes, males lost 35% of their body mass although the females lost only 20% of their body mass despite a greater severity of the disease (bGlc > 22 mM). These results support the suggestion that the effects of diabetes on growth are greater in male rats.

The mechanisms responsible for the enhanced deterioration of growth and body composition in male rats are unknown. Differences in food consumption could, at least in part, account for differences in growth and body composition between genders. However, this is unlikely because diabetic animals are known to be hyperphagic. Cortright[214] previously measured growth, body composition, and food consumption in control and diabetic Sprague-Dawley rats and demonstrated that diabetic animals were hyperphagic. However, there were no differences in food consumption between diabetic females and males when expressed relative to body mass. In addition, because diabetic animals ingest large quantities of food, the amount of digestible energy is reduced as much of their intake passes straight through their gut. Also, even though a significant portion may be digested and absorbed, the amount that actually is taken up by the cells is impaired. Therefore, even if food intake were different, that amount would not reflect the actual energy taken up by the cell due to the physiological impairment in diabetic animals. Thus, it is unlikely that differences in food consumption account for the gender influence on linear growth and body composition.

Similar to endurance exercise, the sexual dimorphic response to type I diabetes also may involve differences in gonadal hormones. It has been demonstrated that the rise in testosterone at puberty is partially responsible for a more severe diabetic state in male than female rats at adult age.[215] Testosterone also has been shown to enhance the hyperglycemic response to streptozotocin in genders and to increase the severity of diabetes in castrated males and females.[216] In contrast, preservation of fat and protein mass in the female may have occurred via mechanisms involving ovarian hormones through alterations in energy balance as described.[19,20,164-166,170]

In conclusion, similar to the effects of a negative energy balance induced by endurance exercise, male diabetic rats are more affected by diabetes with respect to alterations in growth and body composition than are female diabetic rats. Results demonstrate that females respond to diabetes in a metabolically different manner than do males. Although hormonal differences have been suggested to account for the gender dimorphism seen in this study, further studies are needed to understand the relationship(s) of these hormones to the metabolic control of growth and body composition in diabetic animals.

IV. SUMMARY

The purpose of this chapter was to compare and contrast the physiological mechanisms by which males and females regulate growth and body composition (summarized in Figures 9.1 and 9.4). Because the food supply is the single most important extrinsic factor affecting these variables, the control of feeding and nutrient metabolism was first described. Accordingly, a diet insufficient in energy and/or protein adversely will effect the rate of growth in the young and reduce protein and fat mass in adults. The regulation of energy expenditure and amino acid oxidation also was described to facilitate the understanding of how males and females respond to metabolic perturbations in order to maintain energy and protein homeostasis. From our current understanding of the literature, it is apparent that the hormonal milieu orchestrates to a large extent the metabolic response to energy, and protein availability and females differ remarkably in the mechanisms of control and the capacity to adjust to alterations of each. In this regard, examples to illustrate the similarities and differences between the sexes in response to altered energy and protein needs were provided. For example, chronic exercise and diabetes alter the energy and protein status of animals and require metabolic and dietary adjustments to support growth and maintain existing body tissues. Females appear to respond more favorably than males to periods of energy deficit and disease, perhaps due to the presence of ovarian hormones, which create variable differences in the mobilization and cellular utilization of energy substrates, body fat patterning, regulation of food intake, and energy efficiency. As such, females are less affected in terms of growth and loss of body tissues when subjected to chronic periods of negative energy balance. The physiological tradeoff of the sexual dimorphic response to energy imbalance appears to be a stronger propensity of the female toward obesity and the tendency for the female to retain fat mass despite increased energy expenditure due to physical activity. Exercise and overfeeding studies suggest that females gain and retain body and fat mass more efficiently than males.

Finally, several discoveries in the areas of endocrinology and metabolism have provided new insights into the control of food intake and energy conservation. Originally, leptin's function was described as a satiety factor acting centrally to reduce feeding behavior. However, leptin since has been demonstrated to be involved in energy substrate partitioning and thermogenesis in animals. In addition, the cloning of two new uncoupling proteins, one expressed predominately in white adipose tissue (UCP2), the other in skeletal muscle (UCP3), offer potential explanations for the observed gender differences in energy metabolism. In this regard, the regulation and function of both leptin and uncoupling proteins represent exciting new areas of research in metabolism and the study of growth and body composition.

ACKNOWLEDGMENT

The author wishes to thank Drs. G. Lynis Dohm, Stephen E. DiCarlo, Peter W. R. Lemon, Wayne E. Sinning, and Michael Jenkins for their scholarly influence behind the manuscript. Also, special thanks to Dr. James D. Fluckey for his insights into the development of the summary slides.

REFERENCES

1. Food and Agricultural Organization, World Health Organization, and United Nations University, *Energy and Protein Requirements,* Geneva: World Health Organization Technical Report Series 724, 1985.

2. National Research Council, National Academy of Sciences. Nutrient requirements of the laboratory rat, in *Nutrient Requirements of Laboratory Animals,* National Academy Press, Washington DC, 1978, 1.

3. Van Zant, R. S., Influence of diet and exercise on energy expenditure — a review, *Int. J. Sport Nutrition,* 2, 1, 1992.

4. Andersson, B., Xuefan, X., Rebuffe-Scrive, M., Terning, K., Krotkiewski, M., and Bjorntorp, P. A., The effects of exercise training on body composition and metabolism in men and women, *Intern. J. Obes.,* 15, 75, 1991.

5. Stein, T. P., Settle, R. G., Howard, K. A., and Diamond, C. E., Protein turnover and physical fitness in man, *Biochem. Med.,* 29, 207, 1983.

6. Zeman, F. J., Disorders of energy balance and body weight, in *Clinical Nutrition and Dietetics* (2nd ed.), Zeman, F. J., Ed., MacMilllan Publishing Company, New York, NY, 1991, 473.

7. Friedman, J. E. and Lemon, P. W. R., Effect of chronic endurance exercise on retention of dietary protein, *Int. J. Sports Med.,* 10(2), 118, 1989.

8. Phillips, M., Atkinson, S., Tarnopolsky, M. A., and MacDougall, J. D., Gender differences in leucine kinetics and nitrogen balance in endurance athletes, *J. Appl. Physiol.,* 75(5), 2134, 1993.

9. Tarnopolsky, M. A., MacDougal, J. D., and Atkinson, S. A., Influence of protein intake and training status on nitrogen balance and lean body mass, *J. Appl. Physiol.,* 64(1), 187, 1988.

10. Henderson, S. A., Black, A. L., and Brooks, G. A., Leucine turnover and oxidation in trained rats during exercise, *Am. J. Physiol.,* 249, E137, 1985.

11. White, T. P. and Brooks, G. A., [U-^{14}C] glucose, -alanine, -leucine oxidation in rats at rest and during two intensities of running, *Am. J. Physiol.,* 240, E155, 1981.

12. Lemon, P. W. R., Effect of exercise on protein requirements, *J. Sports Sci.,* 9, 53, 1991.

13. Ruby, B. C. and Bobergs, R. A., Gender differences in substrate utilization during exercise, *Sports Med.,* 17(6), 393, 1994.

14. Tarnopolsky, L. J., MacDougall, J. D., Atkinson, S. A., Tarnopolsky, M. A., and Sutton, J. R., Gender differences in substrate for endurance exercise, *J. Appl. Physiol.,* 68, 302, 1990.

15. Cortright, R. N., Chandler, M. P., Lemon, P. W. R., and DiCarlo, S. E., Daily exercise reduces fat, protein and body mass in male but not female rats, *Physiol. Behav.,* 62(1), 105, 1997.

16. Ganong, W. F., The Gonads: Development and function of the reproductive system, in *Review of Medical Physiology* (16th ed.), Lange Medical Publications, Los Altos, CA, 1993, 400.

17. Garn, S. M., Fat weight and fat placement in the female, *Science,* 125, 1091,1957.

18. Guyton, A. C., Female reproduction before pregnancy and the female hormones, in *Textbook of Medical Physiology* (8th ed.), W.B. Saunders, Philadelphia, PA, 1991, 905.

19. Hervey, E. and Hervey, G. R., The effects of progesterone on body weight and composition in the rat, *J. Endocrinol.,* 37, 361, 1967.

20. Wade, G. N., Gray, J. M., and Bartness, T. J., Gonadal influences on adiposity, *Int. J. Obes.,* 9(1), 83, 1985.

21. Hackney, A. C., Endurance training and testosterone levels, *Sports Med.*, 8(2), 117, 1989.

22. Dohm, G. L. and Louis, T. M., Changes in androstenedione, testosterone, and protein metabolism as a result of exercise, *Pro. Soc. Exp. Biol. Med.*, 158, 622, 1978.

23. Axelson, J. F., Forced swimming alters vaginal estrous cycles, body composition, and steroid levels without disrupting lordosis behavior or fertility in rats, *Physiol. Behav.*, 41, 471, 1987.

24. Fisher, E. C., Nelson, M. E., Frontera, W. R., Turksoy, R. N., and Evans, W. J., Bone mineral content and levels of gonadotropins and estrogens in amenorrheic running women, *J. Clin. Endocrinol.*, 62, 1232, 1986.

25. Hoyenga, K. B. and Hoyenga, K. T., Gender and energy balance: sex differences in adaptations for feast and famine, *Physiol. Behav.*, 28(3), 545, 1982.

26. Widdowson, E. M., The response of the sexes to nutritional stress, *Proc. Nutr. Soc.*, 35, 175, 1976.

27. Sinha, M., Human leptin: the hormone of adipose tissue, *Eur. J. Endocrinol.*, 136, 461, 1997.

28. Muoio, D. M., Dohm, G. L., Fiedorek, F. T., Tapscott, E. B., and Coleman, R. A., Leptin directly alters lipid partitioning in skeletal muscle, *Diabetes*, 46, 1360, 1997.

29. Gong, D. W, He, Y., Karas, M., and Reitman, M., Uncoupling protein-3 is a mediator of thermogenesis regulated by thyroid hormone, β3-adrenergic agonists, and leptin, *J. Biol. Chem.*, 272(39), 24129, 1997.

30. Borer, K. T., Hormonal and nutritional determinants of catch-up growth in hamsters, *Growth*, 51(1), 103, 1987.

31. Clutton-Brock, T. H., Harvey, P. H., and Ruder, B., Sexual dimorphism, socioeconomic sex ratio and body weight in primates, *Nature*, 797, 1977.

32. Hoyenga, K. B. and Hoyenga, K. T., *The Question of Sex Differences: Psychological, Cultural and Biological Issues,* Little Brown, Boston, MA, 1979.

33. Hutt, C., *Males and Females,* Penguin, Baltimore, MD, 1972.

34. Houpt, K. A., Houpt, T. R., and Pond, W. G., The pig as a model for the study of obesity and of control of food intake: A review, *Yale J. Biol. Med.*, 52, 307, 1979.

35. Krook, L. S., Larsson, and Rooney, J. R., The interrelationship of diabetes mellitus, obesity, and pyometra in the dog, *Am. J. Vet. Res.*, 21, 120, 1960.

36. Martin, R. J., Beverly, J. L., and Truett, G. E., Energy balance regulation, in *Animal Growth Regulation,* Campion, D. R., Hausman, G. J., and Martin, R. J., Eds., Plenum Press, New York, NY, 1989, 211.

37. Lebowitz, S. F., Brain neurochemistry and eating behavior, in *Advances in Biosciences: Vol. 60. Disorders of Eating Behavior: A Psychoendocrine Approach,* Ferrari, E. and Brambilla, F., Eds., Permagon Press, Oxford, UK, 1986, 65.

38. Ganong, W. F., Central regulation of visceral function, in *Review of Medical Physiology* (16th ed.), Lange Medical Publications, Los Altos, CA, 1993, 213.

39. Vasselli, J. R. and Maggio, C. A., Mechanisms of appetite and body-weight regulation, in *Obesity and Weight Control,* Frankle, R. T. and Yang M. U., Eds., Aspen, Rockville, MD, 1988.

40. Morley, J. E. and Levine, A. S., The pharmacology of eating behavior, *Annu. Rev. Pharm. Toxicol.*, 25, 127, 1985.

41. Morley, J. E. and Mitchell, J. E., Neurotransmitter/neuromodulator influences on eating, in A*dvances in Biosciences: Vol 60. Disorders of Eating Behavior: A Psychoneuro-endocrine Approach,* Ferrari, E. and Brambilla, F., Eds., Permagon Press, Elmsford, 1986, 11.

42. Shmazu, T., Central nervous system regulation of liver and adipose tissue metabolism, *Diabetologia*, 20, 343, 1981.
43. Steffens, A. B., Mogenson, G. J., and Stevenson, A. F., Blood glucose, insulin and free fatty acids after stimulation and lesions of the hypothalamus, *Am. J. Physiol.*, 222, 1446, 1972.
44. Woods, S. C. and Porte, D., Neural control of the endocrine pancreas, *Physiol. Rev*, 54, 596, 1974.
45. Oomura, Y. and Niijima, A., Chemosensitive neurons and neural control of pancreatic secretion, in *Diabetes 1982, Proceedings of the 11th Congress of the National Diabetes Foundation*, Mongola, E. N., Ed., Excerpta Medica, Amsterdam, 1983, 201.
46. Landsberg, L. and Young, J. B., The role of the sympathetic nervous system and catecholamines in the regulation of energy expenditure, *Am. J. Clin. Nutr.*, 38, 1018, 1983.
47. Brooks, G. A. and Fahey, T. D., Neural-endocrine control of metabolism, in *Exercise Physiology: Human Bioenergetics and Its Applications*, MacMillan, New York, NY, 1985, 163.
48. Rhoades, R. and Pflanzer, R., The pituitary gland, in *Human Physiology*, Rhoades, R. and Pflanzer, R., Eds., Saunders College Publishing, Philadelphia, PA, 1989, 403.
49. Press, M., Growth hormone and metabolism, *Diabetes/Metabolism Reviews*, 4(4), 391, 1988.
50. Baxter, J. D. and Rousseau, G. G., Glucocorticoid hormone action: an overview, in *Monographs on Endocrinology*, Baxter, L. D. and Rousseau, G. G., Eds., Springer-Verlag, Berlin, 1979.
51. Hadley, M. E., Thyroid hormones, in *Endocrinology*, Prentice Hall, New Jersey, 1992, 344.
52. Hervey, G. R., The effects of lesions in the hypothalamus in parabiotic rats, *J. Physiol.*, 145, 336, 1958.
53. Kennedy, G. C., The role of depot fat in the hypothalamic control of food intake in the rat, *Proc. R. Soc.*, 140, 578, 1953.
54. Coleman, D. L. and Hummel, K. P., Effects of parabiosis of normal with genetically diabetic mice, *Am. J. Physiol.*, 217, 1298, 1969.
55. Zhang, Y., Proenca, R., Maffei, M., Barone, M. L., and Friedman, J., Positional cloning of the mouse obese gene and its human homologue, *Nature*, 372, 425, 1994.
56. Caro, J. F., Sinha, M. K., Kolaczynski, J. W., Zhang, P. L., and Considine, R. V., Leptin: the tale of an obesity gene, *Diabetes*, 45, 1455, 1996.
57. Considine, R. V., Sinha, M. K., and Heiman, M. L., Serum immunoreactive-leptin concentrations in normal-weight and obese humans, *N. Eng. J. Med.*, 334, 292, 1996.
58. Trayburn, P., Duncan, J. S., and Rayner, D. V., Acute cold-induced suppression of ob (obese) expression in white adipose tissue of mice: mediation by the sympathetic system, *Biochem. J.*, 311, 1995.
59. Cusin, I., Sainsbury, A., Doyle, P., Rohner-Jeanenraud, F., and Jeanenraud, B., The ob gene and insulin: a relationship leading to clues to the understanding of obesity, *Diabetes*, 44, 1467, 1995.
60. De Vos, P., Saladin, R., Auwerx, J., and Staels, B., Induction of ob gene expression by corticosteroids is accompanied by body weight loss and reduced food intake, *J. Biol. Chem.*, 270, 15958, 1995.
61. Rohner-Jeanrenaud, F. and Jeanrenaud, B., Obesity, leptin, and the brain, *New Eng. J. Med.*, 334(5), 324, 1996.

62. Ezzell, C., Fat times for obesity research: tons of new information but how does it all fit together? *J. NIH. Res.,* 7, 39, 1995.

63. Rohner-Jeanrenaud, F., A neuroendocrine reappraisal of dual-center hypothesis: its implications for obesity and insulin resistance, *Int. Natl. J. Ob.,* 19, 517, 1995.

64. Pelleymounter, M. A., Cullen, M. J., Baker, M. B., Hecht, R., Winters, D., Boone, T., and Collins, F., Effects of the obese gene product on body weight regulation in ob/ob mice, *Science,* 269, 540, 1995.

65. Considine, R. V., Considine, E. L., Williams, C. J., Nyce, M. R., Magosin, S. A., Bauer, T. L., Rosato, E. L., Colberg, J., and Caro, J. F., Evidence against either a premature stop codon or the absence of obese gene mRNA in human obesity, *J. Clin. Invest.,* 95, 2986, 1995.

66. Tartaglia, L., Dembski, M., Weng, X. Deng, N., Culpepper, J., Devos, R., Richards, G. J., Campfield, L. A., Clark, F. T., Deeds, J., Muir, C., Sanker, S., Moriarty, A., More, K. J., Smutko, J. S., Mays, G. G., Woolf, E. A., Monroe, C. A., and Teper, R. I., Identification and expression cloning of a leptin receptor, *Cell,* 83, 1263, 1995.

67. Barinaga, M., Researchers nail down leptin receptor, *Science,* 271, 913, 1996.

68. Boston, B. A., Blaydon, K. M., Varnerin, J., and Cone, R. D., Independent and additive effects of central POMC and leptin pathways on murine obesity, *Science,* 278, 1644, 1997.

69. Poehlman, E. T., Exercise and its influence on resting energy metabolism: a review, *Med. Sci. Sports Exerc.,* 21(5), 515, 1989.

70. Westerterp, K. R. and Saris, W. H. M., Limits of energy turnover in relation to physical performance, achievement of energy balance on a daily basis, *J. Sports Sci.,* 9, 1, 1991.

71. Poehlman, E. T. and Horton, E. S., The impact of food intake and exercise on energy expenditure, *Nutr. Reviews.,* 47, 1129, 1989.

72. Sande, K. J. and Mahan, L., Nutritional care for weight management, in *Food, Nutrition, and Diet Therapy* (7th ed.), Krause, M. V. and Mahan, L. K., Eds., W.B. Saunders, Philadelphia, PA, 1984, 514.

73. Apfelbaum, M., Bostsarron, J., and Lacatis, D., Effect of caloric restriction and excessive caloric intake on energy expenditure, *Am. J. Clin. Nutr.,* 24, 1405,1971.

74. Elliot, D. L., Goldberg, L., Kuehl, K. S., and Bennett, W. M., Sustained depression of the resting metabolic rate after massive weight loss, *Am. J. Clin. Nutr.,* 49, 93, 1989.

75. Shibata, H. and Bukowiecki, L. J., Regulatory alterations of daily energy expenditure induced by fasting or overfeeding in unrestrained rats, *J. Appl. Physiol.,* 63, 465, 1987.

76. Keys, A., Brozek, J., Henshel, A., Mickelson, O., and Taylor, H. L., *The Biology of Human Starvation,* University of Minnesota Press, Minneapolis, MN, 1950.

77. Danforth, E., The role of thyroid hormones and insulin in the regulation of energy metabolism, *Am. J. Clin. Nutr.,* 38, 1006, 1983.

78. Saudek, C. D. and Felig, P., The metabolic events of starvation, *Am. J. Med.,* 60, 117, 1976.

79. Felig, P., Pozwfsky, E., Marliss, E., and Cahill, G. F., Alanine: key role in gluconeo-genesis, *Science,* 167, 1003, 1970.

80. Cahill, G. F., Starvation in man, *New Eng. J. Med.,* 282, 668, 1970.

81. Ghilardi, N., Ziegler, S., Wiestner, A., Stoffel, R., Heim, M., and Radek, S. C., Defective STAT signaling by the leptin receptor in diabetic mice, *Proc. Natl. Acad. Sci., USA,* 93, 6231, 1996.

82. Darnell, J. E., Kerr, L. M., and Stark, G. R., Jak-STAT pathways and trancriptional activation in response to IFNs and other extracellular signaling proteins, *Science,* 264, 1415, 1994.

83. Halaas, J. L., Gajiwala, K. S., Maffei, M., Cohen, S. L., Chait, B. T., Rabinowitz, D., Lallone, R. L., Burley, S. K., and Friedman, J. M., Weight-reducing effects of the plasma protein encoded by the obese gene, *Science*, 269, 543, 1995.

84. Levin, N., Nelson, C., Gurney, A., Vandlen, R., and Sauvage, F., Decreased food intake does not completely account for adiposity reduction after ob protein infusion, *Pro. Natl. Acad. Sci., USA,* 93, 1726, 1996.

85. Ahima, R. S., Prabakaran, D., Mantzoros, C., Qu, D., Lowell, B., Maratos-Flier, E., and Flier, J. S., Role of leptin in the neuroendocrine response to fasting, *Nature*, 382, 250.

86. Cortright, R. N. and Dohm, G. L., Mechanisms by which insulin and muscle contraction stimulate glucose transport, *Can. J. Appl. Physiol.,* 22(6), 430, 1997.

87. Cortright, R. N., Muoio, D. M., and Dohm, G. L., Skeletal muscle lipid metabolism: a frontier for new insights into fuel homeostasis, *J. Nutri. Biochem.,* 8, 228, 1997.

88. Shimabukuro, M., Koyama, K., Chen, G., Wang, M. Y., Trieu, F., Lee, Y., Newgard, C. B., and Unger, R., Direct antidiabetic effect of leptin through triglyceride depletion of tissues, *Proc. Natl. Acad. Sci., USA,* 94, 4637, 1997.

89. Walston, J., Silver, K., Bogardus, C., Knowler, W., Celi, F. S., Austin, S., Manning, B., Strosberg, A. D., Stern, M., Raben, N. R., Sorkin, J. D., Roth, J. R., and Shuldiner, A. R., Time of onset of non-insulin dependent diabetes mellitus and genetic variation in the β3-adrenergic-receptor gene, *N. Eng. J. Med.,* 333(6), 343, 1995.

90. Widen, E., Lehto, M., Kanninen, T., Walston, J., Shuldiner, A. R., and Groop, L. C., Association of polymorphism in the β3-adrenergic-receptor gene with features of the insulin resistance syndrome in Finns, *N. Eng. J. Med.,* 333(6), 348, 1995.

91. Collins, S., Daniel, K. W., Rohlfs, E. M., Ramkumar, V., Taylor, I. L., and Gettys, T. W., Impaired expression and functional activity of β_3- and β_1-adrenergic receptors in adipose tissue of congenitally obese (C57BL/6J ob/ob) mice, *Mol. Endocrinol.,* 8, 518, 1994.

92. Kurabayshi, T., Carey, D. G. P., and Morrison, N. A., The β_3-adrenergic receptor gene Trp6Arg mutation is over represented in obese women. Effects on weight, BMI, abdominal fat, blood pressure, and reproductive history in an elderly Australian population, *Diabetes*, 45, 1358, 1996.

93. Campfield, L. A., Smith, F. J., Guisez, Y., Devos, R., and Burn, P., Recombinant mouse ob protein: adiposity and central neural networks, *Science*, 269, 546, 1995.

94. Hickey, M., Houmard, J. A., Considine, R. V., Tyndall, G. L., Midgette, J. B., Gavigan, K. E., Weidner, M. L., McCammon, M. R., Israel, R. G., and Caro, J. E., Gender-dependent effects of exercise training on serum leptin levels in humans, *Am. J. Physiol.,* 272 (*Endocrinol. Metab.,* 35), E562, 1997.

95. Himms-Hagen, J., Role of brown adipose tissue thermogenesis in control of thermoregulatory feeding in rats: a new hypothesis that links thermostatic and glucostatic hypothesis for control of food intake, *Proc. Soc. Exp. Biol. Med.,* 208, 159, 1995.

96. Fleury, C., Neverova, M., Collins, S., Raimbault, S., Champigny, O., Levi-Meyrueis, C., Bouillaud, F., Seldin, M. F., Surwit, R. S., Ricquier, D., and Warden, C. H., Uncoupling protein-2: a novel gene linked to obesity and hyperinsulinemia, *Nature Genetics.,* 15, 269, 1997.

97. Gimeno, R. E., Dembski, M., Weng, X., Deng, N., Shyjan, A. W., Gimeno, C. J., Iris, F., Ellis, S. J., Woolf, E. A., and Tartaglia, L. A., Cloning and characterization of an uncoupling protein homologue, a potential molecular mediator of human thermogenesis, *Diabetes*, 46, 900, 1997.

98. Vidal-Puig, A., Solanes, G., Grujic, D., Flier, J. S., and Lowell, B. B., UCP-3: an uncoupling protein homologue expressed preferentially and abundantly in skeletal muscle and brown adipose tissue, *Biochem. Biophys. Res. Comm.,* 235, 79, 1997.

99. Boss, O., Samec, S., Paoloni-Giacobino, A., Rossier, C., Dullboo, A., Seydoux, J., Uzzin, P., and Giacobino, J. P., Uncoupling protein-3: a new member of the mitochondrial carrier family with tissue-specific expression, *FEBS Letters,* 408, 39, 1997.

100. Sedlock, D. A., Fissinger, J. A., and Melby, C. L., Effect of exercise intensity and duration on postexercise energy expenditure, *Med. Sci. Sports Exerc.,* 26, 662, 1989.

101. Gaesser, G. A. and Brooks, G. A., Metabolic bases of excess post-exercise oxygen consumption: a review, *Med. Sci. Sports Exerc.,* 16, 29, 1984.

102. Hagberg, J. M., Hickson, R. C., Ehsani, A. A., and Holloszy, J. O., Faster adjustments to and recovery from submaximal exercise in the trained state, *J. Appl. Physiol.,* 48, 218, 1980.

103. Poehlman, E. T., Melby, C. L., Badylak, S. F., and Calles, J., Aerobic fitness and resting energy expenditure in young adult males, *Metabolism,* 38, 85, 1989.

104. Bingham, S. A., Goldberg, G. R., and Coward, W. A., The effect of exercise and improved physical fitness on basal metabolism, *Br. J. Nutr.,* 61, 155, 1989.

105. Horton, T. J., Drougas, H., Sharp, T. A., Matinez, L. R., Reed, G. W., and Hill, J. O., Energy balance in endurance-trained females cyclists and untrained controls, *J. Appl. Physiol.,* 76(5), 1937, 1994.

106. Segal, K. R., Gutin, B., Albu, J., and Pi-Sunyer, F. X., Thermic effects of food and exercise in lean and obese of similar lean body mass, *Am. J. Physiol.,* E110, 1987.

107. Bouchard, C. A., Tremblay, A., Nadeau, A., Dussault, J., Despres, J. P., Theriault, G., Lipien, P., Serresse, O., Boulay, M., and Fournier, G., Long term exercise training with constant energy intake. I. Effect on body composition and selected metabolic variables, *Int. J. Obes.,* 14, 57, 1990.

108. U.S. Food and Nutrition Board, Protein and amino acids, in *Recommended Dietary Allowances* (10), National Academy Press, Washington, DC, 1989, 52.

109. Harstook, E. W. and Mitchell, H. H., The effect of age on the protein and methionine requirements in the rat, *J. Nutr.,* 60, 173, 1956.

110. Munro, H. N. and Crim, M., The proteins and amino acids, in *Modern Nutrition in Health and Disease* (7th ed.), Shils, M. E. and Young, V. R., Eds., Lea & Febiger, Philadelphia, PA, 1988, 1.

111. Butterfield, G. E., Amino acids and high protein diets, in *Ergogenics: Perspectives in Exercise Science and Sports Medicine,* Vol. 4, Lamb, D. R. and Williams, M. A., Eds., Brown and Benchmark, Carmel, CA, 1991, 87.

112. Butterfield, G. E. and Calloway, D. H., Physical activity improves protein utilization in young men, *Br. J. Nutr.,* 51, 171, 1984.

113. Hegsted, D. M., Balance studies, *J. Can. Diet Assoc.,* 36, 110, 1976.

114. Oddoye, E. A. and Margen, S., Nitrogen balance studies in humans: long-term effect of high nitrogen intake on nitrogen accretion, *J. Nutr.,* 109, 363, 1979.

115. Calloway, D. H. and Spector, H., Nitrogen balance as related to caloric and protein intake in active young men, *Am. J. Clin. Nutr.,* 2, 405, 1954.

116. Butterfield, G. E., Whole-body protein utilization in humans, *Med. Sci. Sports Exerc.,* 19, (5), S157, 1987.

117. Todd, K. S., Butterfield, G. E., and Calloway, D. H., Nitrogen balance in men with adequate and deficient energy intake at three levels of work, *J. Nutr.,* 114, 1984.

118. Felig, P. and Wahren, J., Amino acid metabolism in exercising man, *J. Clin. Invest.,* 50, 2703, 1971.

119. Yoshimura, H., Adult protein requirements, *Fed. Proc.,* 20, 103, 1961.

120. Haralambie, G. and Berg, A., Serum urea and amino nitrogen changes with exercise duration, *Eur. J. Appl. Physiol.,* 36, 39, 1976.

121. Refsum, H. E. and Stromme, S. B., Urea and creatinine production and excretion in urine during and after prolonged heavy exercise, *Scand. J. Clin. Lab. Invest.,* 33, 247, 1974.

122. Decombaz, J., Reinhardt, P., Anantharaman, K., and von Glutz, G., Biochemical changes in a 100 km run: free amino acids, urea, and creatinine, *Eur. J. Appl. Physiol.,* 41, 1, 1979.

123. Gontzea, I., Sutzescu, P., and Dumitrache, S., The influence of muscular activity on nitrogen balance and on the need of man for proteins, *Nutr. Reports Int.,* 10(1), 35, 1974.

124. Hood, D. A. and Terjung, R. L., Amino acid metabolism during exercise and following endurance training, *Sports Med.,* 9, 23, 1990.

125. Lemon, P. W. R., Does exercise alter dietary protein requirements? in *Advances in Sports Medicine,* Brouns F., Ed., Basel, Karger, 1991, 15.

126. Lemon, P. W. R. and Proctor, D. N., Protein intake and athletic performance, *Sports Med.,* 12(5), 313, 1991.

127. Paul, G. L., Dietary protein requirements of physically active individuals, *Sports Med.,* 8(3), 154, 1989.

128. Hagg, S. A., Morse, E. L., and Adibi, S. A., Effect of exercise on rates of oxidation, turnover, and plasma clearance of leucine in human subjects, *Am. J. Physiol.,* 242, E407, 1982.

129. Lemon, P. W. R., Nagle, F. J., Mullin, J. P., and Benevenga, N. J., *In vivo* leucine oxidation at rest and during two intensities of exercise, *J. Appl. Physiol.,* 53, 947, 1982.

130. Rennie, M. J., Edwards, R. H. T., Krywawych, S., Davies, C. T. M., Halliday, D., Waterlow, J. C., and Millward, D. J., Effect of exercise on protein turnover in man, *Clin. Sci.,* 1, 627, 1981.

131. Wolfe, R. R., Goodenough, R. D., Wolfe, M. H., Royle, F. T., and Nadel, E. R., Isotopic anaylsis of leucine and urea metabolism in exercising humans, *J. Appl. Physiol. (Respirt. Environ. Physiol.),* 52, 470, 1982.

132. Brouns, F., Saris, W. H. M., Stroecken, J., Beckers, E., Thijssen, R., Rehrer, N. J., and ten Hoor, F., Eating, drinking, and cycling. A controlled Tour de France simulation study, part II. Effect of diet manipulation, *Int. J. Sports Med.,* 10(1), S41, 1989.

133. Meredith, C. N., Zackin, M. J., Frontera, W. R., and Evans, W. J., Dietary protein requirements and body protein metabolism in endurance-trained men, *J. Appl. Physiol.,* 66, 2850, 1989.

134. Gontzea, I., Sutzescu, R., and Dumitrache, S., The influence of adaptation to physical effort in nitrogen balance in man, *Nutr. Reports Int.,* 11(3), 231, 1975.

135. Yoshimura, H., Inoue, T., Yamada, T., and Shiraki, K., Anemia during hard physical training (sports anemia) and its causal mechanism with special reference to protein nutrition, *World Rev. of Nutr. and Diet,* 35, 1, 1980.

136. Stein, T. P., Hoyr, R. W., O'Toole, M., Leskiw, M. J., Schluter, M. D., Wolfe, R. R., and Hiller, W. D., Protein and energy metabolism during prolonged exercise in trained athletes, *Int. J. Sports Med.,* 10(5)24, 311, 1989.

137. Young, V. R. and Bier, D. M., A kinetic approach to the determination of human amino acid requirements, *Nutr. Rev.,* 45, 289, 1987.

138. Young, V. R., Bier, D. M., and Pellet, P. L., A theoretical basis for increasing current estimates of the amino acid requirements in adult man, with experimental support, *Am. J. Nutr.,* 50, 80, 1989.

139. Newsholme, E. A., Crabtree, B., and Ardawi, M. S. M., Glutamine metabolism in lymphocytes: its biochemical, physiological and clinical importance, *Q. J. Exp. Physiol.*, 70, 473, 1985.

140. Newsholme, P., Curi, R., Gordon, S., and Newsholme, E. A., *Biochem. J.*, 239, 121, 1986.

141. Consolazio, C. F., Herman, L., Johnson, H. L., Nelson, R. A., Dramise, J. G., and Skala, J. H., Protein metabolism during intensive physical training in the young adult, *Am. J. Clin. Nutr.*, 28, 29, 1975.

142. Cortright, R. N., Rogers, M. E., and Lemon, P. W. R., Does protein intake during endurance training affect growth, nitrogen balance, or exercise performance? *Can. J. Appl. Physiol.*, 18(4), 403, 1993.

143. Baur, L. A., Waters, D. L., Allen, B. J., Blagojevic, N., and Gaskin, K. J., Nitrogen deposition in malnourished children with cystic fibrosis, *Am. J. Clin. Nutr.*, 53, 503,1991.

144. Blizzard, R. M., Martha, P. M., Kerrigan, J. R., Marus, N., and Rogol, A. D., Changes in growth hormone (GH) secretion and in growth during puberty, *J. Endocrinol. Invest.*, 12(Suppl. 3), 65, 1989.

145. Hervey, G. R. and Hutchinson, I., The effects of testosterone on body weight and composition in the rat, *J. Endocrinol.*, 577, XXIV–XXV, 1973.

146. French, V., The control of growth and size during development, in *The Physiology of Human Growth,* J. M., Tanner, J. M., and Preece, M. A., Eds., Cambridge University Press, Cambridge, 1989, 11.

147. Martha, P. M., Rogol, A. D., Veldhius, J. D., Kerrigan, J. R., Goodman, D. W., and Blizzard, R. M., Alterations in the pulsatile properties of circulating growth hormone concentrations during puberty in boys, *J. Clin. Endocr. Metab.*, 69, 563, 1989.

148. Slob, A. K. and Van der Werff Ten Bosch, J. J., Sex differences in body growth in the rat, *Physiol. Behav.*, 14, 353, 1975.

149. Beatty, W. W., Postnatal testosterone treatment fails to alter hormonal regulation of body weight and food intake of female rats, *Physiol. Behav.*, 10, 627,1973.

150. Perry, B. N., McCracken, A., Furr, B. J. A., and MacFie, H. J. H., Separate roles of androgen and estrogen in the manipulation of growth and efficiency of food utilization in female rats, *J. Endocr.*, 81, 35, 1979.

151. Tarttelin, M. F., Shyryne, J. E., and Gorski, R. A., Patterns of body weight change in rats following neonatal hormone manipulation: a "critical period" for androgen-induced growth increases, *Acta Endocrinologica*, 79, 177, 1975.

152. Beatty, W. W., Gonadal hormones and sex differences in nonreproductive behaviors in rodents: organizational and activational influences, *Horm. Behav.*, 12, 112, 1979.

153. Wade, G. N. and Gray, J. M., Gonadal effects of food intake and adiposity: a metabolic hypothesis, *Physiol. & Behav.*, 22, 583, 1979.

154. Ford, J. J. and Klindt, J., Sexual differentiation and the growth process, in *Animal Growth Regulation,* Campion, D. R., Hausman, G. J., and Martin, R. J., Eds., Plenum Press, New York, NY, 1989, 317.

155. Hill, J. O., Latiff, A., and DiGirolamo, M., Effects of variable caloric restriction on utilization of ingested energy in rats, *Am. J. Physiol.* (*Regulatory Integrative Comp. Physiol.*, 17), 248, R549, 1985.

156. Broom, J., Fleck, A., and Davidson, D. F., Biochemical adaptations in early starvation: observations in sex difference, *Proc. Nutr. Soc.*, 37, 92–93, 1978.

157. McPhee, C. P., Trappett, P. C., Neill, A. R., and Duncalfe, F., Changes in growth, appetite, food conversion efficiency and body composition in mice selected for high post-weaning weight gain on restricted feeding, *Theor. Appl. Genet.*, 57, 49, 1980.

158. Widdowson, E. M. and McCance, R. A., The effects of chronic undernutrition and of total starvation in growing and adult rats, *Br. J. Nutr.,* 104, 363, 1956.

159. Williams, J. P., Tanne, G., and Hughes, J. M., Catch-up growth in female rats after growth retardation during the suckling period. Comparison with males, *Pediat. Res.,* 8, 157, 1974.

160. Hall, R. L., Sexual dimorphism for size in seven nineteenth century northwest coast populations, *Human Biology,* 50, 150, 1978.

161. Hill, J. O., Talano, C. M., Nickel, M., and Digirolamo, M., Energy utilization in food-restricted female rats, *J. Nutr.,* 116, 2000, 1986.

162. Merimee, T. J., Misbin, R., and Pulkkinen, A., Sex variations in free fatty acids and ketones during fasting: evidence for a role of glucagon, *J. Clin. Endocrinol. Met.,* 46, 414, 1978.

163. Heymsfield, S. B., Gallagher, D., Poehlman, E. T., Wolper, C., Nonas, K., Nelson, D., and Wang, Z. M., Menopausal changes in body composition and energy expenditure, 29(3–4), 377, 1994.

164. Gavin, M. L., Gray, J. M., and Johnson, P. R., Estrogen-induced effects on food intake and body weight in ovariectomized, partially lipoectomized rats, *Physiol Behav.,* 32(1), 55, 1984.

165. Dudley, S. D., Gentry, T., Silverman, B. S., and Wade, G. N., Estradiol and insulin: independent effects of eating and body weight in rats, *Physiol. Behav.,* 22(1), 63, 1979.

166. Mueller, K. and Hsiao, S., Estrus- and ovariectomized-induced body weight changes: evidence for two estrogenic mechanisms, *J. Comp. Physiol. Psychol.,* 94(6), 1126, 1980.

167. Richard, D., Rochon, L., and Deshaies, Y., Effects of exercise training on energy balance of ovariectomized rats, *Am. J. Physiol.,* 253(22), R740, 1987.

168. Thomas, D. K., Storlien, L. H., Bellingham, W. P., and Gillette, K., Ovarian hormone effects on activity, glucoregulation, and thyroid hormones in the rat, *Physiol. Behav.,* 36(3), 567, 1986.

169. Galletti, F. and Klopper, A., The effect of progesterone on the quantity and distribution of body fat in the female rat, *Acta Endocrin.,* 46, 379, 1964.

170. Guyard, B., Fricker, J., Brigant, L., Betiulle, D., and Apfelbaum, M., Effects of ovarian steroids on energy balance in rats fed a highly palatable diet, *Metabolism*, 40(5), 529, 1991.

171. Gentry, R. T. and Wade, G. N., Androgenic control of food intake and body weight in male rats, *J. Comp. Physiol. Psychol.,* 90, 18, 1976.

172. Rivest, S., Landry, J., and Richard, D., Effect of exercise training on energy balance of orchidectomized rats, *Am. J. Physiol.,* 257(6), R550, 1989.

173. Bartness, T. J. and Wade, G. N., Effects of interscapular brown adipose tissue denervation on body weight and energy metabolism in ovariectomized and estradiol-treated rats, *Behav. Neurosci.,* 98, 674,1984.

174. Laudenslager, M. K. L., Wilkinson, C. W., Carlisle, H. J., and Hammel, H. T., Energy balance in ovariectomized rats with and without estrogen replacement, *Am. J. Physiol.,* 238, R400, 1980.

175. McElroy, J. F. and Wade, G. N., Short- and long-term effects of ovariectomy on food intake, body weight, carcass composition, and brown adipose tissue in rats, *Physiol. Behav.,* 39(3), 361, 1987.

176. Harris, P., Broadhurst, R. B., and Hodgson, D. R., Response of male and female rats to undernutrition: changes in energy utilization, body composition, and tissue turnover during undernutrition, *Br. J. Nutr.,* 52, 289, 1984.

177. Harris, P., Broadhurst, R. B., and Hodgson, D. R., Response of male and female rats to undernutrition: influence of ovariectomy on partition of nutrients by female rats during undernutrition, *Br. J. Nutr.*, 52, 307, 1984.

178. Durnin, J. V. G., Symposium of sex differences in response to nutritional variables, *Proc. Nutr. Soc.*, 35, 145, 1976.

179. Stuart, R. B. and Jacobson, B., Sex differences in obesity, in *Gender and Disordered Behavior*, Gomberg, E. S. and Franks, V., Eds., Brunner/Mazel, New York, NY, 1979, 241.

180. Despres, J. P., Tremblay, A., and Bouchard, C., Sex differences in the regulation of body fat mass with exercise training. *Abstracts 1st European Congress on Obesity*, Stockholm, Sweden, 1988.

181. Mulligan, K. and Butterfield, G. E., Discrepancies between energy intake and expenditure in physically active women, *Br. J. Nutr.*, 64, 23, 1990.

182. Despres, J. P., Bouchard, C., Savard, R., Tremblay, A., Marcotte, M., and Theriault, G., The effect of a 20-week endurance training program on adipose-tissue morphology and lipolysis in men and women, *Metabolism*, 33, 235, 1984.

183. Tremblay, A., Despres, J. P., Leblanc, C., and Bouchard, C., Sex dimorphism in fat loss in response to exercise-training, *J. Obes. Weight Regul.*, 3, 193, 1984.

184. Bjorntorp, P. A., Sex differences in the regulation of energy balance, *Am. J. Clin. Nutr.*, 49, 958, 1989.

185. Applegate, E. A., Upton, D. E., and Stern, J. S., Food intake, body composition and blood lipids following treadmill exercise in male and female rats, *Physiol. Behavior*, 28, 917, 1982.

186. Oscai, L. B., Mole, P. A., Krusack, L. M., and Holloszy, J. O., Detailed body composition analysis of female rats subjected to a program of swimming, *J. Nutr.*, 103, 412, 1973.

187. Crews, E. L., Fuge, K. W., Oscai, L. B., Holloszy, J. O., and Shank, R. E., Weight, food intake, and body composition effects of exercise and of protein deficiency, *Am. J. Physiol.*, 216(2), 359, 1969.

188. Oscai, L. B. and Holloszy, J. O., The effects of exercise training and feeding patterns on rat adipose cell size and number, *Can. J. Appl. Sport Sci.*, 1, 93, 1969.

189. Stevenson, J. A. F., Box, B. M., Feleki, V., and Beaton, J. R., Bouts of exercise and food intake in the rat, *J. Appl. Physiol.*, 21, 118, 1966.

190. Pitts, G. C., Body composition in the rat: interactions of exercise, age, sex, and diet, *Am. J. Physiol. (Regulatory Integrative Comp. Physiol.)*, 246, R495, 1984.

191. Shepard, R. E. and Gollnick, P. D., Oxygen uptake of rats at different work intensities, *Pflugers Arch. Eur. J., Physiol.*, 362, 219, 1976.

192. Nance, D. M., Bromley, R. J., Barnard, R. J., and Gorski, R. A., Sexually dimorphic effects of forced exercise on food intake and body weight in the rat, *Physiol. Behavior*, 19(1), 155, 1977.

193. Oscai, L. B., Mole, P. A., and Holloszy, J. O., Effects of exercise on cardiac weight and mitochondria in male and female rats, *Am. J. Physiol.*, 220(6), 1944, 1971.

194. Tokuyama, K., Saito, M., and Okuda, H., Effects of wheel running on food intake and weight gain of male and female rats, *Physiol. Behavior*, 28(5), 899, 1982.

195. Dohm, G. L., Hecker, A. L., Brown, W. E., Klain, G. J., Puente, F. R., Askew, E. W., and Beecher, G. R., Adaptation of protein metabolism to endurance training. Increased amino acid oxidation in response to training, *Biochem. J.*, 164, 705, 1977.

196. Tapscott, E. B., Kasperek, G. J., and Dohm, G. L., Effect of training on muscle protein turnover in male and female rats, *Biochem. Med.*, 27, 254, 1982.

197. Chatterton, R. T., Hrycyk, L., and Hickson, R. C., Effect of endurance exercise on ovulation in the rat, *Med. Sci. Sport Exerc.*, 27(11), 1509, 1995.

198. Caston, A., Farrell, P. A., and Deaver, D. R., Exercise training-induced changes in anterior pituitary gonadotrope of the female rat, *J. Appl. Physiol.*, 79(1), 194, 1995.

199. Schwartz, S. M., Nunez, A. A., and Axelson, J. F., Effects of voluntary exercise on sexual behavior of female rats, *Physiol. Behav.*, 30(6), 963, 1983.

200. Anantharaman-Barr, G. H. and Decombaz, J., The effect of wheel running and the estrous cycle on energy expenditure in female rats, *Physiol. Behav.*, 46, 259, 1989.

201. Lamb, D. R., Van Huss, W. D., Carrow, R. E., Heusner, W. W., Weber, J. C., and Kertzer, R., Effects of prepubertal physical training on growth, voluntary exercise, cholesterol, and basal metabolism, *The Research Quarterly*, 40(1), 123, 1969.

202. Tipton, C. M., Matthes, R. D., and Maynard, J. A., Influence of chronic exercise in rat bones, *Med. Sci. Sports Exerc.*, 4, 55, 1972.

203. Mondon, C. E., Dolkas, C. B., Sims, C., and Reaven, G. M., Spontaneous running activity in male rats: effect of age, *J. Appl. Physiol.*, 58(5), 1553, 1985.

204. Westerterp, K., Relationship between physical activity related energy expenditure and body composition: a gender difference, *Int. J. Obesity*, 21(3), 184, 1997.

205. Ballor, D. L. and Keesey, R. E., A meta-analysis of the factors affecting exercise-induced changes in body mass, fat mass and fat-free mass in males and females, *Internatl. J. Obes.*, 15(11), 717, 1991.

206. Meijer, G. A. L., Janssen, G. M. E., Westerterp, K. R., Verhoeven, F., Saris, V. H. M., and ten Hoor, F., The effect of a 5-month endurance-training program on physical activity: evidence for a sex-difference in the metabolic response to exercise, *Eur. J. Appl. Physiol.*, 62, 11, 1991.

207. Rolls, B. J. and Rowe, E. A., Dietary obesity: permanent changes in body weight, *J. Physiol.*, 272, 2P, 1977.

208. Rothwell, N. J. and Gorman, A. N., Mechanisms of weight gain and loss in reversible obesity in the rat, *J. Physiol.*, 276, 60P, 1978.

209. Pitts, G. C. and Bull, L. S., Exercise, dietary obesity, and growth in the rat, *Am. J. Physiol.*, 232, R38, 1977.

210. Selafani, A. and Springer, D., Dietary obesity in adult rats: similarities to hypothalamic and human obesity syndromes, *Physiol. Behav.*, 17, 461, 1976.

211. Rolls, B. J. and Rowe, E. A., Exercise and the development and persistence of dietary obesity in male and female rats, *Physiol. Behav.*, 23(2), 241, 1979.

212. Tepper, B. J. and Kanarek, R. B., Dietary self-selection patterns of rats with mild diabetes, *J. Nutr.*, 115, 699, 1985.

213. Friedman, M. I., Hyperphagia in rats with experimental diabetes mellitus: a response to a decreased supply of utilizable fuels, *J. Comp. & Physiol. Psych.*, 92(1), 109, 1978.

214. Cortright, R. N., Collins, H. L., Chandler, M. P., Lemon, P. W. R., and DiCarlo, S. E., Diabetes reduces growth and body composition more in male than in female rats, *Physiol. Behav.*, 60(5), 1233, 1996.

215. Ostenson, C. G., Grill, V., and Roos, M., Studies on sex dependency of β-cell susceptibility to streptozotocin in a rat model of type II diabetes mellitus, *Exp. Clin. Endocrinol.*, 93, 241, 1989.

216. Rossini, A. A., Williams, R. M., Appel, M. C., and Like, A. A., Sex differences in multiple-dose streptozotocin model of diabetes, *Endocrinology*, 103(4), 1518, 1978.

CHAPTER 10

Nutritional Implications of Gender Differences in Metabolism: Energy Metabolism, Human Studies

Klaas R. Westerterp

CONTENTS

I. INTRODUCTION

Women and men show pronounced differences in energy metabolism. On average, women have a lower energy expenditure, mainly as a result of differences in body composition, compared with men. There are indications that the regulation of energy balance, adapting energy intake to expenditure or energy expenditure to intake, are different between women and men as well. Hormonal and behavioral differences might play a role.

Gender differences in energy metabolism may be the result of sexually dimorphic evolutionary pressures,[1] i.e., differences in selection pressures because of sexual selection and differences in reproductive roles. In humans, where women do a large proportion of the initial caretaking of the offspring including pregnancy and lactation, selection has favored small female size with a relatively large energy store as an adaptation to starvation resistance. The same women possibly have preferred large and aggressively active men to protect the offspring.[1] The resultant outcome may be a gender difference in body size and body composition with important consequences for energy metabolism and in the maintenance of energy balance.

This chapter is divided in two main parts: determinants of energy utilization and evidence for and against energy conservation in females. Determinants of energy utilization are presented separately for the three components of daily energy expenditure: sleeping or basal energy expenditure, diet-induced energy expenditure, and activity-induced energy expenditure. Evidence for and against energy conservation in females is illustrated by the response to changes in energy intake and energy expenditure. Additional indicators include the sexual dimorphic response to changes in ambient temperature and the response to energy intake with alcohol.

II. DETERMINANTS OF ENERGY UTILIZATION

Daily energy expenditure consists of four components: the sleeping metabolic rate (SMR), the energy cost of arousal, the thermic effect of food- or diet-induced energy expenditure (DEE), and the energy cost of physical activity (AEE). Sometimes daily energy expenditure is divided into three components, taking sleeping metabolic rate and the energy cost of arousal together as energy expenditure for maintenance or basal metabolic rate (BMR). BMR is usually the main component of average daily metabolic rate (ADMR). The analysis of determinants of energy expenditure and its components will be illustrated with data from a study of the effects of diet composition on energy metabolism in 37 subjects as presented in Table 10.1.[2,3,4] Subjects spent 36 h in a respiration chamber, followed by a two-week observation of ADMR in daily life with doubly labeled water. Body composition

Table 10.1 Subject Characteristics

	Women (n = 17)	Men (n = 20)
Age (y)	25.6 ± 5.1 (20–35)	28.1 ± 5.4 (19–35)
Height (m)	1.67 ± 0.06 (1.56–1.75)	1.81 ± 0.05 (1.72–1.90)**
Body mass (kg)	65.4 ± 7.5 (53.6–79.6)	79.8 ± 10.9 (59.6–101.4)**
Body mass index (kg · m^{-2})	23.6 ± 2.1 (19.4–28.0)	24.4 ± 2.6 (20.0–29.7)
Fat-free mass*	44.5 ± 4.0 (37.7–50.1)	61.5 ± 5.6 (50.3–73.1)**
Body fat (%)*	31 ± 7 (20–42)	22 ± 8 (9–32)**

* As assessed with deuterium dilution.
**Significantly different for women ($p < 0.001$).

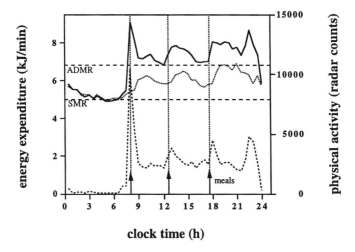

Figure 10.1 Energy expenditure (left axis; upper line: total energy expenditure; intermediate line: resting energy expenditure) and physical activity (right axis; lower line) as measured over a 24 h interval in a respiration chamber. Data are average values of 37 subjects as presented in Table 10.1; ADMR: average daily metabolic rate; SMR: sleeping metabolic rate; arrows on the horizontal axis denote meal times.

was assessed with deuterium dilution. Figure 10.1 shows the average time pattern of energy expenditure and the components and of physical activity, as measured over the 24 h cycle in a respiration chamber in the 37 subjects. Table 10.2 shows the average values over 24 h by gender. Following, the data will be discussed against the presently available information in the literature.

Table 10.2 Data on Energy Expenditure as Measured During a 36 h Stay in a Respiration Chamber

	Women (n = 17)	Men (n = 20)
EI (MJ/d)	8.52 ± 0.53 (7.49–9.03)	10.77 ± 0.90 (8.84–12.52)***
SMR (MJ/d)	6.34 ± 0.48 (5.79–7.04)	7.85 ± 0.81 (6.31–9.69)***
DEE (MJ/d)	0.99 ± 0.27 (0.57–1.65)	1.27 ± 0.33 (0.65–2.01)**
AEE (MJ/d)	1.54 ± 0.55 (0.85–2.59)	1.66 ± 0.48 (0.74–2.73)
24EE (MJ/d)	8.87 ± 0.81 (7.48–10.45)	10.77 ± 1.11 (8.12–12.79)***
ADMR (MJ/d)	11.15 ± 1.57 (7.85–15.28)	13.69 ± 2.13 (10.18–19.68)***
PA (counts/d)	1152 ± 325 (831–2017)*	1004 ± 190 (572–1256)*
ADMR/SMR	1.76 ± 0.26 (1.35–2.52)	1.74 ± 0.16 (1.48–2.05)

Note: Energy intake, EI; sleeping metabolic rate, SMR; diet induced energy expenditure, DEE; activity induced energy expenditure, AEE; 24 h energy expenditure, 24 EE) and energy expenditure as measured over a two week interval under daily living conditions with doubly labeled water (average daily metabolic rate, ADMR) and simultaneous assessment of physical activity with a tri-axial accelerometer (PA).

* Observations in 14 women and 16 men.
**Significantly different with women (p < 0.01).
***Significantly different with women (p < 0.001).

A. Sleeping or Basal Energy Expenditure

Sleeping or basal metabolic rate usually is compared between subjects by standardizing to an estimate of metabolic body size. Fat-free body mass seems to be the best predictor.[5] As stated by the same authors, energy expenditure should not be divided by the absolute FFM value as the relationship between energy expenditure and FFM has a y and x intercept significantly different from zero (Figure 10.2). Comparing SMR per kg FFM between women and men for the subjects as presented in Table 10.1 results in a significant difference: 0.143 ± 0.012 and 0.128 ± 0.080 MJ/kg for women and men, respectively, ($p < 0.0001$). The smaller the FFM the higher the SMR/FFM ratio; thus, the SMR per kg FFM is on average higher in women as compared to men. The accepted method of comparing SMR or BMR data is by regression analysis. Covariates to be included are FFM, fat mass (FM), age, and gender. Given these variables, gender does not emerge as a significant contributor to the explained variation. In a group of 17 women and 20 men (Table 10.1) the significant variables were FFM and FM: SMR (MJ/d) = 1.39 + 0.93 FFM (kg) + 0.039 FM (kg); $r^2 = 0.93$. Apparently, SMR was not different for women and men when corrected for individual differences in body composition. However, there remains a (theoretical) problem with this approach. The covariates are significantly different for the two groups without much overlap as demonstrated by Figure 10.2 for FFM. Ideally, one should compare SMR or BMR in a group of women and men with comparable body composition. However, other systematic differences then will occur. For example, women would have to be very muscular and lean, (i.e., endurance athletes), or men would have to be obese.

Other studies have shown the similarity of SMR and BMR of women and men when properly adjusted for differences in body composition. Klausen et al.[6] compared BMR in 109 women and 53 men, as measured in a respiration chamber. There were no significant differences between the sexes with respect to the regression lines of BMR or adjusted SMR on FFM. However, some studies showed women to have a higher or a lower SMR and BMR compared with men after adjusting for differences in body composition.[7,8,9] The differences were largely a function of the menstrual cycle phase that the women were in at the time of measurement. Bisdee et al.[10] showed that SMR in women was lowest in the late follicular phase and highest in the late luteal phase with an average difference between the two extremes of $6.1 \pm 2.7\%$. The difference was related to luteinizing hormone concentrations in urine. Ferraro et al.[7] also observed higher BMR values in women in the luteal phase compared with women in the follicular phase of the menstrual cycle, resulting in no differences between adjusted BMR, FFM, and FM in a group of 121 men and 114 women, ages 18 to 85. A significantly lower adjusted BMR was found for women in a subgroup analysis of 36 women and men over 50 y of age from the same study.[7] Meijer et al.[9] described SMR with an equation accounting for an effect of the menstrual cycle (MC): SMR (MJ/d) = 0.73 + 0.101 FFM (kg) + 0.023 (FM) + 0.364 MC, where MC is 0 for men and for preovulation women and 1 for postovulation women.

In conclusion, SMR and BMR are comparable for women and men when properly adjusted for body composition. There are indications that postovulation women

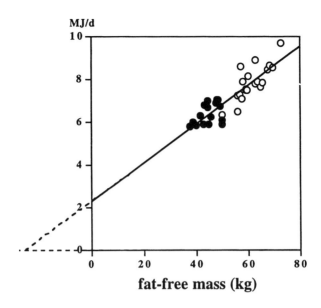

Figure 10.2   Sleeping metabolic rate (SMR) plotted as a function of fat-free mass (FFM) for the subjects described in Table 10.1 (women: closed symbols; men: open symbols) with the calculated linear regression line (SMR (MJ/d) = 2.27 + 0.091 FFM (kg), r^2 = 0.78).

have the same or slightly higher values and preovulation and postmenopausal women have the same or slightly lower values than men.

B. Diet Induced Energy Expenditure

DEE is defined as the increase in energy expenditure above basal fasting level divided by the energy content of the food ingested and is commonly expressed as a percentage. The postprandial rise in energy expenditure lasts for several hours and is often regarded as completely terminated at approximately ten hours after the last meal, but there is still an argument as to when the postabsorptive state is reached. Weststrate et al.[11] did extensive studies on the assessment of DEE. Measuring DEE in postabsorptive subjects and using a meal size of maximally 2.1 MJ in women and 2.6 MJ in men or about 25% of daily energy intake, 90% of the DEE was observed within four hours after the meal. This is about the maximum duration of a ventilated hood measurement where subjects have to be at rest. Using a mixed test meal, DEE was about 8% of the ingested energy. Comparing the measured DEE value with theoretical estimates, DEE comprises hardly more than the obligatory component of digestion and absorption, leaving only 1 to 2% for temporary storage. The facultative component will be negligible in this situation. DEE in the free living condition based upon the observations mentioned previously and is assumed to be 10% of ADMR in subjects consuming the average mixed diet and being in energy balance.

Methodological problems in the measurement of DEE such as the choice of meal size and the length of the measurement interval can be circumvented by measuring

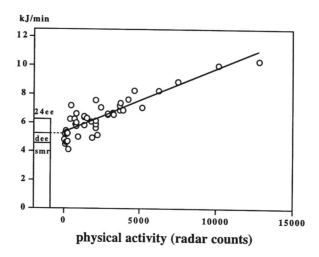

Figure 10.3 Mean energy expenditure over 30 min intervals from a 24 h observation in one subject, plotted as a function of physical activity measured with Dopplar radar. Resting energy expenditure is calculated as the y intercept of the linear regression line, and diet-induced energy expenditure (DEE, including arousal) is the difference between resting energy expenditure and sleeping metabolic rate (SMR).

DEE over 24 h in a respiration chamber.[12] Mean 24 h activity-induced energy expenditure (AEE) is calculated as the product of the mean activity measured by radar and the slope of the regression line between energy expenditure and activity. AEE is subtracted from 24 h EE, leaving SMR, arousal, and DEE (Figure 10.3). Table 10.2 shows the data on DEE in the group of 37 subjects, calculated as described previously. Given lower absolute energy intakes, DEE was expected to be lower in women than in men. However, when DEE was expressed as a percentage of energy intake the values for women and men, 11.7 ± 3.4 and 11.8 ± 2.7, respectively, were the same. The time pattern of DEE throughout the day was comparable for women and men as well (Figure 10.4). In absolute terms, total DEE is lower in females due to the lower absolute and relative total energy intakes. For both genders, the consumption of a progressively lower energy intake (i.e., gymnasts, ballerinas, wrestlers) will result in a proportionately lower total DEE. In conclusion, DEE is comparable for women and men when adjusted for energy intake.

C. Activity-Induced Energy Expenditure

Activity-induced energy expenditure is the most variable component of ADMR. The doubly labeled water method has provided truly quantitative estimates of AEE in free-living humans. Unfortunately, however, there is no consensus on the way to normalize AEE for differences in body size. A frequently used method to quantify physical activity is to express ADMR as a multiple of BMR or SMR.[13] This assumes that the variation in ADMR is due to body size and physical activity. The effect of body size on ADMR is corrected for by expressing ADMR as a multiple of BMR or SMR. Carpenter et al.[14] stated that the expression of ADMR as a multiple of

kJ/min

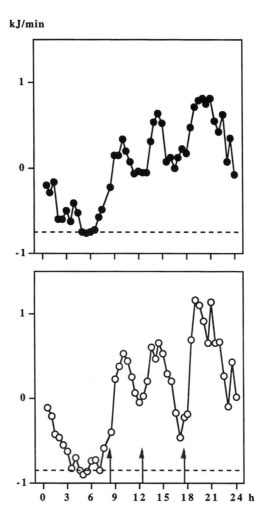

Figure 10.4 The mean pattern of diet-induced energy expenditure throughout the day, calculated by plotting the residual of the individual relationship between energy expenditure and physical activity (Figure 10.3) in time, for women (upper graph) and for men (lower graph). The arrows denote the time of meals.

BMR or SMR for comparison between subjects is precluded by the fact that the nature of the relation between ADMR and BMR or SMR is highly variable between studies and often has a nonzero intercept. They proposed to adjust ADMR for BMR or SMR to correct for the effect of body size in a linear regression analysis. Our results from 37 subjects showed no difference between the two methods; the regression between ADMR and SMR had an intercept not significantly different from zero (Figure 10.5).

An alternative method that studies have used is to adjust AEE for differences in body size has been the expression of AEE per kg body mass, assuming that energy

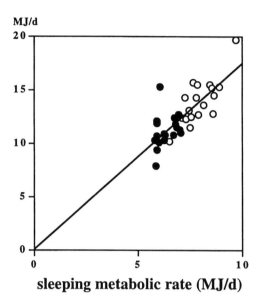

Figure 10.5 Average daily metabolic rate (ADMR) plotted as a function of sleeping metabolic rate (SMR) for the subjects described in Table 10.1 (women: closed symbols; men: open symbols) with the calculated linear regression line (ADMR (MJ/d) = 0.02 + 1.748 SMR (MJ/d), r^2 = 0.61).

expenditure associated with physical activity is weight-dependent. However, not all daily activities are mass-dependent. Prentice et al.[15] proved that normalizing AEE by dividing by body mass to the exponent 1.0 (body mass[1.0]) over-corrects for body size in heavier people, making them appear less active. They suggested that an exponent close to 0.5 is more appropriate for sedentary lifestyles. Alternately, the authors propose that the energy expenditure associated with physical activity be adjusted for differences in body size by expressing BMR or SMR, by using the metabolic body mass as the denominator or body mass to the exponent 0.66 to 0.75. Prentice et al.[15] have stated that it is not always possible to recommend a general coefficient for adjusting AEE and that great caution must be exercised when interpreting AEE data from individuals of markedly different body sizes.

Although respiration chambers can provide excellent quantitation of ADMR, the participant is limited to the confines of the chamber (i.e., not a free-living situation). As stated above, the doubly labeled water method provides an excellent quantification of the AEE in a free living situation; however, the cost is a limitation. Therefore, movement quantification devices such as pedometers, accelerators, and even global positioning satellite (GPS) devises have been used. In the group of 37 subjects studied, the authors obtained the highest correlation of physical activity ADMR/SMR with a body-fixed movement detector (tri-axial accelerometer for movement registration, TRACMOR).[2]

The most elaborate analysis of data on AEE was the analysis of Black et al.[16] of all doubly labeled water estimates of ADMR until the middle of 1994. It included 574 measurements accompanied by direct measurements of BMR in subjects in the

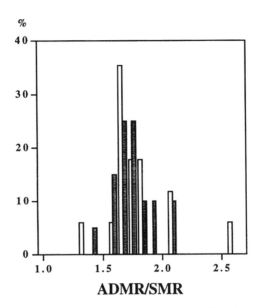

Figure 10.6 Frequency distribution of the activity index ADMR/SMR for the subjects described in Table 10.1 (women: open bars; men: shaded bars).

normal free-living state, namely 319 women and 255 men. There was a constant gender effect on ADMR and the components BMR and AEE, women being 11% lower than men of the same age and body size. Differences between women and men nearly were removed by adjusting for body size by using ADMR/BMR. The distribution of ADMR/BMR had a median value of 1.6 for both women and men. The frequency distribution of activity index ADMR/SMR of the subjects described in Table 10.1 is comparable (Figure 10.6) with a slightly higher median value due to the fact that SMR is slightly lower than BMR.

In conclusion, AEE is comparable for women and men when adjusted for body size and body composition by expressing ADMR as a multiple of BMR. When one examines Table 1.1 from Chapter 1, it is apparent that the AEE when expressed per kilogram LBM is similar between males and females performing endurance exercise.

III. EVIDENCE FOR AND AGAINST ENERGY CONSERVATION IN FEMALES

There is evidence that women and men respond metabolically in a different manner to a disturbance of energy balance. Similar to the data in animals females lose less weight when energy intake is restricted with a weight-reducing diet or when energy expenditure is increased with an exercise program. On the other hand, it was suggested that women do not gain weight, or even lose weight, when alcohol is added to the diet although the opposite seems to hold for men. Finally, further support for a gender difference in energy regulations is given by the finding that women are more sensitive to changes in ambient temperature than men. These phenomena mentioned will be described in more detail.

A. Response to Changes in Energy Intake and Energy Expenditure

The majority of the studies on energy balance in relation to changes in energy intake and energy expenditure were studies on weight reduction, i.e., the effect of a reduction of energy intake or an increase of energy expenditure. The latter usually is accomplished with an exercise program. For obvious reasons there are very few studies on the effects of an increase in energy intake or a restriction of physical activity. Additionally, there is a lack of well-controlled, comparative studies on the effect of changes in energy intake or energy expenditure on energy balance that included both males and females.

In a meta-analysis of the effects of exercise and/or dietary restriction on resting metabolic rate, Ballor and Poehlman[17] reviewed 33 studies, including 491 women and 147 men. The average duration of the weight loss program was 12 weeks in which men lost significantly more weight than women (17.5 vs. 11.5 kg, $p < 0.05$). However, men weighed more and had a higher resting metabolic rate (RMR). Body mass loss as a percentage of the initial value was similar for men (~16%) and women (~12%). There was no statistically significant difference between women and men in the change of RMR following exercise training and/or dietary restriction. The overall RMR decrease was 12% in women as well as men, and exercise training did not affect diet-induced thermogenesis. The lack of significant gender differences in the percentage body mass or RMR might have been a function of the low number of studies that involved males.

Eight of the 33 studies analyzed included male subjects and four included female as well as male subjects. One of the latter studies included as many as 38 women and 40 men and was well-controlled.[18] Subjects were supplied with an individually tailored weight maintenance diet for at least three weeks, followed by a weight reduction period of 13 weeks during which the supplied diet was restricted individually with 4.2 MJ/d. Subjects were encouraged to maintain their habitual physical activity pattern. Body mass loss was the same for women and men (11.7 ± 3.8 and 12.6 ± 3.2 kg) of which 10.3 ± 3.6 and 9.8 ± 3.1 kg, respectively, was fat. However, women lost less FFM than men (1.4 ± 1.3 vs. 2.9 ± 1.7 kg; $p < 0.001$), and consequently the decrease in RMR in women was smaller than in men, (0.27 ± 0.40 and 0.50 ± 0.26 kJ/min; $p < 0.01$). The authors did not discuss the discrepancy between the gender difference in RMR response with regard to the finding of body mass and fat loss being similar. However, the measured difference in RMR response of 0.23 kJ/min would add to a cumulated difference of 15 MJ over the observation interval, assuming a linear change of the difference from 0 at the start to 0.23 kJ/min at 13 weeks. This difference is not detectable with the available technology for the measurement of body composition. More importantly, subjects with an initial abundance of visceral fat (i.e., men) did not lose more body weight, but rather more visceral fat than subjects with less visceral fat. The fact that many studies have reported larger fat losses in subjects with more abdominal fat is explained by larger energy deficits, through the provision of standardized energy-restricted diet (energy deficit of 4.2 MJ/d).

Animal studies have shown that exercise without energy restriction causes an increase in energy expenditure without a proportional increase or even a decrease in EI. Thus, body mass, specifically fat mass, decreases when animals are exercised, despite an increase in FFM. Female rats show a better preservation of body mass through an increase in food intake although a fall in intake has been observed in exercised male rats.[19,20] Similar observations have been made in man.[21,22,23]

Westerterp et al.[22] trained sedentary subjects to run a half marathon after 44 weeks, without controlling EI. ADMR, as measured with doubly labeled water, showed an average increase of 39% in both sexes from the start of the training onward although SMR tended to decrease. EI showed a tendency to increase in the women and a tendency to drop in the men. Body mass did not change in both sexes until the observation at 40 weeks when the mean change in women and men was -0.7 ± 2.0 (ns) and -1.3 ± 1.3 kg; ($p < 0.01$), respectively (Figure 10.7). Fat mass (FM) also changed less in women than in men, -2.8 ± 1.7 ($p < 0.01$) and -4.5 ± 2.2 kg ($p < 0.01$), respectively. There was a close relation between the loss in FM and the initial body fatness in men but not in women (Figure 10.8). The higher the initial fat mass the larger the fat loss. Women tended to preserve their energy balance more strongly than men and consequently loss of FM was significantly less. The gender difference is probably attributable to an increased energy intake in women. The men's reported energy intake after 8-, 20-, and 40-week training was significantly lower than ADMR. In the women, differences between intake and expenditure did not reach significance at any stage of the training program.

Two meta-analyses of the relation between physical activity, as derived from ADMR measured with doubly labeled water and body composition, confirm the gender difference described. Westerterp et al.[24] analyzed 96 existing data sets with observations of FM and habitual activity level (PA). In contrast with females ($r = 0.10$, n.s.), there was an independent relationship between PA and FM in males ($r = -0.41$; $p < 0.05$), such that a higher PA was related to a lower FM. Westerterp and Goran[25] analyzed existing data sets with observations on ADMR, BMR, and % body fat including 290 healthy subjects age 18 to 49 y. PA was quantified by adjustment of ADMR for BMR as suggested by Carpenter et al.[14] The result was a gender difference in the relationship between PA and body composition. In males, there was a significant inverse cross-sectional relationship between activity energy expenditure and % body fat, whereas no such relationship was apparent in females. This suggests that females probably do not lose much fat when they adopt a higher level of PA.

B. Additional Indicators for Gender Differences in Energy Regulation

Examples of gender differences in energy regulation are evident in the relationship between alcohol intake and body weight and between ambient temperature and heat production. Briefly, in women there is an inverse relation between alcohol intake and body mass index although in men there is no such association.[26] With regard to

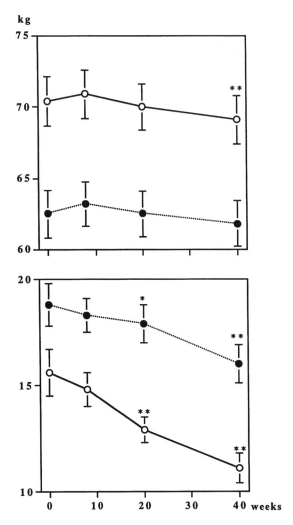

Figure 10.7 Mean body mass (upper figure) and fat mass (lower figure) with the standard error of estimate in 23 novice athletes (11 women: closed symbols; and 12 men: open symbols) before and 8, 20, and 40 weeks after the start of a training period in preparation for the half-marathon (adapted from Westerterp et al.[22]). Value significantly different from pretraining value: * p <0.05; ** p < 0.01.

ambient temperature, women compared with men showed earlier signs of thermal discomfort when the ambient temperature was lowered or raised.[27]

Colditz et al.[26] studied relations between alcohol intake, body mass index, and diet in 89,538 women and 48,493 men in two cohort studies. Total energy intake increased with alcohol consumption in women with the increase being even more pronounced in men. However, energy intake without the contribution of alcohol showed a small inverse relation with alcohol intake in women but not in men. There are indications that alcohol energy is wasted. The result was a clear inverse relation

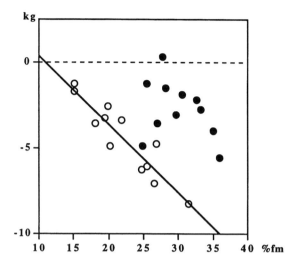

Figure 10.8 Fat mass change in novice athletes from before until 40 weeks after the start of a training period in preparation for the half-marathon, plotted against the initial body fatness in women (closed symbols) and men (open symbols) with the calculated linear regression line for men (adapted from Westerterp et al.[22]).

between alcohol consumption and body mass index among women but not among men. The difference in associations between alcohol intake and body mass index was not explained by differences in cigarette smoking or type of beverage consumption. One explanation could be a decrease in the prevalence of use and total intake of sugar added to food and beverages with increasing alcohol consumption in women but not in men. The overall impression was that women compensated more for an increase in energy intake with alcohol than men. Paradoxically this resulted in an inverse relation between alcohol intake and body mass index for women but not for men,[28] perhaps due to differing metabolic pathways for alcohol metabolism from carbohydrates, protein, and fat.

Differences in thermoregulation between women and men are linked closely to gender differences in body size and body composition. The greater fat content, enhancing insulation, may not provide women with a thermoregulatory advantage over men. First, women generally have a smaller total body mass resulting in a greater surface area per unit body mass. Second, a smaller lean body mass, the source of metabolic heat production, limits the female's capacity for heat production, compared to a male of comparable total body mass. In a comparative study on the thermoregulatory responses of women and men, Cunningham et al.[27] observed that women's responses were shifted to higher values. Females showed earlier signs of discomfort and an earlier increase in metabolic rate at a falling ambient temperature. At a rising ambient temperature, the thermal sensation and response with an increase in evaporative heat loss came later in females. The shift was about 0.6°C for responses to cold and about 0.3°C for response to heat, together resulting in a narrower thermoneutral zone in women compared with men. All evidence presented indicates that women react more to a disturbance of energy balance than men.

IV. ONGOING CONTROVERSY AND FUTURE DIRECTIONS

Points of interest for future research include the mechanisms for energy conservation in women and the control of these mechanisms. A limitation in the present analysis of the mechanisms is the measurement of energy intake. The measurement of habitual food consumption is one of the more difficult methodological barriers to the study of energy balance in men. Basic problems include the accurate determination of a subject's customary food intake and the conversion of this information to nutrient and energy intake. Any technique used to measure food intake should not be so intensely applied as to interfere with the subject's dietary habits and thus alter the variable being measured. Another problem concerns the length of time of the measured food intake. The doubly labeled water method is considered the gold standard to validate records of energy intake in free-living subjects. Unfortunately the availability and costs of ^{18}O labeled water and the need for an expensive isotope mass spectroscopy unit for sample analysis restrict widespread application. An alternative method is to estimate energy requirements from estimated resting/basal metabolic rate and estimated physical activity, the two main components of daily energy expenditure. Currently there are several devices to monitor physical activity. Bouten et al.[2] validated a triaxial accelerometer as an objective method that can be used to quantify physical activity-related energy expenditure. The TRACMOR now has been miniaturized to a 30 gram instrument measuring $7 \times 2 \times 0.8$ cm, which can be worn invisibly and without hindrance. Estimated or measured resting metabolic rate in combination with TRACMOR-assessed physical activity allows large scale validation of energy intake measurements. An interesting development in research on control mechanisms of energy balance is the isolation of ob gene product leptin. Leptin is secreted from adipocytes and acts as a feedback signal to the central nervous system, in particular to the satiety center in the hypothalamus.[29] Several studies have shown that leptin levels are reduced after exercise training[30] and some studies have shown a gender-dependent effect of exercise training on serum leptin.[31] It remains to be shown whether exercise and leptin levels are related causally and whether the gender difference in energy conservation is based upon a gender difference in leptin sensitivity for disturbances in energy balance. A detailed discussion about the potential role of leptin and gender differences in metabolism can be found in Chapter 9.

V. SUMMARY

The analysis of determinants of energy expenditure in relation to gender shows pronounced differences between women and men, but the differences become less apparent when the components of energy expenditure are corrected for gender differences in body size, body composition, and energy intake. On average, women have a lower energy intake and a lower average daily metabolic rate due to a lower body mass, fat-free mass, and a higher % body fat. There is a clear gender difference in the maintenance of energy balance. Women adjust energy intake to energy expenditure energy expenditure to energy intake better than men. Thus, weight loss in response to a restricted energy intake or an increased energy expenditure is lower in women than in men. This implies a greater ability for females to preserve body mass in the face of an energy deficit. This observation is consistent with the hypothesis of a phylogenetic advantage for females during periods of starvation.[1]

REFERENCES

1. Hoyenga, K. B. and Hoyenga, K. T., Gender and energy balance: sex differences in adaptations for feast and famine, *Physiol. Beh.,* 28, 545, 1982.
2. Bouten, C. V. C., Verboeket-van de Venne, W. P. H. G., Westerterp, K. R., Verduin, M., and Janssen J. D., Physical activity assessment: comparison between movement registration and doubly labeled water, *J. Appl. Physiol.,* 81, 1019, 1996.
3. Verboeket-van de Venne, W. P. H. G., Westerterp, K. R., Hermans-Limpens, T. J. F. M. B., de Graaf, C., van het Hof, K. H., and Weststrate, J. A., Long-term effects of consumption of full-fat or reduced-fat products in healthy non-obese volunteers; assessment of energy expenditure and substrate oxidation, *Metabolism,* 45, 1004, 1996.
4. Westerterp, K. R., Verboeket-van de Venne, W. P. H. G., Bouten, C. V. C., de Graaf, C., van het Hof, K. H., and Weststrate, J. A., Energy expenditure and physical activity in subjects consuming full- or reduced-fat diets, *Br. J. Nutr.,* 76, 785, 1996.
5. Ravussin, E. and Bogardus, C., Relationship of genetics, age, and physical fitness to daily energy expenditure and fuel utilization, *Am. J. Clin. Nutr.,* 49, 968, 1989.
6. Klausen, B., Toubro, S., and Astrup, A., Age and sex effects on energy expenditure, *Am. J. Clin. Nutr.,* 65, 895, 1997.
7. Ferraro, R., Lillioja, S., Fontvieille, A-M., Rising, R., Bogardus, C., and Ravussin, E., Lower sedentary metabolic rate in women compared with men, *J. Clin. Invest.,* 90, 780, 1992.
8. Arciero, P. J., Goran, M. I., and Poehlman, E. T., Resting metabolic rate is lower in women than in men, *J. Appl. Physiol.,* 75, 2514, 1993.
9. Meijer, G. A. L., Westerterp, K. R., Saris, W. H. M., and ten Hoor, F., Sleeping metabolic rate in relation to body composition and the menstrual cycle, *Am. J. Clin. Nutr.,* 55, 637, 1992.
10. Bisdee, J. T., James, W. P. T., and Shaw, M. A., Changes in energy expenditure during the menstrual cycle, *Br. J. Nutr.,* 61, 187, 1989.
11. Weststrate, J. A., Weys, P. J. M., Poortvliet, E. J., Deurenberg, P., and Hautvast, J. G. A. J., Diurnal variation in postabsorptive resting metabolic rate and diet-induced thermogenesis, *Am. J. Clin. Nutr.,* 50, 908, 1989.
12. Tataranni, P. A., Larson, D. E., Snitker, S., and Ravussin, E., Thermic effect of food in humans: methods and results from the use of a respiratory chamber, *Am. J. Clin. Nutr.,* 61, 1013, 1995.
13. World Health Organization, *Energy and protein requirements, report of a joint FAO/WHO/UNU expert consultation,* Technical Report Series 724, Geneva 1985.
14. Carpenter, W. H., Poehlman, E. T., O'Connell, M., and Goran, M. I., Influence of body composition and resting metabolic rate on variation in total energy expenditure: a meta-analysis, *Am. J. Clin. Nutr.,* 61, 4, 1995.
15. Prentice, A. M., Goldberg, G. R., Murgatroyd, P. R., and Cole, T. J., Physical activity and obesity: problems in correcting energy expenditure for body size, *Int. J. Obes.,* 20, 688, 1996.

16. Black, A. E., Coward, W. A., Cole, T. J., and Prentice, A. M., Human energy expenditure in affluent societies: an analysis of 574 doubly-labelled water measurements, *Eur. J. Clin. Nutr.*, 50, 72, 1996.

17. Ballor, D. L. and Poehlman, E. T., A meta-analysis of the effects of exercise and/or dietary restriction on resting metabolic rate, *Eur. J. Appl. Physiol.*, 71, 535, 1995.

18. Leenen, R., van der Kooy, K., Deurenberg, P., Seidell, J. C., Weststrate, J. A., Schouten, F. J. M., and Hautvast, J. G. A., Visceral fat accululation in obese subjects: relation to energy expenditure and response to weight loss, *Am. J. Physiol.*, 263, E913, 1992.

19. Nance, D., Bromley, B., Barard, R. J., and Gorski R., Sexually dimorphic effects of forced exercise on food intake and body weight in the rat, *Physiol. Beh.*, 19, 155, 1977.

20. Applegate, E., Upton, D., and Stern, J., Food intake, body composition and blood lipids following treadmill exercise in male and female rats, *Physiol. Beh.*, 28, 917, 1982.

21. Tremblay, A., Després, J-P., Leblanc, C., and Bouchard, C., Sex dimorphism in fat loss in response to exercise-training, *J. Obes. Weight Reg.*, 3, 193, 1984.

22. Westerterp, K. R., Meijer, G. A. L., Janssen, G. M. E., Saris W. H. M., and ten Hoor, F., Long-term effect of physical activity on energy balance and body composition, *Br. J. Nutr.*, 68, 21, 1992.

23. Westerterp, K. R., Meijer, G. A. L., Schoffelen, P., and Janssen, E. M. E., Body mass, body composition and sleeping metabolic rate before, during and after endurance training, *Eur. J. Appl. Physiol.*, 69, 203, 1994.

24. Westerterp, K. R., Meijer, G. A. L., Kester, A. D. M., Wouters, L., and ten Hoor, F., Fat-free mass as a function of fat mass and habitual activity level, *Int. J. Sports. Med.*, 13, 163, 1992.

25. Westerterp, K. R. and Goran M., Relationship between physical activity related energy expenditure and body composition: a gender difference, *Int. J. Obes.*, 21, 184, 1997.

26. Colditz, G. A., Giovannucci, E., Rimm, E. B., Stampfer, M. J., Rosner, B., Speizer, F. E., Gordis, E., and Willettt, W. C., Alcohol intake in relation to diet and obesity in women and men, *Am. J. Clin. Nutr.*, 54, 49, 1991.

27. Cunningham, D. J., Stolwijk, J. A. J., and Wenger, C. B., Comparative thermoregulatory responses of resting men and women, *J. Appl. Physiol.*, 45, 908, 1978.

28. Westerterp, K. R., Alcohol calories do not count the same as other calories, *Int. J. Obes.*, 19(S2), 14, 1995.

29. Campfield, L. A., Smith, F. J., Guisez, Y., Devos, R., and Burn, P., Recombinant mouse OB protein: evidence for a peripheral signal linking adiposity and central neural networks, *Science*, 269, 546, 1995.

30. Pasman, W. J., Westerterp-Plantenga, M. S., and Saris, W. H. M., The effect of exercise training on leptin levels in obese males, *Am. J. Physiol.*, in press.

31. Hickey, M. S., Houmard, J. A., Considine, R. V., Tyndall, G. L., Midgette, J. B., Gavigan, K. E., Weidner, M. L., McCammon, M. R., Israel, R. G., and Caro, J. F., Gender-dependent effects of exercise training on serum leptin levels in humans, *Am. J. Physiol.*, 272, E562, 1997.

CHAPTER 11

Nutritional Implications of Gender Differences in Metabolism: Estrogen and Oxygen Radicals: Oxidative Damage, Inflammation, and Muscle Function

Peter M. Tiidus, Ph.D.

CONTENTS

I. INTRODUCTION

Recent exercise-related studies have highlighted a number of physiological and biochemical differences between genders. Some of these differences, particularly as they relate to muscular responses to exercise and training, have been associated with the relatively large divergences in circulating steroid hormone concentrations

**Table 11.1   Some Potential Effects of Estrogen on Skeletal
              Muscle**

	References
1. Decreased postexercise membrane disruption	41, 42, 43
2. Decreased postexercise structural damage	46
3. Increased maximum voluntary force	82, 83, 84
4. Increased resistance to fatigue	84
5. Increased resistance to oxidative stress	2, 37

between the sexes. Considerable research has been performed examining the effects of the primary male steroid hormone, testosterone, on skeletal muscle responses to exercise and training.[1] However, until recently relatively little was known about the potential effects of the primary female steroid hormone, estrogen, on exercising skeletal muscle. It is possible that estrogen affects skeletal muscle function in females by alternate, but complementary, mechanisms to testosterone, such that female muscle function and protection is optimized.

This chapter will review the current understanding of the effects of estrogen as an antioxidant in muscle during exercise and its potential to modify the postexercise inflammatory response in muscle. Estrogen also may positively affect muscle force generation and fatigability. Table 11.1 summarizes some of the reported potential effects of estrogens on skeletal muscle. Many of the potential physiological effects of estrogen on skeletal muscle function and inflammation may be related to its role as an antioxidant and membrane stabilizer. Hence, this chapter will present a brief overview of the biochemistry of oxygen free radicals and estrogens as they relate to exercise and muscle oxidative stress. The final part of this chapter will review the current controversy regarding the potential for estrogen to modify voluntary and involuntary muscle force generation and delay muscle fatigue. The capacity for estrogen to modify muscle force and fatigue may also, in part, be related to its ability to protect muscle from oxygen radical-induced oxidative stress.

The potential for estrogen to protect muscle from exercise-induced peroxidative damage and postexercise inflammatory damage may result in female muscle being less susceptible to exercise damage than male muscle. Depending on the stage of their ovarian cycle, females may have up to 10 times more circulating estrogen than males.[2] The potential for estrogen to affect force generation and to protect muscle from oxygen radical-induced damage may have significant implications for all females. In addition, females on postmenopausal estrogen replacement therapy and those using oral contraceptives may conceivably experience further positive effects on skeletal muscle. These possibilities and their implications in gender differences will be discussed.

II. OXYGEN RADICALS AND ESTROGEN BIOCHEMISTRY

A. Oxygen Radicals in Exercise

The elevated production of oxygen free radicals as byproducts of strenuous muscular exercise has been documented well. A free radical can be defined as any atom, group of atoms, or molecule in a particular state with one unpaired electron occupying an outer orbital.[3] Because of this extra electron, free radicals usually are charged. They can be distinguished from ions, which, although charged (due to an unequal amount of electrons and protons), do not have an unpaired electron in their outer orbital.[4]

Muscular exercise, which elevates mitochondrial oxygen consumption, results in increased generation of the oxygen free radical, superoxide. It has been suggested that up to 2 to 4% of mitochondrial oxygen consumption can result in the generation of superoxide (O_2^{*-})[5] (reaction 1).

$$O_2 + e^- \rightarrow O_2^{*-} \tag{1}$$

The formation of superoxide during exercise is due primarily to increased electron leakage at intermediary steps in electron transport.[6] The most likely site is the ubiquinone (coenzyme Q10) and cytochrome b electron transfer point in the electron transport chain, which is located on the inner mitochondrial membrane.[7] It recently was demonstrated that *in vitro* disruption of mitochondrial complex I electron transport leads to elevated superoxide production that is also characteristic of patients with hereditary complex I deficiency.[8] Subsequent reactions between superoxides give rise to other reactive oxygen species, notably hydrogen peroxide (H_2O_2) (superoxide dismutase) and ultimately the highly reactive hydroxyl free radical (OH*) (reaction 3).[9]

$$2O_2^{*-} + 2H^+ \rightarrow H_2O_2 + O_2 \tag{2}$$

$$Fe^{2+} + H_2O_2 \rightarrow Fe^{3+} + OH^* + OH^- \tag{3}$$

The presence of a transition metal ion such as iron or copper is required to react with superoxide and hydrogen peroxide in the formation of the hydroxyl radical.[3] During exercise it is possible that iron ions from hemoglobin, myoglobin, transferrin, or ferritin may be temporarily available to catalyze the formation of hydroxyl radicals.[3,6] It is the hydroxyl radical that is the most potent and likely cause of oxygen radical-induced tissue damage.[3,9]

When the generation of oxygen radicals exceeds the ability of tissue antioxidants to detoxify them, the resultant oxidative stress can cause muscle damage.[6,9] Because oxygen radicals (particularly the hydroxyl radical) are unstable in biological systems they tend to react with nearby macromolecules such as lipids and proteins. These reactions damage and denature the macromolecules via peroxidation, which ultimately leads to their breakdown and removal.[6] In particular the oxidative modification of proteins is an important mechanism in targeting certain proteins for proteolytic degradation.[10]

Using electron spin resonance, Davies et al.[11] were the first to report increased free radical presence in exercised rat skeletal muscle. Subsequent studies have provided direct evidence for increased intermuscular superoxide, hydrogen peroxide, and hydroxyl radical formation during muscular contraction.[12,13]

Oxygen radicals generated during exercise have been implicated directly in muscular fatigue[14] and associated muscle damage.[6] Exercise-induced peroxidative damage of muscle phospholipids, membranes, proteins, and DNA have been related directly to increased levels of oxygen radical production.[6,15] Exercise-related muscle fatigue may, in part, be due to oxygen radicals disrupting sarcoplasmic reticulum stability and consequently may affect calcium homeostasis[16,17] (see Section IV.A). Oxygen radicals also may play an important role in the postexercise muscle inflammatory response (see Section III.A).

B. Estrogen as an Antioxidant and Membrane Stabilizer in Muscle

Antioxidants react with oxygen radicals and detoxify them. Skeletal muscle possesses several lines of antioxidant defense. These include the antioxidant enzymes superoxide dismutase (Mn SOD as the primary mitochondrial isozyme and Cu/Zn SOD as the primarily cytosolic isozyme), catalase, and glutathione peroxidase as well as vitamins E and C, the tripepeptide-reduced glutathione (GSH), and iron-binding proteins.[6,15] Antioxidant enzymes such as superoxide dismutase or glutathione peroxidase work by reacting directly with oxygen radicals or their peroxide byproducts and thereby catalyze reactions to yield unreactive products such as H_2O.[3,6] Antioxdant vitamins and peptides also can react with specific oxygen radicals or peroxides in various cell locations to yield neutral byproducts. However, unlike enzymes, they are often altered and subsequently degraded in the process.[3,6,18]

It recently has been suggested that estrogens may possess antioxidant and cell membrane stabilization characteristics.[2,19] The term estrogens refers to three structurally similar steroid hormones: estradiol-17β, estrone, and estriol. Of these, estradiol is the primary human estrogen and the one with the highest estrogenic properties.[2] Unless specifically referring to one of these estrogens, this chapter will use the term estrogen generically. The exact mechanism(s) by which estrogen may act as an antioxidant have yet to be demonstrated experimentally. Nevertheless, as seen in Figure 11.1, estrogens do possess a hydroxyl group on their A ring in the same position and configuration as found in the A ring of vitamin E.[20] It is by oxidation or reduction of this phenolic hydroxyl group that vitamin E acts as an antioxidant.[21] It has been suggested that estrogens may act in a similar manner.[2,20] Other natural steroids (i.e., testosterone, progesterone), which do not possess this hydroxyl group, exhibit no *in vitro* antioxidant properties.[20] Recently, Lacourt et al.[22] demonstrated that estrogens are most potent as antioxidants when they interfere with iron-associated free radical production.

It is well-known that estrogens can inhibit LDL and cholesterol oxidation.[19,23,24] This antioxidant property of estrogen may be a significant factor in the lower incidence of atherosclerosis in premenopausal women as compared to men of the same age.[25] Other potential mechanisms by which estrogens may reduce the risk of heart disease in women include their ability to increase HDL cholesterol, prevent cholesterol deposition, increase production of prostacylin, increase nitric oxide production in endothelial cells, and interfere with thromboxane effects on blood vessels.[26,27]

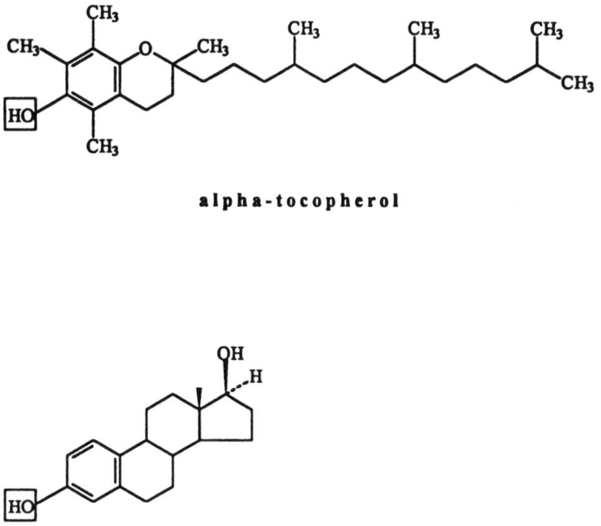

alpha-tocopherol

Figure 11.1 α-Tocopherol and estradiol-17β with similar location of OH group highlighted in box. The antioxidant properties of both molecules may be due to this OH group.

Although its direct effects on skeletal muscle are not as well-documented, the ability of estrogens to act as antioxidants are well-known. Using various methodologies, several *in vitro* studies also have demonstrated the considerable antioxidant potential of various forms of estrogens in various media.[20,28-30] Yagi and Komura[28] reported that estradiol was a significantly more effective antioxidant than the other natural forms of estrogen (estrone and estriol). Nakano et al.[31] further reported that the catechol derivatives of estrogens (2-hydroxy estradiol and 2-hydroxy estrone) had significantly higher antioxidant properties in their *in vitro* model than their corresponding estrogens. Because estrogen target tissues generally convert estrogens to their catachol analogues,[20] this suggests that the potential for tissue level antioxidant activity is optimized.[2,20] Recently, Tang et al.[32] also have reported that the estradiol metabolite 4-hydroxyestrone was superior to other estrogen forms and metabolites in inhibiting peroxidation of lipoproteins. It appears that various forms of estrogen, its metabolites, and its derivatives may have differing effectiveness as antioxidants depending on the source of oxidative stress and the targets for peroxidative damage.[32] Further clarification of the antioxidant efficacy of various forms of estrogen awaits further research.

Because vitamin E can act as an important intermembrane antioxidant in skeletal muscle, it has been postulated that exercise-induced increases in oxygen radical production will result in decreased muscle vitamin E concentration.[33] In several studies, acute exercise has been reported to decrease muscle vitamin E concentrations in male and sexually immature female rats.[34,35] However, acute exercise did not affect muscle vitamin E levels in sexually mature female rats.[36] These results indirectly suggested that gender differences, possibly due to different circulating levels of estrogen, may render skeletal muscle less susceptible to exercise-induced oxidative damage.[2,36] However, other preliminary work from the laboratory could not confirm consistently reduced postexercise muscle damage induced specifically by oxidative stress in estrogen-injected male and female animals.[37] Thus, the mechanisms by which estrogen may act to diminish exercise-induced muscle damage need to be investigated further.

Wiseman et al.[38] have suggested that estrogen also may protect membranes from peroxidative damage by decreasing membrane fluidity and increasing membrane stability in ways similar to cholesterol and the anticancer drug tamoxifen. It is possible that this type of membrane stabilization also involves direct interaction between membrane phospholipids and estrogen in ways similar to the membrane-stabilizing mechanisms of vitamin E and cholesterol.[2] Among other mechanisms, vitamin E acts to increase the orderliness of membrane lipid packing, via London-Van der Waals force effects on cis-double bonds of the membrane polyunsaturated fatty acids.[33] In addition, estrogen also may affect muscle membrane stability via estrogen receptor mediated reactions. Although skeletal muscle does possess estrogen receptors, their concentration is relatively low.[39] Thus it seems more likely that estrogen may exert its membrane-stabilizing effect via direct interaction with muscle membrane phospholipids.[2,38]

In a series of studies, Bär and co-workers used *in vitro* and *in vivo* creatine kinase (CK) release as a measure of the effect of estrogen on membrane stability.[40-44] They demonstrated that, following exercise or *in vitro* muscle stimulation, female rats and rats treated with estrogen had significantly greater membrane stability (as determined by muscle CK release) than male and untreated rats. A strong inverse relationship existed between estrogen levels and *in vitro* muscle CK release following electrical stimulation.[43] It was suggested that estrogen theoretically could be protecting muscle membranes through any of its potential actions as an antioxidant, a membrane stabilizer, or via estrogen receptor mediation.[2,41,45]

Another study compared exercise-induced muscle damage (as determined by electron micrographs) from vitamin E-deprived male and female rats.[46] This study reported that vitamin E-deficient male rats exhibited significant histological evidence of morphological muscle damage following treadmill running, and female rats did not. They attributed this lack of postexercise muscle damage in female rats to their higher estrogen levels.[46] In contrast, Van der Meulen et al.[47] reported little difference in histological evidence of muscle damage between normal diet male and female rats following treadmill running. This may imply that gender differences in exercise-induced muscle damage may be amplified by elevated oxidative stress experienced when tissue vitamin E levels are reduced concurrent with exercise.[2] In support of this hypothesis, Tiidus and Houston[48,49] also reported that vitamin E-deprived female rats were as fatigue-resistant and trainable as normal diet female rats and that they exhibited few blood or muscle indices of postexercise oxidative stress or damage. These results contrast with those of other studies using male rats where vitamin E deprivation resulted in increased fatigue and oxidative stress.[11,50]

Taken collectively, the preceeding studies suggest that due to significantly higher levels of circulating estrogens, female muscle may be less susceptible to exercise-induced damage and/or oxidative stress than male muscle. However, the exact mechanisms of the effect of estrogen on skeletal muscle await further experimental evidence.

III. ESTROGEN, GENDER AND POSTEXERCISE MUSCLE INFLAMMATION

A. Free Radicals and Postexercise Muscle Inflammation

Subsequent to exercise-induced muscle damage, an acute inflammatory response occurs at the initial stage of the repair process. Acute postexercise muscle inflammatory response is a complex series of events associated with the influx of various leukocytes, fluids, and proteins into damaged muscle to promote ultimately the clearance of damaged tissue and subsequent repair.[17,51] Inflammation also may be an important part of the specific immune response to bacterial infection.[52] The inflammatory response to exercise-induced muscle damage is remarkably similar to the inflammatory immune response to sepsis and infection.[52]

Neutrophils and macrophages are the two main cellular infiltrates in exercise-damaged muscle. Within hours of exercise termination, circulating neutrophil concentration can increase several-fold.[53] Neutrophil infiltration into muscle can begin before the end of an unaccustomed exercise bout.[54] Belcastro et al.[55] reported a 75% increase in neutrophil accumulation in rat skeletal muscle immediately following one hour of treadmill exercise. Similar findings also have been reported following ischemia-reperfusion-induced skeletal muscle injury.[56] Elevated muscle neutrophil accumulation has been reported to persist for at least five days following unaccustomed eccentric exercise in humans.[57] Macrophages constitute the other predominant muscle infiltrate cell during the inflammation repair cycle. Macrophages can be present in damaged muscle within one to two days postexercise and may peak as late as seven days postexercise (depending on the extent of damage).[58]

Neutrophils, and to a lesser extent macrophages, generate superoxide via a respiratory burst catalyzed by the enzyme NADPH oxidase, located in its plasma membrane.[51,54] In activated neutrophils, NADPH oxidase shuttles electrons from cytosolic NADPH to dissolved oxygen in the extracellular fluid, thereby forming superoxide (reaction 4).

$$2O_2 + NADPH \rightarrow 2O_2^{*-} + NADP^+ + H^+ \tag{4}$$

Neutrophils also have the capacity to generate the powerful oxidant hypochlorous acid (HOCl), via the myeloperoxidase reaction[59] (reaction 5).

$$H_2O_2 + Cl^- + H^+ \rightarrow HOCl + H_2O \tag{5}$$

The generation of free radicals along with the release of proteases and hypochlorous acid by neutrophils and macrophages are critical in removing damaged tissues following exercise-induced damage.[17,51] The neutrophil and macrophage invasion of damaged muscle is critical for the subsequent repair process to occur. In fact, blocking neutrophil infiltration will prevent subsequent muscle repair.[53] However, McCord[60] has stated that the neutrophil is programmed for overkill, not caution, because so much is at risk if it fails to carry out its mission. Hence neutrophil infiltration has the potential to destroy healthy as well as damaged tissue. In the exercise-damaged muscle, neutrophil- and macrophage-generated oxygen radicals have the capacity to further peroxidise undamaged muscle membrane phospholipids as well as structural and functional proteins. If their generation is not regulated tightly, oxygen radicals produced by neutrophils theoretically can become propagators of further postexercise muscle damage and inflammatory response (secondary to the initial exercise-induced damage).[51] Studies by Fielding et al.[57] and Cannon et al.[61,62] demonstrate a relationship between muscle neutrophil infiltration, muscle ultrastructural damage, and alterations in muscle membrane permeability and stability. It also has been suggested that the neutrophil-associated postexercise inflammatory response also can contribute to the decreased capacity of the muscle to generate force[17,58] (see Section IV.A).

In addition to direct participation in the removal of exercise-damaged muscle tissue, oxygen radicals also may mediate other factors related to the postexercise muscle inflammatory response. Cannon et al.[62] have suggested a relationship between exercise-induced elevations in oxygen radicals and the production of inflammation-mediating cytokines, interleukin-1 (IL-1), and tumor necrosis factor (TNF). Both IL-1 and TNF also are capable of increasing macrophage-mediated superoxide production,[63] although exercise itself may stimulate myeloperoxidase activity.[64] Furthermore, Cannon and Dinarello[65] have reported that females in the luteal phase of their menstrual cycle have significantly higher circulating levels of IL-1 than males or females in the follicular phase of the menstrual cycle. It has been suggested that differences in the regulation of IL-1 secretion between genders may play a role in the lower susceptibility of females to infection and possibly their greater susceptibility to autoimmune disease.[66] However, it is unclear if changes in IL-1 levels are related directly to changes in circulating estrogen or progesterone levels.[66]

Very few studies have examined directly the effect of modified muscle antioxidant status on the postexercise inflammatory response. Antioxidants such as superoxide dismutase have been reported to inhibit tissue neutrophil accumulation in several inflammation models in animals.[67] By potentially reducing initial damage induced by exercise,[68] superoxide dismutase may be able to diminish neutrophil and macrophage infiltration into muscle postexercise. Duarte et al.[69] also have reported a decrease in 48-hour postexercise muscle damage, when neutrophil-induced oxidative stress was inhibited in exercised mice. In contrast to these studies, Warren et al.[70] found no effect of elevated muscle vitamin E on indices of exercise-induced muscle injury immediately or 48 hours postexercise in rats.

B. Estrogen and Postexercise Muscle Inflammation

If estrogen has the capacity to attenuate exercise-induced muscle damage and to act as an antioxidant, it potentially can act to diminish postexercise muscle inflammatory response and the associated postexercise muscle damage and strength loss.[2,51] As previously discussed, antioxidants clearly have the theoretical capacity to diminish exercise-induced muscle damage and postexercise muscle inflammation. However, there is little experimental information as to their actual *in vivo* effect on the inflammatory process.[51] Nevertheless, if, as previously suggested, exercise-induced muscle damage or oxidative stress were to be diminished by estrogens[2] it would seem logical that the degree of postexercise muscle inflammation also should decrease accordingly.

The specific effects of estrogen (and consequently gender) on the magnitude and process of postexercise muscle inflammatory response and resultant damage remain purely speculative at this time. As previously discussed, oxygen radicals can play a significant role in postexercise muscle inflammation and damage.[51] It also has been demonstrated that antioxidants have the potential to attenuate postexercise muscle damage[3,6,15] and the general tissue inflammatory response.[52] Therefore, it is theoretically attractive to suggest that due to its potential as a membrane stabilizer and antioxidant, estrogen could play an important role in modifying postexericse muscle inflammation and damage.[2] If prolonged postexercise disruption of muscle force generation also is related in part to the postexercise inflammatory response,[17] then estrogen may play a role in protecting muscle force-generating capacity during recovery.[71]

In addition, it has been demonstrated that estrogen and gender can affect positively macrophage and neutrophil function in endotoxemic rats.[72] Gender differences in immune response and autoimmune diseases also may be related partially to sex steroid influence on various immunological factors that are related to the inflammatory response.[72,73] Hence, the potential for estrogens and gender to influence the postexercise muscle damage and inflammatory response certainly exists.

IV. ESTROGEN, MUSCLE FORCE, FATIGUE, AND FREE RADICALS

A. Free Radicals in Muscle Force and Fatigue

The reduction in ability of a muscle to produce force following exercise is called fatigue and may be due to disruption in the excitation/contraction coupling process, muscle damage, or both.[17] A common form of muscle fatigue related to eccentric or prolonged exercise is termed low frequency fatigue and refers to fatigue associated with low or physiological levels of neural stimulation.[74] This type of fatigue can last for several days and may be associated with exercise-induced muscle damage and the postexercise inflammatory response.[17,53]

Several lines of evidence have suggested that oxygen radicals can play a role in muscle fatigue and force generation. O'Neill et al.[13] have demonstrated a direct relationship between hydroxyl radical generation during *in vivo* static muscle contraction in cats and the rate of muscle fatigue. Reid et al.[12] and Barcley and Hansel[75] have also reported a similar relationship between oxygen radical generation and fatigue with *in vitro* diaphragm and skeletal muscle, respectively.

Barclay and Hansel[75] have reported that infusion of the antioxidant superoxide dismutase can delay the onset of fatigue in canine gastrocnemius/plantaris muscles contracting *in vitro.* Novelli et al.[76] noted that rats injected with vitamin E or antioxidant spin trappers were able to swim longer than rats not given any antioxidant supplementation. However, not all studies using antioxidant supplementation have noted prolonged exercise endurance times.[18] Nevertheless, the aforementioned studies do suggest that oxygen radicals may play a role in muscle force generation and fatigue.

The mechanisms by which muscle fatigue may be accelerated by oxygen radicals are not understood fully. Muscle sarcoplasmic reticulum (SR) and the SR calcium ATPase are highly susceptible to oxygen radical attack and denaturation.[77] Exercise-induced muscle damage also may be related in part to exercise-induced disruption of SR function.[78] Muscle fatigue, particularly low frequency fatigue, is characterized by a decreased ability of the SR to uptake calcium.[79] Favero et al.[80] have reported that oxygen radicals also may inhibit calcium release from the sarcoplasmic reticulum. Reid et al.[14] have demonstrated that oxygen radicals induce low frequency fatigue in rat diaphragm. Oxygen radical-induced peroxidation of SR membrane phospholipids or denaturation of the calcium ATPase enzyme itself may be factors in limiting the ability of SR to sequester calcium during muscle contraction.[81] Alternatively, Brotto and Nosek[16] have demonstrated that the reactive oxygen species, hydrogen peroxide (H_2O_2) disrupts SR calcium uptake in rat muscle. However, hydrogen peroxide apparently had little effect on muscle isometric force in this experiment.[16]

Several studies have reported a biphasic decline in postexercise muscle force.[17,58] The initial postexercise decline in force is followed by a brief (two to four hour) partial recovery and then a subsequent second decline that can persist for several days.[17,58] The second decline in force (or low frequency fatigue) may be associated with inflammatory and oxygen radical-related damage to muscle SR or contractile proteins.[17,58]

In addition to its ability to induce peroxidative damage, the hydroxyl radical may interfere in other ways with muscle excitation-contraction coupling to cause decreased muscle force generation.[13] O'Neill et al.[13] noted that the hydroxyl radical was associated with a reduced capacity of cat skeletal muscle to generate force prior to detectable oxidative damage. Hence, oxygen radicals also may interfere with the ability of muscle to produce maximal force by affecting various aspects of excitation-contraction coupling.

B. Estrogen, Gender, and Muscle Force

Three recent studies have suggested that estrogens may be able to enhance muscle force development and affect fatiguability and relaxation times in human females.[82-84] These studies have renewed research interest in the potential for estrogens to affect skeletal muscle. It has been documented well that estrogens can have significant effects on the contractility, function, and mass of smooth and cardiac muscle.[85-87] Estrogen also has been reported to have anabolic effects on muscle in cattle.[88] However, the potential for estrogen to affect skeletal muscle function has yet to be documented fully.

Phillips et al.[83] measured age-related changes in maximal voluntary isometric force per cross-sectional area of adductor pollicis muscle in males and females 17 to 90 years of age. There was no difference between age-matched males and females until female menopause, when a significant decline in force relative to males occurred. This decline was not evident in females taking postmenopausal estrogen replacement therapy.[83] A subsequent study reported that in 20- to 30-year-old females, voluntary isometric adductor pollicis force was higher around ovulation (when circulating estrogen levels are highest) than at other times during the menstrual cycle.[82] Sarwar et al.[84] found similar results with menstrual cycle-related variations in forearm and quadriceps muscle strength, fatiguability, and relaxation time in 19- to 24-year old females, with peak responses corresponding to peak circulating estrogen levels. Females taking oral contraceptives exhibited no variation in muscle function throughout their menstrual cycle.

Preliminary findings from the authors' laboratory also suggest that estrogen and gender may affect positively the rate of *in vitro* muscle force recovery following fatiguing contractions mouse muscles.[71] Soleus muscles from male and female mice injected with estrogen for 14 days exhibited significantly faster recovery of peak tetanic tension and rate of peak tension development following a fatiguing protocol than those from untreated mice.[71]

Not all studies have reported a relationship between estrogen levels and muscle force or fatigue. Using survey data from England, Bassey et al.[89] found no difference in quadriceps or hand grip strength (expressed as an index of fat-free mass) between pre- and postmenopausal women aged 45 to 54 years. Seeley et al.[90] reported no difference in current muscle strength in elderly (over 65 years old) females who had taken estrogen supplements at any time after reaching menopause. This finding suggests that, as seen with the reports on menstrual cycle strength variations, the effect of estrogen on muscle force may be acute and not sustainable significantly beyond circulatory peaks. In addition, there is little indication of variation in sports performance in female athletes during different menstrual cycle phases or with oral contraceptive use.[91,92] Greeves et al.[93] recently reported on voluntary strength and fatiguability of the first dorsal interosseus muscle in women undergoing *in vitro* fertilization. They found no effect of estrogen administration on these variables and suggested that progesterone rather than estrogen might be responsible for the previously reported positive findings. Another recent study found that estrogen supplementation did not seem to protect mouse EDL muscle from isometric strength loss following electrically stimulated lengthening induced injury.[94] It is evident that more experiments are needed to clarify the conflicting findings and to describe more fully the effects of estrogen and other female steroid hormones on muscle force and postexercise injury and fatigue.

If estrogen does have an effect on muscle force or fatiguability, its physiological mechanisms of action are unknown. As has been suggested throughout this chapter, the effect of estrogen on skeletal muscle function may be due in part to its effects as an antioxidant and/or membrane stabilizer. These effects may diminish oxygen radical-induced muscle damage incured either by the exercise protocol *per se* or the postexercise inflammatory response.

V. SUMMARY AND CONCLUSIONS

Experimental evidence clearly indicates that estrogen possesses antioxidant and membrane-stabilizing properties. There is also strong evidence that oxygen radicals are important factors in exercise-induced muscle damage and the postexercise inflammatory response. The degree to which estrogen influences skeletal muscle function, and therefore gender differences in muscle strength, protection from exercise induced muscle damage as well as fatiguability, needs to be further investigated. Although estrogen has the potential to act as an antioxidant, the extent to which it is capable of protecting muscle from exercise or inflammation-induced oxidative stress needs to be quantified further. The compelling possibilities suggested by the current literature for estrogen to act in diminishing exercise-induced muscle damage and to positively affect muscle strength need to be investigated further. In addition, estrogen replacement therapy and possibly oral contraceptives could be used to enhance female muscle strength, function, and protection from exercise-induced damage. The potential effects and mechanisms of estrogen action on skeletal muscle need to be investigated further.

REFERENCES

1. Bär, P., The influence of sex hormones on the plasma activity of muscle enzymes, *Int. J. Sports Med.,* 11, 409, 1990.
2. Tiidus, P. M., Can estrogens diminish exercise induced muscle damage? *Can. J. Appl. Physiol.,* 20, 26, 1995.
3. Yu, B. P., Cellular defenses against damage from reactive oxygen species, *Physiol. Rev.,* 74, 139, 1994.
4. Jenkins, R. R., Free radical chemistry: relationship to exercise, *Sports Med.,* 5, 156, 1988.
5. Cadenas, E., Biochemistry of oxygen toxicity, *Annu. Rev. Biochem.,* 58, 79, 1989.
6. Ji, L. L., Exercise and oxidative stress: role of the cellular antioxidant systems, in *Exercise and Sport Science Reviews 23,* Holloszy, J. O., Ed., Williams & Wilkins, Baltimore, MD, 1995, 135.
7. Feher, J., Csomos, G., and Verecki, A., *Free Radicals Reactions in Medicine,* Springer-Verlag, Berlin, 1988, 4.
8. Pitkänen, S. and Robinson, B., Mitochondrial complex I deficiency leads to increased production of superoxide radicals and induction of superoxide dismutase, *J. Clin. Invest.,* 98, 345, 1996.
9. Jaeschke, H., Mechanisms of oxidant stress-induced acute tissue injury, *P.S.E.M.B.,* 209, 104, 1995.
10. Starke-Reed, P. and Oliver, C., Protein oxidation and proteolysis during aging and oxidative stress, *Arch. Biochem. Biophys.,* 275, 559, 1989.
11. Davies, K. A., Quintanilha, A., Brooks, G., and Packer, L., Free radicals and tissue damage produced by exercise, *Biochem. Biophys. Res. Comm.,* 107, 1198, 1982.
12. Reid, M. B., Shoji, T., Moody, M., and Entman, M., Reactive oxygen in skeletal muscle II: Extracellular release of free radicals, *J. Appl. Physiol.,* 73, 1805, 1992.

13. O'Neill, C. A., Stebbins, C., Bonigut, S., Halliwell, B., and Longhurst, J., Production of hydroxyl radicals in contracting skeletal muscle of cats, *J. Appl. Physiol.,* 81, 1197, 1996.

14. Reid, M. B., Haak, K., Franchek, K., Valberg, P., Kobzink, L., and West, M., Reactive oxygen in skeletal muscle I: Intracellular oxidant kinetics and fatigue *in vitro, J. Appl. Physiol.,* 73, 1797, 1992.

15. Sen, C. K., Oxidants and antioxidants in exercise, *J. Appl. Physiol.,* 79, 675, 1995.

16. Brotto, M. and Nosek, T., Hydrogen peroxide disrupts calcium release from the sarcoplasmic reticulum of rat skeletal muscle fibers, *J. Appl. Physiol.,* 81, 731, 1996.

17. MacIntyre, D. L., Reid, W. D., and McKenzie, D., Delayed muscle soreness. The inflammatory response to muscle injury and its clinical implications, *Sports Med.,* 20, 24, 1995.

18. Tiidus, P. M. and Houston, M. E., Vitamin E status and response to exercise training, *Sports Med.,* 20, 12, 1995.

19. Subbiah, M., Kessel, B., Agrawal, M., Rajan, R., Abplnalp, W., and Rymaszeski, Z., Antioxidant potential of specific estrogens on lipid peroxidation, *J. Clin. Endocrin. Metabol.,* 77, 1095, 1993.

20. Sugioka, K., Shimosegawa, Y., and Nakano, M., Estrogens as natural antioxidants of membrane phospholipid peroxidation, *FEBS Lett.,* 210, 37, 1987.

21. Burton G. and Ingold, K., Vitamin E as an *in vivo* and *in vitro* antioxidant, *Annal. N.Y. Acad. Sci.,* 570, 7, 1989.

22. Lacourt, M., Leal, A., Liza, M., Martin, C., Martinez, R., and Ruiz-Larrea, M., Protective effect of estrogens and catecholestrogens against peroxidative membrane damage *in vitro, Lipids,* 30, 141, 1995.

23. Huber, L., Scheffler, E., Poll, T., Zeigler, R., and Dresel, H., 17β-estradiol inhibits LDL oxidation and cholesteryl ester formation in cultured macrophages, *Free Rad. Res. Comm.,* 8, 167, 1990.

24. Maziere, C., Anclair, M., Ronveaux, M., Salmon, S., Santus, R., and Maziere, J., Estrogen inhibits copper and cell-mediated modification of low density lipoprotein, *Atherosclerosis*, 89, 175, 1991.

25. Barrett-Connor, E. and Bush, T., Estrogen and coronary heart disease in women, *J.A.M.A.,* 265, 1861, 1991.

26. Schwartz, J., Freeman, R., and Frishman, W., Clinical pharmacology of estrogens: cardiovascular actions and cardioprotective benefits of replacement therapy in post-menopausal women, *J. Clin. Pharmacol.,* 35, 1, 1995.

27. Hayashi, T., Fukuto, J., Ignarro, L., and Chaudhuri, G., Basal release of nitric oxide from aerotic rings is greater in female rabbits than in male rabbits: Implications for atherosclerosis, *Proc. Natl. Acad. Sci., USA*, 89, 11259, 1992.

28. Yagi, K. and Komura, S., Inhibitory effect of female hormones on lipid peroxidation, *Biochem. Int.,* 13, 1051, 1986.

29. Niki, E. and Nakano, M., Estrogens as antioxidants, *Methods Enzymol.,* 186, 330, 1990.

30. Ruiz-Larrea, B., Garrido, J., and Lacourt, M., Estradiol-induced effects on glutathione metabolism in rat hepatocytes, *J. Biochem.,* 113, 563, 1993.

31. Nakano, M., Sugioka, K., Naito, I., Susumu, T., and Niki, E., Novel and potent biological antioxidants on membrane phospholipid peroxidation: 2-hydroxy estrone and 2-hydroxy estradiol, *Biochem. Biophys. Res. Comm.,* 142, 919, 1987.

32. Tang, M., Abplanalp, W., Ayers, S., and Subbiah, M. T. R., Superior and distinct antioxidant effects of selected estrogen metabolites on lipid peroxidation, *Metabolism*, 45, 411, 1996.

33. Kagan, V. E., Spirichev, V., Serbinova, E. Witt, E., and Packer, L., The significance of vitamin E and free radicals in physical exercise, in *Nutrition in Exercise and Sport* 2nd Ed., Wolinkski, I. and Hickson, J. F., Eds., CRC Press, Boca Raton, FL, 1994, 185.

34. Bowles, D. K., Torgan, C., Ebner, S., Kehrer, J., Ivy, J., and Starnes, J., Effects of acute, submaximal exercise on skeletal muscle vitamin E, *Free Rad. Res. Comm.,* 14. 139, 1991.

35. Sen, C., K., Atalay, M., Agren, J., Laaksonen, D., Roy, S., and Hänninen, O., Fish oil and vitamin E supplementation in oxidative stress at rest and after physical exercise, *J. Appl. Physiol.,* 83, 189, 1997.

36. Tiidus, P. M., Behrens, W., Madere, R., and Houston, M. E., Muscle vitamin E levels following acute submaximal exercise in female rats, *Acta Physiol. Scand.,* 147, 249, 1993.

37. Tiidus, P. M., Bombardier, E., Hidiroglou, N., and Madere, R., Tissue ascorbate, tocopherol and glutathione status: effects of estrogen administration and exercise, *The Physiologist,* 39, A15, 1996.

38. Wiseman, H., Quinn, P., and Halliwell, B., Tamoxifan and related compounds decrease membrane fluidity in liposomes, *FEBS Letts.,* 330, 53, 1993.

39. Dahlberg, E., Characterization of the cytosolic estrogen receptor in rat skeletal muscle, *Biochim. Biophys. Acta,* 717, 65, 1982.

40. Amelink, G. and Bär, P., Exercise-induced muscle damage in the rat: Effects of hormonal manipulation, *J. Neurol. Sci.,* 76, 61, 1986.

41. Bär, P., Amelink, G., Oldenburg, B., and Blankenstein, M., Prevention of exercise induced muscle damage by oestadiol, *Life Sci.,* 42, 2677, 1988.

42. Amelink, G., Kamp, H., and Bär, P., Creatine Kinase isoenzyme profiles after exercise in the rat: Sex linked differences in leakage of CK-MM, *Pflügers Arch.,* 412, 417, 1988.

43. Amelink, G., Koot, R., Erich, W., Van Gijn, J., and Bär, P., Sex-linked variation in creatine kinase release, and its dependence on oestradiol can be demonstrated in an *in vitro* rat skeletal muscle preparation, *Acta Physiol. Scand.,* 138, 115, 1990.

44. Koot, R., Amelink, G., Blankenstein, M., and Bär, P., Tamoxifan and oestrogen both protect the rat muscle against physiological damage, *J. Steroid Biochem. Molec. Biol.,* 40, 689, 1991.

45. Bär, P., Radboud, W., Koot, R., and Amelink, G., Muscle damage revisited: does tamoxifan protect by membrane stabilisation or radical scavenging, rather than via the E2-receptor? *Biochem. Soc. Trans.,* 23, 236S, 1995.

46. Amelink, G., Van der Waal, Wokke, J., Van Asbeck, B., and Bär, P., Exercise induced muscle damage in the rat: The effect of vitamin E deficiency, *Pflügers Arch.,* 419, 304, 1991.

47. Van der Meulen, J., Kuipers, J., and Drukker, J., Relationship between exercise-induced muscle damage and enzyme release in rats, *J. Appl. Physiol.,* 71, 999, 1991.

48. Tiidus, P. M. and Houston, M. E., Vitamin E status does not affect the responses to exercise training and acute exercise in female rats, *J. Nutr.,* 123, 834, 1993.

49. Tiidus, P. M. and Houston, M. E., Antioxidant and oxidative enzyme adaptations to vitamin E deprivation and training, *Med. Sci. Sports Exerc.,* 26, 354, 1994.

50. Gohil, K., Packer, L., DeLumen, B., Brooks, G., and Terblanche, S., Vitamin E deficiency and vitamin C supplements: exercise and mitochondrial oxidation, *J. Appl. Physiol.,* 60, 1986, 1986.

51. Tiidus, P. M., Radical species in inflammation and overtraining, *Can. J. Physiol. Pharmacol.,* (in press).

52. Shephard, R. J. and Shek, P., Physical activity and immune changes: A potential model of subclinical inflammation and sepsis, *Critical Rev. Phys. Rehab. Med.,* 8, 153, 1996.
53. Evans, W. and Cannon, J., Metabolic effects of exercise-induced muscle damage, in *Exercise and Sports Sciences Reviews 18,* Holloszy J. O., Ed., Williams & Wilkins, Baltimore, MD, 1991, 99.
54. Pyne, D., Regulation of neutrophil function during exercise, *Sports Med.,* 17, 245, 1994.
55. Belcastro, A., Arthur, G., Albisser, T., and Raj, D., Heart, liver and skeletal muscle myeloperoxidase activity during exercise, *J. Appl. Physiol.,* 80, 1331, 1996.
56. Smith, J. K., Grisham, M., Granger, N., and Korthuis, R., Free radical defence mechanisms and neutrophil infiltration in postischemic skeletal muscle, *Am. J. Physiol.,* 256, H789, 1989.
57. Fielding, R., Manfredi, T., Ding, W., Fiatarone, M., Evans, W., and Cannon, J., Acute phase response to exercise III. Neutrophil and IL-β accumulation in skeletal muscle, *Am. J. Physiol.,* 265, R166, 1993.
58. Faulkner, J. A., Brooks, S., and Opiteck, J., Injury to skeletal muscle fibers during contractions: conditions of occurrence and prevention, *Phys. Ther.,* 73, 911, 1993.
59. Weiss, S. J., Tissue destruction by neutrophils, *N. Eng. J. Med.,* 320, 365, 1989.
60. McCord, J., Superoxide radical: Controversies, contradictions, and paradoxes, *P.S.E.B.M.,* 209, 112, 1995.
61. Cannon, J., Orencole, S., Fielding, R., Meydani, M., Meydani, S., Fiatarone, M., Blumberg, J., and Evans, W., Acute phase response in exercise: interaction of age and vitamin E on neutrophils and muscle enzyme release, *Am. J. Physiol.,* 259, R1214, 1990.
62. Cannon, J., Meydani, S., Fielding, R., Meydani, M., Farhengmehr, M., Orencole, S., Blumberg, J., and Evans, W., Acute phase response in exercise II: Associations between vitamin E, cytokines, and muscle proteolysis, *Am J. Physiol.,* 260, R1235, 1991.
63. Ward, P., Warren, J., and Johnson, K., Oxygen radicals, inflammation, and tissue injury, *Free Rad. Biol. Med.,* 5, 403, 1988.
64. Suzuki, K., Sato, H., Kikuchi, T., Abe, T., Nakaji, S., Sugawara, K., Totsuka, M., Sato, K., and Yamaya, K., Capacity of circulating neutrophils to produce reactive oxygen species after exhaustive exercise, *J. Appl. Physiol.,* 81, 1213, 1996.
65. Cannon, J. and Dinarello, C., Increased plasma interleukin-1 activity in women after ovulation, *Science*, 227, 1247. 1985.
66. Lynch, E., Dinarello, C., and Cannon, J., Gender differences in IL-1, IL-1β, and IL-1 receptor antagonist secretion from mononuclear cells and urinary excretion, *J. Immunol.,* 153, 300, 1994.
67. McCord, J., Wong, K., Stokes, S., Petrone, W., and English, D., Superoxide and inflammation: a mechanism for the anti-inflammatory activity of superoxide dismutase, *Acta Physiol. Scand.,* 492S, 25, 1980.
68. Radak, Z., Katsumi, A., Inoue, M., Kizika, T., Shuji, O., Suzuki, K., Taniguchi, N., and Ohno, H., Superoxide dismutase derivative reduces oxidative damage in skeletal muscle of rats during exhaustive exercise, *J. Appl. Physiol.,* 79, 129, 1995.
69. Duarte, J., Carvalho, F., Bastos, M., Soares, J., and Appell, H., Do invading leucocytes contribute to the decrease in glutathione concentrations indicating oxidative stress in exercising muscle, or are they important for its recovery?, *Eur. J. Appl. Physiol.,* 68, 45, 1994.

70. Warren, J., Jenkins, R., Packer, L., Witt, E., and Armstrong, R., Elevated muscle vitamin E does not attenuate eccentric exercise-induced muscle injury, *J. Appl. Physiol.*, 72, 2168, 1992.

71. Bestic, N. M., Tiidus, P. M., and Houston, M. E., Estrogen effects on mouse muscle contractile parameters, *Med. Sci. Sports Exerc.*, 29S, S93, 1997.

72. Spitzer, J. A. and Zhang, P., Gender differences in neutrophil function and cytokine-induced neutrophil chemoattractant generation in endotoxic rats, *Inflammation*, 20, 485, 1996.

73. Grossman, C., Possible underlying mechanisms of sexual dimorphism in the immune response; fact and hypothesis, *J. Steroid Biochem.*, 34, 241, 1989.

74. Fitts, R. H., Cellular mechanisms of muscle fatigue, *Physiol. Rev.*, 74, 49, 1994.

75. Barclay, J. K. and Hansel, M., Free radicals may contribute to oxidative skeletal muscle fatigue, *Can. J. Physiol. Pharmacol.*, 69, 279, 1991.

76. Novelli, G., Bracciotti, G., and Falsini, S., Spin-trappers and vitamin E prolong endurance to muscle fatigue in mice, *Free Rad. Biol. Med.*, 92, 211, 1986.

77. Kukreja, R., Okabe, E., Schrier, G., and Hess, M., Oxygen radical-mediated lipid peroxidation and inhibition of calcium-ATPase activity of cardiac sarcoplasmic reticulum, *Arch. Biochem. Biophys.*, 261, 447, 1988.

78. Byrd, S. K., Alterations in the sarcoplasmic reticulum: a possible link to exercise-induced muscle damage, *Med. Sci. Sports Exerc.*, 24, 531, 1992.

79. Allen, D., Lannergen, L., and Westerblad, H., Muscle cell function during prolonged activity: cellular mechanisms of fatigue, *Exp. Physiol.*, 80, 497, 1995.

80. Favero, T., Zable, A., Bowman, M., Thompson, A., and Abramson, J., Metabolic end products inhibit sarcoplasmic reticulum Ca^{2+} release and [^{3}H]ryanodine binding, *J. Appl. Physiol.*, 78, 1665, 1995.

81. Chin, E. R. and Green, H. J., Effects of tissue fractionation on exercise-induced alterations in SR function in rat gastrocnemius muscle, *J. Appl. Physiol.*, 80, 940, 1996.

82. Phillips, S. K., Gopinathan, J., Meehan, K., Bruce, S., and Woledge, R., Muscle strength changes during the menstrual cycle in human adductor pollicis, *J. Physiol.*, 473, 125P, 1993.

83. Phillips, S. K., Rook, K., Siddle, N., Bruce, S., and Woledge, R., Muscle weakness in women occurs at an earlier age than in men, but strength is preserved by hormone replacement therapy, *Clin. Sci.*, 84, 95, 1993.

84. Sarwar, R., Beltran-Niclos, B., and Rutherford, O., Changes in muscle strength, relaxation rate and fatiguability during the human menstrual cycle, *J. Physiol.*, 493, 267, 1996.

85. Scheuer, J., Malhotara, A., Schaible, T., and Capasso, J., Effects of gonadectomy and hormonal replacement on rat hearts, *Circ. Res.*, 61, 12, 1987.

86. Elliott, R. and Castledon, C., Effect of progestogens and oestrogens on the contractile response of rat detrusor muscle to electrical field stimulation, *Clin. Sci.*, 87, 337, 1994.

87. Zhang, F., Ram, J., Standley, P., and Sowers, J., 17β-estradiol attenuates voltage-dependant calcium currents in A7r5 vascular smooth muscle cell line, *Am. J. Physiol.*, 266, C975, 1994.

88. Hayden, J., Bergen, W., and Merkel, R., Skeletal muscle protein metabolism and serum growth hormone, insulin, and cortisol concentrations in growing steers implanted with estradiol-17β, tenbolone acetate, or estradiol-17β plus trenbolone acetate, *J. Anim. Sci.*, 70, 2109, 1992.

89. Bassey, E. J., Mockett, S., and Fentem, P., Lack of variation in muscle strength with menstrual status in healthy women aged 45–54 years: data from a national survey, *Eur. J. Appl. Physiol.,* 73, 382, 1996.

90. Seeley, D., Cauley, J., Grady, D., Browner, W., Nevitt, M., and Cummings, S., Is postmenopausal estrogen therapy associated with neuromuscular function or falling in elderly women? *Arch. Int. Med.,* 155, 293, 1995.

91. Lebrun, C. M., Effect of the different phases of the menstrual cycle and oral contraceptives on athletic performance, *Sports Med.,* 16, 400, 1993.

92. Lebrun, C. M., McKenzie, D., Prior, J., and Taunton, J., Effects of menstrual cycle phase on athletic performance, *Med. Sci. Sports Exerc.,* 27, 437, 1995.

93. Greeves, J. P., Cable, N., Luckas, M., Reilly, T., and Biljan, M., Effects of acute changes in oestrogen on muscle function of the first dorsal interosseus muscle in humans, *J. Physiol.,* 500, 265, 1997.

94. Warren, G., Lowe, D., Inman, C., Orr, O., Hogan, H., Bloomfield, S., and Armstrong, R., Estradiol effect on anterior crural muscles-tibial bone relationship and susceptibility to injury, *J. Appl. Physiol.,* 80, 1660, 1996.

CHAPTER 12

Gender Differences in Exercise-Induced Muscle Damage

Priscilla M. Clarkson and Stephen P. Sayers

CONTENTS

I. INTRODUCTION

Strenuous, unaccustomed exercise results in damage to muscle fibers as observed through morphological analysis of muscle tissue in both human and rodent models. Other manifestations of damage include prolonged losses in muscle strength,

increased activity of muscle enzymes in the blood, and delayed onset muscle soreness.[1-4] Damage to skeletal muscle can result in the efflux of several intramuscular
enzymes and proteins, e.g., creatine kinase (CK), lactate dehydrogenase (LDH),
aspartate aminotransferase (AST), and myoglobin, into the blood, but the most
commonly measured is creatine kinase.[5,6]

This chapter first will review studies that assessed blood levels of muscle
enzymes at rest and after exercise in human males and females. Studies using rodent
models to examine gender differences in muscle enzymes in the blood at rest and
after exercise, as well as morphological changes in muscle after exercise, will then
be reported. Because estrogen has been suggested to affect membrane permeability
at rest and may function to protect muscle from exercise damage, the role of estrogen
and muscle damage will be discussed.

II. GENDER DIFFERENCES: HUMAN STUDIES

Muscle enzyme activity in the blood at rest appears to be lower in females
compared to males, and some, but not all, studies have found that females show an
attenuated increase in muscle proteins in the blood in response to strenuous exercise.
No studies were uncovered that compared morphological changes in muscle of males
and females after damage-inducing exercise, although muscle damage has been
observed in females who perform strenuous exercise.

A. Resting Enzyme Activity in Blood

Resting activity of blood CK appears to be lower for females compared with
males.[7,8] It was suggested that estrogen may play a role in prevention of CK leakage
from skeletal muscle.[9,10] Examination of resting serum CK activity in females of
varying ages showed that serum CK activity was highest in premenarchal girls and
lowest in pregnant women, and then appeared to rise again in postmenopausal
women.[11] Also, Lane and Roses[12] found that serum CK activity was significantly
higher in premenarchal girls than in postmenarchal girls and adult women.

Norton et al.[8] found that differences in serum CK activity between males and
females could not be accounted entirely for by differences in lean body mass and
suggested that estrogen may play a role. When diethylstilbestrol was administered
to 11 boys with Duchenne muscular dystrophy, the elevated levels of serum CK and
LDH were reduced significantly, and this was reversed when the hormone was
discontinued.[10]

The difference in resting serum CK activity between males and females has been
suggested to be due to the activity level of the subjects.[13] The higher level of physical
activity in males may result in higher blood CK activity. Spitler et al.,[14] however,
found that even when males and females were categorized by fitness level, males
still had higher serum CK activity. The resting CK activities for high and low fitness
men were 158.8 and 139.3 U/L, and the corresponding values for the women were
97.8 and 94.8 U/L.[14] Also, Staron et al.[15] reported that resting CK levels taken over
an eight-week high-intensity resistance-training program were consistently lower

for females compared to the males. The amount of CK in muscle also may explain different resting plasma or serum CK levels as males have been found to have higher CK activity in muscle compared with females,[16] but this finding is equivocal.[17]

Of interest, Staron et al.[15] reported that resting CK activity over nine weeks was significantly lower for both trained and untrained females compared with males and that the CK-MB fraction was also significantly lower for females compared with males. Because CK-MB is found predominantly in heart muscle (although it has been identified to a small extent in skeletal muscle) it might be suggested that the smaller resting total CK activity in the blood of females is due to effects more on cardiac rather than skeletal muscle. At present there is no clear explanation for the gender difference in resting CK activity.

B. Exercise-Induced Changes

Whether exercise in humans results in an attenuated increase in activity of muscle enzymes in the blood for females, and whether this lower response is related to estrogen is not clear. Early studies examined changes in the activity of muscle enzymes in the blood of males and females after exercise and reported that females had a smaller response, suggesting that females were protected from damage. However these studies generally used exercises that were not likely to cause significant damage and were not well controlled. Studies using exercises that produced evidence of profound muscle damage showed that females had large increases in CK activity in the blood postexercise.

1. Studies Using Moderate Intensity Exercise

In 1968, Fowler et al.[18] assessed male and female serum enzyme response to exercise, but unfortunately not much can be obtained from the data because the absolute exercise intensity was the same for all subjects (5 mph with increasing grades on a treadmill). The females stopped the exercise at a slope of five degrees, and the males stopped at eleven degrees. It appeared that the females had slightly higher increases in aspartate aminotransferase (AST), alanine aminotransferase (ALT), lactate dehydrogenase, malate dehydrogenase, and aldolase at the five-degree slope, but this may be due to a higher relative workload for the females.

In 1979, Shumate et al.[9] examined serum CK activity in 11 men and 9 women who performed a cycle ergometer test. The intensity of the exercise was about 50% max VO_2 for 120 minutes. The increase in CK from pre- to 24 hours postexercise was 541 U/L for the males and 81 U/L for the females. Brooke et al.[19] examined CK response after an endurance cycle ergometer exercise in two untrained males, two untrained females, three trained males, and three trained females. The CK increases for the 2 untrained males were 1603 and 8 U/L, and for the two untrained females were 28 and 111 U/L. The CK increases for the three trained males were 17, 8, and 108 U/L, and for the trained females were 17, 0, and 32 U/L. Thus, the responses were variable and, although males tended to have a larger response, there appeared to be no distinct difference between males and females. Clearly, the small sample size was a concern in the latter study.

Bär et al.[20] reported that the change from pre- to postexercise (2 hr, 50% max VO_2, cycle ergometer) for females and males, respectively, was −9% and +47% for CK, −9% and +49% for myoglobin, and +13% and +46% for aldolase. Furthermore, the increase in both serum total CK and CK-MB after a marathon in women runners was 5.5 and 7.6 times less than that found in the male runners.[16]

The effect of isometric exercise was examined in a group of postmenopausal (mean age 52.8 yrs), older premenopausal (mean age 43.6 yrs), and younger pre-menopausal (mean age 24.6 yrs) women (21). Serum CK, isometric strength, and muscle soreness were assessed before and 6, 24, 48, and 72 hours after 40 maximal isometric contractions. There was a significant increase in CK and muscle soreness and a significant decrease in isometric strength, but no significant difference in the response among groups. However, the sample size was small in each group (only 6 subjects in the postmenopausal group), postmenopausal subjects would be classi-fied as in an early stage of menopause, and inspection of the data showed a somewhat higher mean increase in CK activity for the postmenopausal group. Thus, further studies of exercise stress in pre- vs. postmenopausal subjects are warranted.

2. Studies Using Strenuous or Eccentric Exercise

Few studies have compared the response of males and females to exercises that are thought to cause significant muscle damage. Of these studies, four have used exercises containing an aerobic component, one used weight lifting, and another used high force eccentric contractions. Eccentric or muscle lengthening contractions are known to result in more muscle damage than concentric or isometric contrac-tions.[1] Additionally, one study examined muscle damage during the course of a resistance-training program.

Janssen et al.[17] assessed plasma CK and AST after a 15, 25, and 42 km race in males and females and found that the changes were generally greater for males. Miles and Schneider[22] had 15 college-aged females perform a bench-stepping exer-cise that required eccentric actions of the leg muscles. They found that the increase in serum CK activity was not related to either lean body mass or blood estradiol levels. The authors suggested that all subjects may have had sufficient estradiol levels to attain a maximum protective effect. Only when estrogen levels vary widely (e.g., males vs. females, pre- vs. postmenopausal) might there be a relationship between estrogen and CK activity. Webber et al.[23] assessed serum CK activity and muscle soreness after downhill running and found that the males had a significantly higher CK response (mean change of 292 U/L) compared with the females (mean change 70 U/L). However, perceived soreness did not show a gender difference. Last, Apple et al.[16] reported that female runners had a 5.5-fold smaller increase in serum CK after a marathon race compared with men.

Nuttal and Jones[24] found that females had higher peak CK activity in response to weight-lifting exercise, which the authors attribute to women having performed more work in relation to their muscle mass because the weights lifted were based on total body weight. However, no statistical analysis was performed, and inspection of the data showed that the peak CK activity for the females was about 42 U/L and for the males was 38 U/L. The slightly higher peak for the females could be attributed to one high responder in that group. Miles et al.[25] examined the CK response of nonweight-trained females and males who performed 50 maximal eccentric actions of the forearm flexor muscles. The females had a lower baseline CK (81 U/L) compared with males (139 U/L), but the females had a greater peak and relative increase in serum CK in response to the exercise. When the contralateral limb was exercised 21 days later the same patterns were found. Thus, contrary to the results for an aerobic-type exercise, the females had a greater CK responses. Other studies that examined high force eccentric exercise in females found that they demonstrated very high CK responses and prolonged losses in range of motion and strength.[1]

Muscle damage has been assessed from biopsy samples taken from males and females during an eight-week high-intensity resistance-training program consisting of concentric and eccentric actions.[15] Subjects were preconditioned for one week prior to the training. No analysis was performed between males and females, but both genders showed small diameter (atrophic) and degenerating fibers, and the most common intracellular change was Z-line streaming. Females appeared to show a higher frequency of atrophic and degenerating fibers compared with the males. This is interesting in light of the (nonsignificant) finding of lower serum CK activity for the females. Staron et al.[26] also reported evidence of muscle damage in another group of females after a six-week resistance exercise program; however, no gender comparisons were assessed.

III. GENDER DIFFERENCES: ANIMAL STUDIES

Many studies of animal models reported an increase in muscle proteins (CK, LDH, and AST) in the blood following unaccustomed strenuous exercise.[27-35] However, studies that have assessed morphological changes in muscle fibers of male and female animals after damage-inducing exercise consistently have not shown gender differences.[32,34] This section will examine gender differences in protein leakage from muscle at rest and review morphological changes in muscle and protein leakage following exercise damage. The role of estrogen in these processes also will be discussed.

A. Blood Protein Profiles at Rest

Proteins released from resting muscle (CK, LDH, AST) have been assessed by both *in vivo* and *in vitro* studies. *In vivo* studies examined muscle proteins in the blood of intact, living animals.[27,30,32,33] *In vitro* studies examined dissected animal muscle under resting conditions[35,36] and constant tension or nonstimulated conditions.[28] In the *in vitro* studies, the muscles were dissected, placed in glass tubes, incubated in a Krebs-Ringer buffer[28,35] or a balanced salt solution,[36] and muscle proteins then were assessed in the bathing medium.

1. In Vivo Studies

In vivo studies found that resting serum or plasma CK activity was significantly lower in female compared with male rats.[27,30,32,33] However, AST activity in the blood was not significantly different between males and females.[27,33] Studies investigated whether the lower resting CK level in females was due to the presence of estrogen.[27,30,32,33] Amelink and Bär[27] examined four groups of rats: males, females, and early (before sexual maturity) and late (mature) ovariectomized females (OVX); Bär et al.[30] included two additional groups, males supplemented with estradiol (E_2) and early OVX females supplemented with E_2. Both studies observed a significantly larger resting serum CK activity in male rats compared to females. In the Amelink and Bär[27] study, early OVX female rats had significantly higher resting serum CK values than did intact females. However, the late OVX females had significantly lower serum CK activity than did the early OVX females (levels were more similar to intact females). It was hypothesized[27] that late OVX female rats benefited from their longer exposure to estrogen, thereby maintaining lower serum CK activity as compared to early OVX females. Similarly, Bär et al.[30] found that early OVX females had significantly higher serum CK activity than either intact females or early OVX females supplemented with E_2. These researchers suggested that the low serum CK activities observed in OVX females supplemented with E_2 may be due to an estrogen-linked decrease in muscle membrane permeability at rest.

When male rats were supplemented with E_2, however, there was no attenuation of the efflux of CK from the muscle.[30] No significant differences were observed between male rats supplemented with E_2 and male rats not supplemented with E_2. This is interesting in light of the fact that following strenuous exercise, male rats supplemented with E_2 had an attenuation of CK efflux from the muscle compared with male rats not supplemented with E_2. The mechanism for the release of CK into the blood at rest may differ from the mechanism of CK release during exercise. However, CK in the blood is being released not only from the muscle at rest, but also from other organs in the body, and it is the release from other organs that may explain differences in total CK activity between males and females.

CK is comprised of three isoenzymes, CK-MM, found predominantly in muscle, CK-MB, found predominantly in cardiac tissue, and CK-BB, found in the brain, liver, and blood platelets.[33] Amelink et al.[33] reported no significant differences in the plasma CK-MM isoenzyme profile of male and female rats at rest. In a subsequent study, Amelink et al.[32] reported no significant differences in the plasma CK-MM isoenzyme profile between normal male and female rats or vitamin E-deficient male and female rats at rest. If females have an estrogen-linked decrease in muscle membrane permeability and male rats do not, as suggested by Bär et al.,[30] males would have significantly greater resting plasma CK-MM values than females, but this was not observed. Instead, larger plasma CK-BB isoenzyme activity was reported in male rats at rest in both Amelink et al. studies[32,33] contributing to higher total resting plasma CK levels in male rats (Figure 12.1).

2. In Vitro Studies

The isoenzyme profiles described suggest that the attenuation of resting blood CK activities in the female rat might be due to the effect of estrogen on organs such as the brain, liver, or blood platelets, instead of skeletal muscle, as suggested previously. However, *in vitro* studies examining excised animal muscles do not

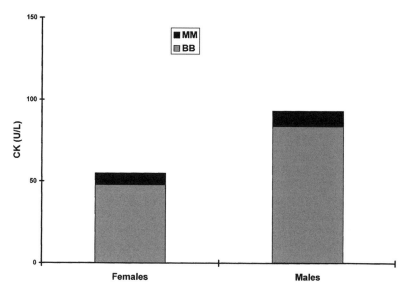

Figure 12.1 CK Isoenzyme distribution at rest in female and male rats. (Data modified from Amelink et al.[33])

support this hypothesis. CK release from the muscle into the bathing medium was significantly greater for males than females under non-stimulated conditions, suggesting that it is the muscle itself that is being influenced by estrogen and not other organs in the body. Amelink et al.[28] also observed significantly lower CK activity in the bathing medium for the isolated soleus muscles of OVX females treated with E_2 than for the isolated soleus muscles of OVX females not treated with E_2 (Figure 12.2). When the possible effects of circulating estrogen on other organs of the body have been eliminated by *in vitro* muscle analysis, it is the muscle itself that appears to be affected predominantly by E_2.

In another *in vitro* study, Warren et al.[35] examined two groups of OVX female mice, one group supplemented with E_2 for 21 days and one without. After a one-hour incubation, LDH release from the resting isolated extensor digitorum longus (EDL) muscle was greater, although not significantly, in the E_2-deficient mice. It appears that CK release for male and female rats is significantly different, although LDH release is not significantly different for male and female mice under resting conditions *in vitro*. Whether this reflects a difference between species, methodology, or LDH vs. CK release from the muscle is not known. With regard to the latter explanation, studies finding significant differences in resting serum or plasma CK activity between males and females have not found significant differences in the resting serum activity of another muscle protein, AST.[27,33]

One explanation for the nonsignificant difference in LDH efflux between male and female mice may be obtained from an earlier study[36] that examined LDH efflux from the isolated gastrocnemius muscle of mice. In one group of mice, the efflux of LDH was small after one hour (similar to the nonsignificant changes observed in the Warren et al.[35] study after one hour). However, after five hours, the efflux of

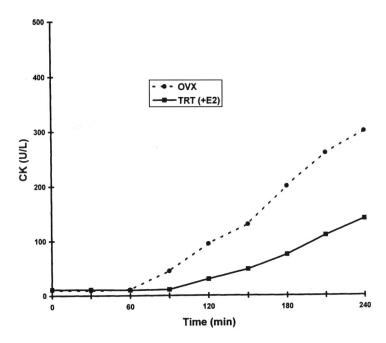

Figure 12.2 Basal CK release from isolated soleus muscle *in vitro* in ovariectomized rats who were pretreated *in vivo* with estradiol (Trt+E$_2$) or control (OVX). (Data modified from Amelink et al.[28])

LDH was large, approximately six times that of LDH efflux after one hour. This suggests that a longer incubation time may be necessary for significant increases in LDH to be observed, as well as possible gender differences to manifest themselves. Amelink et al.[28] also reported that significant increases in CK efflux for both males and females were observed as incubation time increased.

In summary, *in vivo* studies of isoenzyme profiles have raised new questions about whether the attenuation of plasma CK efflux in females is due to estrogen's effect on the muscle or its effect on other organs in the body. *In vitro* studies, however, appear to provide support for estrogen's effect on the muscle. Further research is needed regarding the role of estrogen on muscle protein leakage at rest.

B. Blood Protein Profiles Postexercise

In vivo studies examined muscle proteins in the blood of intact, living animals exposed to an exercise bout of treadmill running,[27,30,32,33] and *in vitro* studies examined dissected animal muscle under conditions of electrical stimulation.[28,29,35] Two methods were used to assess differences between males and females in response to electrical stimulation. In one method, the muscles were dissected and adjusted to a length to give maximal twitch tensions and stimulated with impulse trains at 30-minute intervals for four hours.[28,29] In the other method, muscles were given an isometric twitch 57.5 minutes into the 60-minute incubation, an isometric tetanus

30 seconds later, followed by another isometric tetanus at 60 minutes.[35] Muscle proteins then were assessed in the bathing medium.

1. In Vivo Studies

Several *in vivo* studies assessed gender differences in the efflux of muscle proteins following strenuous exercise. The protocol involved exercising male and female rats on a treadmill for two hours on a zero-degree incline at 19 m/min.[27,30,32,33] These studies all found large, significant increases in blood CK activity in male rats immediately following exercise. Amelink and Bär[27] and Bär et al.[30] found no significant increase in serum CK activity in female rats following exercise (Figure 12.3), although Amelink et al.[33] observed significant, albeit very small, postexercise increases in plasma CK activity in female rats. Amelink and Bär[27] and Amelink et al.[33] also found that males had a significantly greater increase in AST compared with females.

Van Der Meulen et al.[34] used a more aggressive treadmill protocol with two groups of rats running for either 90 or 150 minutes on a ten-degree incline at a speed of 30 m/min. The researchers observed significant increases in plasma CK activity for both male and female rats immediately after 150 minutes of exercise, although male plasma CK values were significantly higher than females. In the group of rats running for 90 minutes, only male rats had significant increases in plasma CK

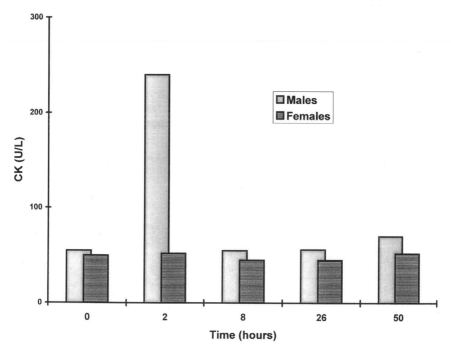

Figure 12.3 Serum CK activity in rats before (0) and 2, 8, 26, and 50 hours after 2 hours of treadmill running. (Data modified from Amelink and Bär.[27])

activity,[34] which was similar to other studies.[27,30] Males also demonstrated significantly higher levels of AST and LDH compared with females. The uphill protocol and increased exercise time in the Van Der Meulen et al.[34] study may have induced greater damage than in other less vigorous treadmill protocols.[27,30,32,33]

The effect of estrogen on the muscle following strenuous exercise has been observed directly in several studies using E_2 supplementation, ovariectomization, or both.[27,30] In these studies, early OVX female rats exhibited significantly greater serum CK activity after exercise than the intact female rats. Removing the source of estrogen made the early OVX female rat as susceptible to exercise-induced muscle damage as the male rat. Bär et al.[30] found that postexercise serum CK values of the E_2-supplemented OVX females were significantly less than the OVX females, although E_2-supplemented males demonstrated lower postexercise serum CK levels as compared with normal males.

There also may be a long-lasting protective effect of estrogen. Late OVX rats, who previously had been exposed to estrogen, did not show as large an increase in CK as early OVX females.[27] Moreover, Bär et al.[30] reported that when E_2 was administered to males only one hour before exercise, there was no reduction of CK efflux from the muscle. As the duration of E_2 treatment increased (from 24 hours to 21 days), the protective effect was increased, with progressively lower CK values observed by the 21st day (Figure 12.4). The same pattern was found for AST. The extended presence of estrogen in the late OVX females prior to ovariectomization acted to protect the muscles of these animals, even after the removal of estrogen-producing organs.[27,30]

Examining the isoenzyme profile of male and female rats, Amelink et al.[33] observed a change in the CK-MM profile, but not the CK-BB profile, following

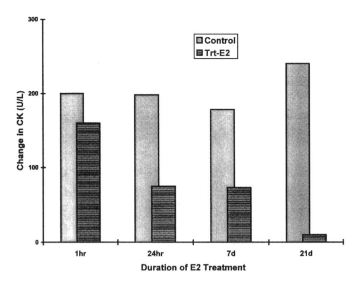

Figure 12.4 CK increase in male rats immediately after two hours of treadmill exercise. On the X-axis is the length of time the Trt-E_2 rats were pretreated with estradiol before the treadmill run. (Data modified from Bär et al.[30])

exercise. The increase in CK-MM was significantly different between male and female rats. CK-MM showed a highly significant increase in males, although females showed a smaller, but significant increase. CK-BB increases were modest and not significantly different between males and females. Amelink et al.[32] also observed significant increases in plasma CK-MM of normal males, vitamin E-deficient males, and vitamin E-deficient females following exercise. The CK-BB increases in the Amelink et al.[32] study were similar to the increases found in the Amelink et al.[33] study and again were not significantly different between the males and females. These data suggest that the increases in plasma total CK in male rats following exercise were provided predominantly by the CK-MM isoenzyme. Thus, lower postexercise increases in plasma total CK and CK-MM activity in female rats imply that estrogen may be exerting a protective effect on the muscle membrane, inhibiting efflux of CK from the muscle following strenuous exercise.

Vitamin E was examined in the Amelink et al.[32] study because it is believed to stabilize membrane integrity and arrest lipid peroxidation by interacting with the membrane and quenching unpaired electrons generated from free radical species.[37] Several studies have reported that exercise results in an increase in lipid peroxidation.[38] A vitamin E-deficient diet caused greater exercise-induced muscle damage than a normal diet.[32] Because both E_2 and vitamin E are structurally similar, it has been thought that E_2 also may interrupt lipid peroxidation of the membrane,[39] reducing oxidative stress to the muscle. Koot et al.[29] examined the effects of E_2 and Tamoxifen, an estrogen antagonist with antioxidant properties,[40] on the efflux of CK from the muscle. The researchers found that muscles treated with E_2 and Tamoxifen, separately and in combination, caused significant decreases in CK leakage from the muscle compared with untreated muscles (Figure 12.5). It was suggested that E_2 and Tamoxifen both exert a protective effect on the membrane because of their antioxidant capabilities.[41] Thus, estrogen may exert a protective effect on the muscle membrane of females following strenuous exercise by its actions as an antioxidant.

2. In Vitro Studies

Results of *in vitro* exercise studies are similar to results observed in the aforementioned *in vivo* studies. Amelink et al.[28] examined gender differences in CK release following electrical stimulation of the isolated soleus and found that CK release was significantly greater for males than for females. Koot et al.,[29] using a similar protocol, reported that males released a greater absolute amount of CK than females, although no statistical analysis was reported.

The Amelink et al.[28] study also revealed that the longer the duration of the treatment period with E_2, the less CK efflux from the exercised muscle, similar to the *in vivo* studies previously discussed.[27,30] Both Amelink et al.[28] and Koot et al.[29] observed that the pretreatment of male rats with E_2 and OVX female rats with E_2 for three weeks attenuated CK efflux from the exercised soleus muscle *in vitro* (Figure 12.6). However, Amelink et al.[28] found that a 24-hour pretreatment did not attenuate this efflux. As suggested by *in vivo* studies[27,30] and supported by *in vitro*

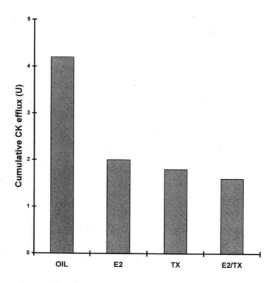

Figure 12.5 Effect of tamoxifen (TX), estradiol (E$_2$), a combination of tamoxifen and estradiol (E$_2$/TX), and control (OIL) on CK release from isolated soleus muscles of ovariectomized rats. Muscles were electrically stimulated prior to assessing CK release *in vitro*. (Data modified from Koot et al.[29])

research,[28,29] estrogen may exert a long-lasting effect that provides protection from exercise-induced muscle damage.

Despite strong evidence for estrogen's protective effect on the muscle following exercise stress, one study refutes this supposition.[35] Warren et al.[35] examined OVX mice and OVX mice treated with E$_2$ after an *in vivo* eccentric contraction protocol. The researchers found no difference of LDH levels between groups following eccentric exercise contractions of the EDL muscle *in vitro*, suggesting that muscle damage was unaffected by the presence of E$_2$. Moreover, E$_2$ treatments were found to worsen muscle injury as determined by muscle contractility decrements. The differences observed may have been due to the method of determination of muscle damage. The Warren et al.[35] study did not rely on muscle proteins in the blood but examined the contractile properties of the muscle, which were suggested to be a more valid index of injury.[35,42,43] However, many factors could contribute to changes in contractile properties so that these data do not negate a potential effect of estrogen on muscle damage *per se*. Other explanations could be in the different effects that E$_2$ is known to have on rats and mice[35] or in the methodological differences employed between the Warren et al.[35] study compared to previous studies.[28,29] However, the weight of the evidence for rat muscle *in vivo* and *in vitro* studies suggests that estrogen plays a role in the attenuation of release of muscle proteins into the blood.

C. Morphological Changes Following Strenuous Exercise

Only two studies have examined differences between male and female animals in both morphological indices of muscle damage and muscle protein release to the blood.[32,34] Morphological changes in the muscle following strenuous exercise were

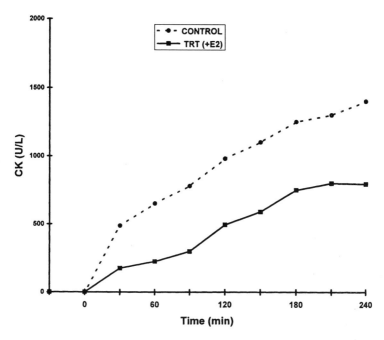

Figure 12.6 CK release after electrical stimulation of isolated soleus muscle *in vitro* in male rats who were pretreated *in vivo* with estradiol (Trt+E$_2$) or control. (Data modified from Amelink et al.[28])

determined in two ways. First, muscle damage was determined by the total volume of observed damage determined from central nuclei, hyaline aspect, vacuoles, and inflammatory cell infiltration, compared to the total volume of muscle (light microscopy).[34] Second, muscle damage was determined by the ratio of A-band widening, z-line streaming, and myofibrillar disruption to the total muscle area (electron microscopy).[32]

Van Der Meulen et al.[34] observed that a 150-minute uphill treadmill protocol resulted in significantly greater amounts of morphological muscle damage compared to a 90-minute protocol for both males and females. However, no significant difference in damage was found between males and females following either of the strenuous exercise protocols. Amelink et al.[32] observed that, in vitamin E-deficient and in vitamin E-normal rats, there was significantly greater morphological damage in male as compared to female rats postexercise. Moreover, the amount of damage in the vitamin E-normal rats was not as extensive as in the vitamin E-deficient rats.

One explanation for the differences observed between the studies could be in the timing of the dissection of the muscles following the exercise protocol. Amelink et al.[32] extracted the muscles from the rats 48 hours postexercise, and Van Der Meulen et al.[34] waited an additional 24 hours before dissection. It is unlikely, however, that morphological changes would have disappeared in only 24 hours, even though it has been reported that indices of muscle damage are most pronounced in rats approximately 48 hours postexercise.[44] It also is interesting to note that, despite examination of the entire muscle, Van Der Meulen et al.[34] observed no significant differences in morphological damage between males and females. Amelink et al.[32] observed only sections from the middle of the muscle yet found significant gender differences.

The lack of differences between males and females in muscle morphology following strenuous exercise found by Van Der Meulen et al.[34] is interesting in light of the fact that the researchers did find a significant difference between males and females when examining muscle proteins in the plasma following the 150-minute treadmill protocol. Van Der Meulen et al.[34] suggested that greater muscle protein clearance rates in female rats postexercise might account partly for the findings in their study. Postexercise protein release from the muscle can occur without the presence of morphological damage.[45] Amelink et al.[32] observed a significant increase in CK-MM activity of both the vitamin E-normal and vitamin E-deficient females following strenuous exercise, but no corresponding evidence of morphological damage.

It remains unclear why Van Der Meulen et al.[34] found no significant differences in morphological damage between males and females after the less strenuous exercise protocol in their study. This exercise was more aggressive than the protocol employed by Amelink et al.,[32] who observed significant differences in muscle morphology between males and females, albeit the damage after exercise in the normal vitamin E rats was more subtle than damage found in the vitamin E-deficient rats after exercise. Possibly the effects of estrogen are sufficient to protect females against morphological damage when using a mild treadmill protocol,[32] but not when using a more damaging protocol with greater speeds and an uphill component.[34] Further research is needed to uncover the discrepancies in the findings observed between morphological indices of muscle damage and muscle protein activity in the blood following exercise stress.

IV. SUMMARY AND CONCLUSIONS

In studies of both humans and animals, resting muscle enzyme activity in the blood, particularly creatine kinase (CK), has been found to be lower in females. CK isoenzyme profiles suggested that lower resting levels of total CK in females may be due to lower levels of the BB fraction (rodents) or the MB fractions (humans), indicating less of a release of CK from tissues other than skeletal muscle. However, *in vitro* studies of animal models support the contention that estrogen has a direct effect on skeletal muscle. Further research is needed to determine the role of estrogen on muscle protein leakage at rest.

It appears that aerobic or endurance-type exercise results in a lower CK response, and possibly less muscle damage, in females compared to males. Of the two studies that examined morphological changes after exercise in animal models, one reported more damage in males compared with females after a more mild exercise stress of level running,[32] and the other reported no difference between genders after a more intense (faster speed) endurance exercise protocol of uphill running.[34] One possible explanation for less damage in females after mild to moderate endurance exercise may be the protective role that estrogen plays as an antioxidant and membrane stabilizer during exercise with a relatively high oxidative stress.[38,46-49] (The role of estrogen as an antioxidant will be covered in the next chapter.) Also, estrogen may exert a greater protective role during moderate endurance exercise by sparing muscle glycogen. Trained females have been shown to oxidize more lipid and less carbohydrate and protein during exercise than trained males.[50-52]

Although several studies have examined gender differences in response to exercise-damage, the results are not conclusive. Estrogen appears to play some role in the protection of muscle against damage, but how and under what circumstances this occurs are still unclear.

REFERENCES

1. Clarkson, P. M., Nosaka, K., and Braun, B., Muscle function after exercise-induced muscle damage and rapid adaptation, *Med. Sci. Sports Exerc.*, 24, 512, 1992.
2. Clarkson, P. M. and Newham, D. J., Associations between muscle soreness, damage, and fatigue, *Adv. Exper. Med. Biol.*, 384, 457, 1995.
3. Ebbeling, C. B. and Clarkson, P. M., Exercise-induced muscle damage and adaptation, *Sports Med.*, 7, 207, 1989.
4. MacIntyre, D. L., Reid, W. D., and McKenzie, D. C., Delayed muscle soreness: the inflammatory response to muscle injury and its clinical implications, *Sports Med.*, 20, 24, 1995.
5. Nosaka, K., Clarkson, P. M., and Apple, F. S., Time course of serum protein changes after strenuous exercise of the forearm flexors, *J. Lab. Clin. Med.*, 119, 183, 1992.
6. Mair, J., Koller, A., Artner-Dworzak, E., Haid, C., Wicke, K., Judmaier, W., and Puschendorf, B., Effects of exercise on plasma myosin heavy chain fragments and MRI of skeletal muscle, *J. Appl. Physiol.*, 72, 656, 1992.
7. Harris, E. K., Wong, E. T., and Shaw, Jr., S. T., Statistical criteria for separate reference intervals: race and gender groups in creatine kinase, *Clin. Chem.*, 37, 1580, 1991.
8. Norton, J. P., Clarkson, P. M., Graves, J. E., Litchfield, P., and Kirwan, J., Serum creatine kinase activity and body composition in males and females, *Human Biol.*, 57, 591, 1985.
9. Shumate, J. B., Brooke, M. H., Carroll, J. E., and Davis, J. E., Increased serum creatine kinase after exercise: A sex-linked phenomenon, *Neurology*, 29, 902, 1979.
10. Cohen, L. and Morgan, J., Diethylstilbestrol effects on serum enzymes and isoenzymes in muscular dystrophy, *Arch. Neurol.*, 33, 480, 1976.
11. Bundey, S., Crawley, J. M., and Edward, J. H., Serum creatine kinase levels in pubertal, mature, pregnant and post menopausal women, *J. Med. Genet.*, 16, 117, 1979.
12. Lane, R. J. and Roses, A. D., Variation of serum creatine kinase levels with age in normal females: implications for genetic counseling in Duchenne muscular dystrophy, *Clin. Chim. Acta*, 113, 75, 1981.
13. Hortobágyi, T. and Denahan, T., Variability in creatine kinase: methodological, exercise, and clinically related factors, *Int. J. Sports Med.*, 10, 69, 1989.
14. Spitler, D. L., Alexander, W. C., Hoffler, G. W., Doerr, D. F., and Buchanan, P., Haptaglobin and serum enzyme responses to maximal exercise in relation to physical fitness, *Med. Sci. Sports Exerc.*, 16, 366, 1984.
15. Staron, R. S., Hikida, R. S., Murray, T. F., Nelson, M. M., Johnson, P., and Hagerman, F., Assessment of skeletal muscle damage in successive biopsies from strength-trained and untrained men and women, *Eur. J. Appl. Physiol.*, 65, 258, 1992.

16. Apple, F. S., Rogers, M. A., Casal, D. C., Lewis, L., Ivy, J. L., and Lampe, J. A., Skeletal muscle creatine kinase-MB alterations in women marathon runners, *Eur. J. Appl. Physiol.*, 56, 49, 1987.

17. Janssen, G. M. E., Kuipers, H., Willems, G. M., Does, R. J. M. M., Janssen, M. P. E., and Geurten, P., Plasma activity of muscle enzymes: Quantification of skeletal muscle damage and relationship with metabolic variables, *Int. J. Sports Med.*, 10, S160, 1989.

18. Fowler, W. M., Gardner, G. W., Kazerunian, H. H., and Lauvstad, W. A., The effect of exercise on serum enzymes, *Arch. Phys. Med. Rehab.*, 49, 554, 1968.

19. Brooke, M. H., Carroll, J. E., Davis, J. E., and Hagberg, J. M., The prolonged exercise test, *Neurology*, 29, 636, 1979.

20. Bär, P. R., Driessen, M., Rikken, B., and Jennekens, F. G. I., Muscle protein leakage after strenuous exercise: sex and chronological differences, *Neurosci. Lett.*, 22, S288, 1985.

21. Buckley-Bleiler, R., Maughan, R. J., Clarkson, P. M., Bleiler, T. L., and Whiting, P. H., Serum creatine kinase activity after isometric exercise in premenopausal and postmenopausal women, *Exp. Aging Res.*, 15, 195, 1989.

22. Miles, M. P. and Schneider, C. M., Creatine kinase isoenzyme MB may be elevated in healthy young women after submaximal eccentric exercise, *J. Lab. Clin. Med.*, 122, 197, 1993.

23. Webber, L. M., Byrnes, W. C., Rowland, T. W., and Foster, V. L., Serum creatine kinase activity and delayed onset muscle soreness in prepubescent children: a preliminary study, *Ped. Exerc. Sci.*, 1, 351, 1989.

24. Nuttall, F. Q. and Jones, B., Creatine kinase and glutamic oxalacetic transaminase activity in serum: kinetics of change with exercise and effect of physical conditioning, *J. Lab. Clin. Med.*, 71, 847, 1968.

25. Miles, M. P., Clarkson, P. M., Smith, L. L., Howell, J. N., and McCammon, M. R., Serum creatine kinase activity in males and females following two bouts of eccentric exercise, *Med. Sci. Sports Exerc.*, 26, S168, 1994.

26. Staron, R. S., Leonardi, M. J., Karapondo, D., Malicky, E. S., Falkel, J. E., Hagerman, F. C., and Hikida, R. S., Strength and skeletal muscle adaptations in heavy resistance-trained women after detraining and re-training, *J. Appl. Physiol.*, 70, 631, 1991.

27. Amelink, G. J. and Bär, P. R., Exercise-induced muscle protein leakage in the rat: Effects of hormonal manipulaion, *J. Neurol. Sci.*, 76, 61, 1986.

28. Amelink, G. J., Koot, R. W., Erich, W. B. M., Gijn Van, J., and Bär, P. J., Sex-linked variation in creatine kinase release, and its dependence on oestradiol, can be demonstrated in an *in-vitro* rat skeletal muscle preparation, *Acta Physiol. Scand.*, 138, 115, 1990.

29. Koot, R. W., Amelink, G. J., Blankenstein, M. A., and Bär, P. J., Tamoxifen and oestrogen both protect the rat muscle against physiological damage, *J. Steroid Biochem. Molec. Biol.*, 40, 689, 1991.

30. Bär, P. R., Amelink, G. J., Oldenburg, B., and Blankenstein, M. A., Prevention of exercise-induced muscle membrane damage by oestradiol, *Life Sci.*, 42, 2677, 1988.

31. Armstrong, R. B., Oglivie, R. W., and Schwane, J. A., Eccentric exercise-induced injury to rat skeletal muscle, *J. Appl. Physiol.: Respirat. Environ. Exercise Physiol.*, 54, 80, 1983.

32. Amelink, G .J., van de Wal, W. A. A., Wokke, J. H. J., van Asbeck, B. S., and Bär, P. R., Exercise-induced muscle damage in the rat: the effect of vitamin E deficiency, *Pflugers Arch.*, 419, 304, 1991.

33. Amelink, G. J., Kamp, H. H., and Bär, P. R., Creatine kinase isoenzyme profiles after exercise in the rat: sex-linked differences in leakage of CK-MM, *Pflug. Arch.,* 412, 417, 1988.
34. Van Der Meulen, J. H., Kuipers, H., and Drukker, J., Relationship between exercise-induced muscle damage and enzyme release in rats, *J. Appl. Physiol.,* 71, 999, 1991.
35. Warren, G. L., Lowe, D. A., Inman, C. L., Otto, M. O., Hogan, H. A., Bloomfield, S. A., and Armstrong, R. B., Estradiol effect on anterior crural muscles-tibial bond relationship and susceptibility to injury, *J. Appl. Physiol.,* 80, 1660, 1996.
36. Dempsey, B. S., Morgan, J., and Cohen, L., Reduction of enzyme efflux from skeletal muscle by diethylstilbestrol, *Clin. Pharm. Ther.,* 18, 104, 1975.
37. Capel, I., Jenner, M., and Williams, D., The effect of prolonged oral contraceptive steroid use on erythrocyte glutathione peroxidase activity, *J. Steroid Biochem.,* 14, 729, 1981.
38. Clarkson, P. M., Antioxidants and physical performance, *Clin. Rev. Food Sci. Nutr.,* 35, 131, 1995.
39. Ji, L. L., Exercise and oxidative stress: role of cellular antioxidative systems, *Exerc. Sports Ssi. Rev.,* 23, 135, 1995.
40. Jenkins, R. R., Drause, D., and Schofield, L. S., Influence of exercise on clearance of oxidant stress products and loosely bound iron, *Med. Sci. Sports Exerc.,* 25, 213, 1993.
41. Bär, P. R., Koot, R. W., and Amelink, G. J., Muscle damage revisited: does tamoxifen protect by membrane stabilisation or radical scavenging, rather then via the E2 receptor? *Biochem. Soc. Trans.,* 23, 236S, 1995.
42. Lowe, D. A., Warren, G. L., Ingalls, C. P., Boorstein, D. B., and Armstrong, R. B., Muscle function and protein metabolism after initiation of eccentric contraction-induced injury, *J. Appl. Physiol.,* 79, 1260, 1995.
43. Warren, G. L., Hayes, D. A., Lowe, D. A., and Armstrong, R. B., Mechanical factors in the initiation of eccentric contraction-induced injury in rat soleus muscle, *J. Physiol.,* 464, 457, 1993.
44. Kuipers, H., Drukker, J., Frederik, P. M., Geurten, P., and van Kranenburg, G., Muscle degeneration after exercise in rats, *Int. J. Sports Med.,* 4, 45, 1983.
45. Jones, D. A., Jackson, M. J., and Edwards, R. H. T., Release of intracellular enzymes from an isolated mammalian skeletal muscle preparation, *Clin. Sci.,* 65, 193, 1983.
46. Ji, L. L., Oxidative stress during exercise: Implication of antioxidant nutrients, *Free Radic. Biol. Med.,* 18, 1079, 1995.
47. Sen, C. K., Oxidants and antioxidants in exercise, *J. Appl. Physiol.,*79, 675, 1995.
48. Dekkers, J. C., van Doornen, L. J. P., and Kemper, H. C. G., The role of antioxidant vitamins and enzymes in the prevention of exercise-induced muscle damage, *Sports Med.,* 21, 213, 1996.
49. Tiidus, P. M., Can estrogens diminish exercise induced muscle damage? *Can. J. Appl. Physiol.,* 20, 26, 1995.
50. Phillips, S. M., Atkinson, S. A., Tarnopolsky, M. A., and MacDougall, J. D., Gender differences in leucine kinetics and nitrogen balance in endurance athletes, *J. Appl. Physiol.,* 75, 2134, 1993.
51. Tarnopolsky, L. T., MacDougall, J. D., Atkinson, S. A., Tarnopolsky, M. A., and Sutton, J. R., Gender differences in substrate for endurance exercise, *J. Appl. Physiol.,* 68, 302, 1990.
52. Tarnopolsky, M. A., Atkinson, S. A., Phillips, S. M., and MacDougall, J. D., Carbo-hydrate loading and metabolism during exercise in men and women, *J. Appl. Physiol.,* 78, 1360, 1995.

CHAPTER 13

Gender Differences in the Metabolic Responses to Caffeine

Terry E. Graham and Cyndy McLean

CONTENTS

I. INTRODUCTION

This chapter will not review fundamental aspects of caffeine's effects on metabolism during exercise (there are many reviews that address this[1,2,3,4]), but will focus on the potential for men and women to have different responses to caffeine ingestion. Caffeine is clearly a potent ergogenic drug (Figure 13.1), but as in most areas of metabolic and exercise physiology the studies almost exclusively have used male subjects. This is highlighted by a recent text by Spiller[5] on caffeine. There is a very wide range of topics addressed in the text (including the metabolism of methylxan-

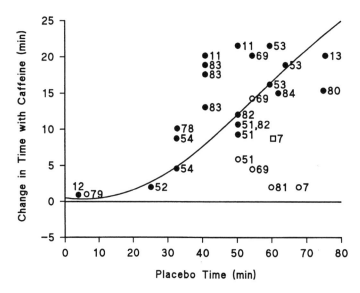

Figure 13.1   The impact of caffeine ingestion on endurance time. Data from studies in which endurance was measured using protocols in which the power output was not varied. The number beside the data point indicates the reference number. The horizontal solid line indicates where a data point would be placed if there was no change from the placebo condition. Filled symbols represent data that was significantly different from placebo and an open symbol represents a nonsignificant finding. The square represents the one study that presented for women.[7] In those cases where the same study is presented more than once this is because different caffeine doses,[51,69,83] methylxanthines,[54] days of withdrawl,[53] exercise modes,[11] or genders[7] were studied.

thines, caffeine as a ergogenic agent, caffeine's effects on metabolism), but women, estrogen, progesterone etc. are not considered except in the brief final chapter on reproductive function. This is unfortunate both for practical reasons and because caffeine is potentially a very valuable research tool to explore a wide range of possible gender differences. Caffeine and other methylxanthines are metabolized within the hepatic P450 system. Caffeine has been suggested as a probe to study the integrity of this system and thus it also could be used to examine potential male/female differences in the metabolic pathway.

As reviewed in other chapters of this text, there may be gender differences in fat mobilization. Caffeine is a potent lipolytic agent and could be used to examine gender differences in regulation of fat metabolism. In the area of sport there are several practical issues; little is known about possible male/female differences in its ergogenic properties. In addition, if the hepatic metabolism of caffeine is gender-specific, sport organizations should have different acceptable caffeine levels for men and women.

In a comprehensive review of the metabolism of caffeine, Arnaud[6] stated that there are no gender differences in caffeine metabolism, but he also stated that menstrual cycle phase, oral contraceptive (OCS) use, and pregnancy alter the metabolism of caffeine. How is this possible if there are no gender differences? A close examination of this literature reveals several important limitations. First, many of these definitive statements are based on very few studies. Second, several of the studies are not internally consistent in their pharmacological data, suggesting either unusual physiological responses or experimental error. In addition, most of the studies examining the reproductive status of women have not included a group of male subjects for comparison. There is such a wide range among studies in such pharmacokinetic data as the half-life of caffeine that it would be very difficult to show that a given group of women in a single study differ from this range. To test the possibility that there are gender differences, direct comparisons within a single protocol are necessary with well-matched groups and the menstrual status of the women needs to be evaluated clearly.

The topic of whether or not there are differences between women and men in the responses to caffeine ingestion is a difficult issue. As all of the chapters in this text have demonstrated, it is very difficult to conduct studies comparing men and women for any aspect of metabolism and feel confident that differences are due to gender and not the lifestyle — exercise history, menstrual cycle "status" (use of OCS, amenorrhea, position within the cycle, etc.), nutritional status, etc. — of the individuals tested. Rarely have men and women been compared for any aspect of caffeine's effects, and it is disappointing that of the few studies that have included female subjects there are several in which menstrual status of the women was not documented or considered[7,8,9,10] and where male subjects were not included for comparison.[8,9,10] The authors too are not immune to this criticism as there are several studies from their laboratory in which some women subjects were included and there was no documentation or control for menstrual cycle.[11,12,13] In addition, in several cases[7,14] an absolute amount of caffeine was administered to both the men and women, resulting in the latter receiving a greater dose per kg body wt. Furthermore, rarely, if ever, have the groups been matched for factors that can alter caffeine metabolism such as dietary habits, fat mass, or exercise habits. Even if these are controlled for, there could be male/female differences due to (a) the pharmacokinetics of caffeine's metabolism leading to different exposures to circulating caffeine and its metabolites, (b) the possible innate differences between genders in carbohydrate and fat metabolism, and (c) the sensitivity of key tissues to the metabolic or ergogenic signal(s) associated with caffeine.

II. THE PHARMACOKINETICS OF CAFFEINE

A number of factors are associated with variations in the pharmacokinetics of caffeine. Although caffeine absorption is unaffected by these factors, the metabolism and excretion of caffeine may be altered. Elevated sex hormones associated with pregnancy, OCS use, and menstrual cycle position are associated with a decrease in caffeine metabolism. Furthermore, smoking, obesity, dietary factors, and exercise habits have been shown to alter the levels and activities of the cytochrome P450 enzymes responsible for the metabolism of caffeine. Plasma caffeine concentration and the concentrations of its metabolites may be affected by these factors (Tables 13.1 and 13.2). This then could lead to differences in responses in various tissues.

Table 13.1 Factors Affecting CYP1A2 and Drug Metabolism

Factor	Ref. #	Subjects	Parameter	Effect	Comment
Dietary					
• charcoal-broiled meat	35	8 m (NS/ND)	theophylline kinetics	$\downarrow t_{1/2}$, $\uparrow Cl_{AUC}$	ENV
• cruciferous vegetables	16	4 m/5 f	CYP1A2 activity	± 12%	ENV, no MC
	34	7 m/3 f (NS)	antipyrine kinetics	$\downarrow t_{1/2}$, $\uparrow Cl_{AUC}$	no MC or ENV, AD
Smoking	16	335 m/f	CYP1A2 activity	↑ 68%	no gender difference
	32	14 m/14 f (S & NS)	theophylline kinetics	$\downarrow t_{1/2}$, $\uparrow Cl_{AUC}$	MC, gender difference, no DIET, AD
	33	63 f	antipyrine kinetics	$\uparrow Cl_{AUC}$	AD, MC, OCS negate effect of smoking
Obesity	23	15 f (4 S) (5 m (2 S)	caffeine kinetics	$\downarrow Vd$	ENV, no MC or DIET, AD
	22	3 lean m, 3 obese m (NS)	caffeine kinetics	$\uparrow t_{1/2}$, caffeine absorption	ENV
Exercise	36	6 f (2 OCS) (8 m (1 S)	antipyrine kinetics	relationship between $\uparrow VO_{2max}$ and $\uparrow Cl_{AUC}$ and $\downarrow t_{1/2}$	DIET, AD
• training	16	23 m	CYP1A2 activity	↑ 70%	training consisted of 8-11 h/d for 30 d, no ENV or DIET
	37	12 rats	P450 content/activity	≠	14 days, 30 min/day
	38	rats	P450 content/activity	Ø	8 weeks, 4×/week
	39	20 m rats	P450 content/activity	no effect	11 weeks, 5×/week

• acute			no effect	14 days, 30 min/day
37	12 rats	P450 content/activity	↑ peak [caffeine], ↓ $t_{1/2}$, Vd	results internally inconsistent, AD, ENV, no MC
42	6 m/6 f (NS)	caffeine kinetics	↑ Vd, ↓ $t_{1/2}$ in high caffeine users	results internally inconsistent, ENV
	(5/6 f high caffeine users)	theophylline kinetics	↓ clearance, Vd	ENV
43	6 m (NS)	caffeine kinetics	↓ peak [caffeine], AUC	
22	3 lean, 3 obese (NS)	caffeine kinetics	no gender difference	ENV, MC, DIET
McLean and Graham	6 m/8 f		no effect of exercise	

Note: Cl_{AUC} — plasma clearance, Vd — volume of distribution, $t_{1/2}$ — elimination half-life, CYP1A2 — cytochrome P450 1A2 enzymes, S — smokers, NS — nonsmokers, NOCS — nonoral contraceptive steroid users, ND — nondrug users, DIET — controls (caffeine intake, crusiferous vegetables, charcoal-broiled meat), E NV — Environmental controls (e.g., smoking, exercise, level of training, body composition), MC — Menstrual cycle controls (e.g., OCS, menstrual cycle position, pregnancy), AD — absolute dosage of caffeine, SH — sex hormone measurements, EUM — eumenorrheic.

Table 13.2   Effect of Gender on CYP1A2 activity and Caffeine Kinetics

Factor		Ref. #	Subjects	Parameter	Effect	Comment
Gender	• males vs. females	18	309 m/f	CYP1A2 activity	↓ f	no ENV, AD
		19	26 m/14 f	CYP1A2 activity	↓ in chinese f but not caucasian f	no DIET or MC, AD
			NS/ND			
		20	59 m/61 f	CYP1A2 activity	↓ f	AD, no MC, greater incidence of toxic side effects in f
			(S & NS)			
		15	186 m/f	CYP1A2 activity	no gender difference (after control for OCS)	subjects ingested 1–4 c coffee or tea
		17	113 m/f	CYP1A2 activity	no gender difference	nulliparous f < parous f
		85	4 m/4 EUM f/4 OCS	caffeine kinetics	no gender difference (after control for OCS)	
		21	245 m/f	CYP1A2 activity	no gender difference	MC, ENV, no DIET, AD
	• menstrual cycle	24	10 EUM	caffeine kinetics	↓ Cl$_{AUC}$	MC, SH, no DIET, ENV. AD
	• OCS	27	9 OCS	caffeine kinetics	↑ AUC, mean residence time	no SH or DIET, AD
			2/9 – S			
		28	9 OCS/9 NOCS/13 m	caffeine kinetics	↑ t$_{1/2}$ and ↓ Cl$_{AUC}$ with OCS	NS, ENV, no DIET, AD
		29	9 OCS users 9 f controls	caffeine kinetics	↑ t$_{1/2}$ and ↓ Cl$_{AUC}$ with OCS	NS, ENV, no SH, AD
	• pregnancy	30	15 f	caffeine kinetics	↑ t$_{1/2}$ and ↓ Cl$_{AUC}$	no ENV, SH or DIET, AD

Note: Cl$_{AUC}$ — plasma clearance, Vd — volume of distribution, t$_{1/2}$ — elimination half-life, CYP1A2 — cytochrome P450 1A2 enzymes, S — smokers, NS — nonsmokers, NOCS — nonoral contraceptive steroid users, ND — nondrug users, DIET — controls (caffeine intake, crusiferous vegetables, charcoal-broiled meat), E NV — Environmental controls (e.g., smoking, exercise, level of training, body composition), MC — Menstrual cycle controls (e.g., OCS, menstrual cycle position, pregnancy), AD — absolute dosage of caffeine, SH — sex hormone measurements, EUM — eumenorrheic.

III. CAFFEINE METABOLISM

In humans, caffeine is metabolized mostly by three-demethylation to form the dimethylxanthine, paraxanthine. This biotransformation is catalyzed by cytochrome P450 1A2 (CYP1A2) and accounts for 83.9 ± 5.4 percent of the primary degradation of caffeine. Theobromine, and, to a minor extent, theophylline, also accumulate in plasma following caffeine ingestion. These metabolites account for 12.2 ± 4.1 percent and 3.7 ± 1.3 percent of caffeine demethylation, respectively. The major pathway for caffeine 1- and 7-demethylations is mediated by CYP1A2, yet a small amount is attributed to the ethanol-inducible cytochrome P450 2E1 (CYP2E1). Each of the primary demethylation products is metabolized further to form a variety of xanthines, uric acids, and uracils.[15] The urinary fate of caffeine will be discussed later.

The P450 enzymes responsible for caffeine metabolism are also important for the bioactivation and/or detoxification of many drugs, carcinogens, and endogenous compounds (e.g., estrogen). As a result, caffeine has been used as a test compound to assess liver function and the foreign compound metabolizing capacity of CYP1A2 and CYP2E1. The measurement of the pharmacokinetics of caffeine provides a simple method for the assessment of enzyme activities important for the metabolic activation of carcinogens.[16] This has practical application to the assessment of cancer susceptibility. Horn et al.[17] examined the possibility that gender differences in CYP1A2 are associated with a higher incidence of bladder cancer in males. Although this study found no statistical difference between males and females in CYP1A2 activity (as assessed by the caffeine breath test), nulliparous women had significantly lower CYP1A2 activity than parous women. No other study has evaluated the impact of a previous pregnancy on CYP1A2 activity or caffeine metabolism.

A. Gender and CYP1A2

As previously mentioned, the enzymes responsible for caffeine metabolism are also responsible for the metabolism of estrogen. Estrogen may have an inhibitory effect on CYP1A2 activity and/or levels. Although sex differences in CYP1A2 may be expected, studies evaluating the impact of gender on the activity of these enzymes have produced conflicting results. Relling et al.[18] demonstrated in a group of children that that females had lower CYP1A2 activity and lower concentrations of all caffeine metabolites than males. Similarly, low CYP1A2 activity was noted in Chinese women but not Caucasian women compared with their male counterparts.[19] Lower CYP1A2 activity also has been associated with a greater self-reported incidence of toxic effects in both nonsmoking and smoking females.[20] However, after controlling for OCS use, both Kalow et al.[15] and Catteau et al.[21] demonstrated no difference between men and women in CYP1A2 activity.

Although there is evidence that suggests a gender difference in CYP1A2 activity, limitations in the preceding studies confound the results. A number of the studies[18,20,21] have used an absolute caffeine dosage rather than a dosage based on the subject's body weight. This may explain partially an increased incidence of toxic effects following caffeine ingestion in female subjects (dose for females = 5.4 mg/kg vs. dose for males = 4 mg/kg).[20] Additionally, there is new evidence suggesting that chronic caffeine ingestion may be associated with higher caffeine breath test levels and enhanced caffeine metabolism.[17] A number of the previously mentioned studies did not account for chronic caffeine usage.[18,19] Furthermore, the failure of the studies to control for OCS use,[20] menstrual cycle position (and hormonal status) and previous pregnancies,[19,21] and lifestyle (e.g., dietary and physical fitness) and environmental factors (e.g., smoking) in both sexes[18] may have an impact on CYP1A2 activity and thus the metabolism of caffeine.

It has been suggested that drug metabolism might be affected by the elevated body fat associated with obesity. This factor seldom is accounted for in pharmacokinetic studies. Because women generally have a larger percentage of their body weight from adipose tissue than men, failure to control for this factor may confound the evaluation of gender differences in caffeine metabolism. This observation may however be considered a potential mechanism for an observed gender difference. There is evidence demonstrating that extreme obesity (BMI > 39 kg/m^2) enhances the absorption of caffeine[22] and reduces the apparent volume of distribution (Vd) (corrected for body weight).[23] However, plasma clearance (Cl_{AUC}) is unaffected and the elimination half-life ($t_{1/2}$) has been shown to be both longer in obese individuals[22] and not different[23] from lean controls. If obesity has an affect on the pharmacokinetics of caffeine it is minimal. Thus, observed gender differences in caffeine may only be partially attributable to body fat differences.

IV. SEX HORMONES AND CAFFEINE METABOLISM

In healthy individuals, the reported $t_{1/2}$ ranges from 3.1 to 6.4 h, Cl_{AUC} from 0.98 to 1.82 ml/min/kg, and Vd from 0.52 to 0.60 l/kg (Table 13.3). Part of the variability in these measurements may be due to environmental and lifestyle factors of the subjects; however, gender, menstrual status, pregnancy, and OCS use also have been reported to alter the pharmacokinetics of caffeine. Elevated levels of sex hormones are believed to be responsible for the inhibition of caffeine metabolism because no evidence of alterations in caffeine absorption or hepatic extraction have been demonstrated.

Lane et al.[24] noted the increase in estradiol and progesterone associated with the luteal phase of the menstrual cycle was correlated with a significant reduction in the systemic clearance of caffeine. Similarly, a 25 percent decrease in caffeine elimination (and a corresponding increase in $t_{1/2}$) during the luteal phase of a normal menstrual cycle was noted by Balogh and coworkers.[25] Although they have not been studied, one might expect that amenorrheic women would have similar caffeine pharmacokinetics to eumenorrheic women in the follicular phase because amenorrheic women have comparable concentrations of both estradiol and progesterone but do not experience a cyclical increase in these sex hormones (Chapter 2). In female subjects, it has been suggested that menstrual cycle variables may account for 25 to 50 percent of the total variability in the measures of caffeine elimination at rest.[24]

The use of OCS and pregnancy consistently alter caffeine kinetics. The administration of levonorgestrel (a synthetic progesterone) has been shown to have no independent effect on caffeine metabolism; however, the administration of ethinyl

Table 13.3 Summary of Previous Methylxanthine Pharmacokinetic Literature at Rest and During Exercise With and Without Heat

Condition	Ref. #	Subjects	Methylxanthine Dose	K_{el} (h^{-1})	V_d (l/kg)	CL_{AUC} $(ml/min/kg)$	$t_{1/2}$ (h)	Comments
Rest	86	4 m	5 mg/kg caffeine	0.11	0.56	1.01	6.3	DIET, no ENV
	87	6 (1 f/5 m) NS	50, 300, 500, 750 mg caffeine	0.12	0.52	0.98	6.0	DIET, no ENV or MC, no effect of dose on CL_{AUC}
	88	13 (4 f/9 m) (1 S/12 NS)	70, 200, 300 mg caffeine	0.12 ◆	0.55	1.08	6.4	DIET, no ENV or MC, ↓ CL_{AUC} with ↑ dose
	23	14 (9 f/5 m)	200 mg caffeine	0.11 ◆	0.59	1.23	6.1	ENV, no MC or DIET
	42	6 m/6 f (NS) (5/6 f high caffeine users)	250 mg caffeine	0.18 ◆	0.60	1.82	4.0	results internally inconsistent, ENV, no MC
	44	6 m (NS)	200 mg/m2 body surface area theophylline	0.12	0.52	0.99	6.4	results internally inconsistent, ENV
	89	5 m (2 smokers)/7 f	250, 500 mg caffeine	0.15 ◆	0.53	1.64	4.7	↓ CL_{AUC} and ↑ $t_{1/2}$ with ↑ dose
	McLean and Graham	6 m/8 f (NS, NOCS)	6 mg/kg caffeine	0.12	0.61	1.19	6.4	ENV, MC, DIET
Exercise	42 (	6 m/6 f (NS) (5/6 f high caffeine users)	250 mg caffeine	0.31 ◆	0.34	1.76	2.3	results internally inconsistent, ENV, no MC
	43 *	6 m (NS)	200 mg/m2 body surface area theophylline	0.08	0.51	0.70	8.5	results internally inconsistent, ENV
	43 ◆	6 m (NS)	200 mg/m2 body surface area theophylline	0.10	0.45	0.75	7.2	results internally inconsistent, ENV
	McLean and Graham Ψ	6 m/8 f (NS, NOCS)	6 mg/kg caffeine	0.12	0.60	1.14	6.9	ENV, MC, DIET

Table 13.3   Summary of Previous Methylxanthine Pharmacokinetic Literature at Rest and During Exercise With and Without Heat *(continued)*

Condition	Ref. #	Subjects	Methylxanthine Dose	Kel (h⁻¹)	Vd (l/kg)	Cl_AUC (ml/min/kg)	t₁/₂ (h)	Comments
Exercise with heat	43 *	6 m (NS)	200 mg/m2 body surface area theophylline	0.09	0.43	0.62	8.0	results internally inconsistent, ENV
	McLean and Graham Ψ	6 m/8 f (NS, NOCS)	6 mg/kg caffeine	0.10	0.64	1.05	8.3	ENV, MC, DIET

Note: ♠ — data was not provided by the author. Calculations were based on the data provided, # — exercise performed at 30 percent VO₂max for 1 h, * — exercise performed at 30 percent VO₂max for 2 h, ♦ — exercise performed at 50 percent VO₂max for 2 h, Ψ — exercise performed at 65 percent VO₂max for 1.5 h, S — smokers, NS — nonsmokers, NOCS — nonoral contraceptive steroid users, ND — nondrug users, DIET — Diet controls (caffeine intake, cruciferous vegetables, charcoal-broiled meat), E NV — Environmental controls (e.g., smoking, exercise, level of training, body composition), MC — Menstrual cycle controls (e.g., OCS, menstrual cycle position, pregnancy), AD — absolute dosage of caffeine, SH — sex hormone measurements, EUM — eumenorrheic.

estradiol with and without progesterone markedly reduced the elimination of caffeine.[26] The use of OCS increases $t_{1/2}$ from 5.8 h to 11.1 h,[27] decreases Cl_{AUC} by 50 percent,[28] and prolongs the time to reach peak caffeine concentration ([caffeine]).[29] Aldridge et al.[30] demonstrated no difference in Cl_{AUC} during the first trimester of pregnancy, yet a progressive reduction in Cl_{AUC} during the second and third trimester. The $t_{1/2}$ increased from 5.3 h to 18.1 h during the last two trimesters.

It has been suggested that elevated estradiol concentrations inhibit caffeine metabolism due to substrate competition or the impairment of CYP1A2 activity. Ironically, the majority of studies have not measured sex steroid levels.[27,28,29,30] Furthermore, based on *in vitro* studies, the hormone concentrations required for enzyme inhibition are higher than those achieved by OCS use and menstrual cycle fluctuations.[31]

Similar to studies evaluating the impact of gender on CYP1A2 activity, the majority of studies evaluating the effect of sex hormones on caffeine kinetics suffer from methodological problems. These studies have not evaluated a homogeneous group of women, have included women of a wide reproductive age (for example, 18 to 35 years[27]), and have not controlled for the reproductive (or hormonal concentrations) status of the subjects. In two studies,[27,29] five of the non-OCS controls were tested during the luteal phase although four were tested during the follicular phase. Additionally, the subjects in OCS studies have been on a variety of OCS for varying durations. The OCS can vary in chemical form and concentrations.[27,28] The impact of these factors on blood hormone concentrations and caffeine metabolism has not been evaluated. Furthermore, two out of nine subjects in one study evaluating the effects of OCS were cigarette smokers.[27] Cigarette smoking has been demonstrated to increase the activity and hepatic content of CYP1A2 by four percent per cigarette/day.[16] The effect of smoking on hepatic metabolism might be gender-specific because Jennings et al.,[32] demonstrated an enhanced Cl_{AUC} and shorter $t_{1/2}$ of theophylline in eumenorrheic, non-OCS female smokers (tested in the follicular phase) compared with men. Additionally, moderate cigarette smoking has been shown to counteract the inhibition of OCS on antipyrine (a drug that also is metabolized by CYP1A2) metabolism.[33] Finally, none of the previously mentioned studies have considered the physical fitness levels of the subjects.

Recently, the authors investigated the effect of both gender and exercise on caffeine metabolism in six men and eight eumenorrheic women. All subjects were nonsmokers and nondrug users (including OCS), were matched for level of fitness (VO_{2max}) (females: 50.6 ± 1.2 ml/kg/min versus males: 50.7 ± 1.7 ml/kg/min) and caffeine intake (females: 80 mg/d versus males: 100 mg/d), and were asked to follow a controlled diet excluding cruciferous vegetables and charbroiled meat (both shown to alter caffeine kinetics (34 and 35, respectively) prior to testing. Although not matched for body composition, the female and male subjects were similar in their percentage body fat (females: 21.0 ± 0.7 percent versus males: 16.4 ± 1.8 percent). All subjects were tested for eight hours at rest following the ingestion of 6 mg/kg caffeine (3 to 9 mg/kg has been shown to be ergogenic). The female subjects were tested during the early follicular phase (as confirmed by estradiol and progesterone measures) of the menstrual cycle. Although peak [caffeine] (women = 47.3 ± 2.5 µM vs. men = 40.3 ± 2.9 µM) approached significance (p = 0.09), there were no gender differences in time to peak [caffeine] (women = 1.79 ± 0.26 h vs. men = 1.92 ± 0.08 h), $t_{1/2}$ (women = 6.95 ± 1.05 h vs. men = 5.70 ± 0.75 h), Cl_{AUC} (women = 1.10 ± 0.19 ml/min/kg vs. men 1.30 ± 0.12 ml/min/kg) or Vd (women = 0.60 ± 0.03 l/kg vs. men = 0.61 ± 0.05 l/kg). These results demonstrate that gender has no effect on the absorption, distribution, and metabolism of caffeine when male and female subjects are matched for level of fitness and lifestyle habits and when menstrual cycle variables (tested in the midfollicular phase) are controlled so that estrogen and progesterone are low.

V. GENDER, EXERCISE AND CAFFEINE METABOLISM

Enhanced hepatic drug metabolism is associated with improvements in physical fitness. Boel et al.[36] reported a significant positive correlation between improvements in maximal oxygen uptake (VO_{2max}) following a three-month training period and the metabolism of antipyrine. In animal studies, an increase,[37] a decrease,[38] and no change[39] in hepatic microsomal enzymes or their activity has been found following endurance training. Interestingly, it has been proposed that amenorrhea in highly trained females may be associated with an enhanced hepatic metabolism of estrogens by CYP1A2.[40] Caffeine could be a valuable tool to assess this possible relationship.

The hepatic metabolism of some drugs also may be affected by an acute bout of physical exercise. Hepatic clearance is the product of hepatic blood flow and hepatic extraction. Unlike high clearance drugs (such as indocyanine green), the clearance of drugs with enzyme-limited metabolisms (such as caffeine) is independent of hepatic blood flow.[41] It is for this reason that caffeine metabolism should not be affected by exercise-induced changes in hepatic blood flow, and the measurement of caffeine pharmacokinetics can be used as an indicator of hepatic drug-metabolizing activity. Although in animals no effect of an acute bout of exercise on P450 content has been observed,[37] there is evidence suggesting that acute exercise alters caffeine pharmacokinetics.

Collomp et al.[42] examined caffeine kinetics in a group of men and women over an eight-hour period both at rest (R) and with mild (30 percent VO_{2max}) exercise (E) during the first hour. In contrast to previous investigations of drugs similar to caffeine,[41] exercise raised the maximal plasma [caffeine] (R = 37.5 μM vs. E = 53.8 μM) and reduced the $t_{1/2}$ (R = 4.0 h vs. E = 2.29) and Vd (R = 0.60 l/kg vs. 0.34 l/kg). Caffeine Cl_{AUC} appeared not to be altered by exercise. The authors suggested the increase in peak [caffeine] and the decrease in Vd were linked to the cardiocirculatory adjustments associated with exercise. However, there were no measurements that could confirm this hypothesis. It is unlikely that exercise of such a mild intensity would reduce liver blood flow drastically and/or cause a sweat loss extreme enough to account for the dramatic alterations in caffeine pharmacokinetics observed with exercise in this study.

The pharmacokinetic data for the male and female subjects in this investigation appeared similar at rest and responded the same to exercise, with the exception of Vd. The Vd (corrected for body weight) both at rest and with exercise was approximately 50 percent greater in the female subjects. Similarly, Patwardhan et al.,[28] found that women (non-OCS users) had a higher Vd than men at rest, but there were no other gender differences in caffeine kinetics. However, in the Collomp study,[42] five out of the six female subjects were heavy coffee drinkers, and regular heavy coffee intake was shown by these researchers to increase Vd and decrease caffeine elimination. Therefore, it is difficult to assess whether the differences observed in these women reflected habitual coffee consumption or gender differences. Also, it is tempting to suggest that the gender difference in Vd is the result of greater body fat in the female subjects; however, as previously mentioned, higher body fat with obesity has been associated with a lower Vd (corrected for body weight) in both men and women[23] and could not account for the large difference between genders. Finally, the lack of dietary controls and the failure to control for the menstrual cycle phase of the female subjects (6 out of 12 subjects) could have confounded the results.

In contrast, acute exercise in male subjects has resulted in an extended $t_{1/2}$ yet a reduction in Vd and Cl_{AUC} of theophylline.[43] The authors concluded that the change in Vd was evidence of dehydration with exercise. However, there were no measurements that could confirm that dehydration had occurred. Furthermore, Kaminori et al.[22] demonstrated that acute exercise consistently decreased maximal [caffeine] (31.9 μM vs. 30.3 μM) and the area under the concentration-time curve (AUC) in obese but not lean men. The results of this study are questionable because each group consisted of only three subjects.

Although there is evidence to suggest methylxanthine pharmacokinetics may be affected by exercise, limitations in the preceding studies confound the results. Failure to control for factors that alter the intrinsic ability of the liver to metabolize caffeine (level of fitness, diet, the menstrual status of female subjects, etc.) may have an impact on the pharmacokinetic results. Furthermore, it is difficult to interpret these studies[42,43] because the results are contradictory and internally inconsistent. For example, Collomp et al.[42] noted a decrease in Vd and $t_{1/2}$, yet paradoxically no effect of exercise on Cl_{AUC}. Because Cl_{AUC} is calculated as the product of hepatic clearance (Kel) and Vd, in their study Kel must have increased to a similar extent as Vd decreased in response to exercise (e.g., 40 to 50 percent). The exercise intensity was only 30 percent VO_{2max}, and even maximal fluid losses equivalent to 6 to 10 percent body weight reported with intense exercise in the heat[44] could not account for the large reductions in Vd that must have occurred in this study.

In the authors' previously described study of the pharmacokinetics of caffeine, the eight-hour protocol was repeated with an exercise component. Ninety minutes of cycling at 65 percent VO_{2max} was performed one hour following caffeine ingestion in the exercise trial. As with the resting trial, the women were tested in the midfollicular phase of their menstrual cycle. Weight loss due to sweating during the exercise was not different between females (1.25 ± 0.13 kg) and males (1.82 ± 0.29 kg). Furthermore, exercise had no effect on any of the pharmacokinetic measures. Similar to the resting trial, there were no gender differences in time to reach peak [caffeine] (women = 2.06 ± 0.26 h vs. men = 1.83 ± 0.25), $t_{1/2}$ (women = 6.92 ± 0.85 h vs. men = 6.28 ± 0.55 h), Cl_{AUC} (women = 1.14 ± 0.19 ml/min/kg vs. men = 1.27 ± 0.11 ml/min/kg), or Vd (women = 0.60 ± 0.03 vs. men = 0.67 ± 0.04) in the exercise trial. However, peak [caffeine] was significantly higher in the females than the males (women = 47.0 ± 1.82 μM vs. men = 37.4 ± 2.37 μM).

To investigate the impact of exercise with an additional thermal stress, female subjects completed one additional eight-hour trial, which included 90 minutes of cycling at 65 percent VO_{2max}, one hour following caffeine ingestion. In this trial, the subjects wore additional clothing to create a heat stress. Rectal and abdominal skin temperatures and weight loss due to sweating were significantly greater with exercise and heat ($39.4 \pm 0.22°C$, $36.5 \pm 0.41°C$, and 1.51 ± 0.09 kg, respectively) than with exercise alone ($38.6 \pm 0.11°C$, $32.6 \pm 0.84°C$, and 1.25 ± 0.13 kg, respectively). Although the thermal stress was greater in the exercise with heat trial, this had no effect on peak [caffeine] (44.2 ± 1.71 μM), time to peak [caffeine] (2.00 ± 0.16 h), $t_{1/2}$ (8.27 ± 1.15 h), Vd (0.64 ± 0.03), or Cl_{AUC} (1.05 ± 0.18 ml/min/kg).

From the data, it is difficult to explain the higher peak [caffeine] in females compared to males both at rest and with exercise particularly because there were no gender differences in Vd. However, the data appear to be quite reproducible because in the male group the peak [caffeine] was 40 μM and 37 μM in the resting and exercise trials, respectively, and in the female group the peak [caffeine] was 47 μM, 47 μM, and 44 μM in the resting, exercise, and exercise with heat trials, respectively. Although not significant, there was a trend for the area under the concentration-time curves (AUC) to be higher in the female subjects than the male subjects both at rest (women = 104.9 (g/ml · h ± 14.7 vs. men = 81.5 ± 9.79 μg/ml · h) and with exercise (women = 99.9 ± 11.1 μg/ml · h vs. men = 82.3 ± 8.93 μg/ml · h). AUC reflects the exposure to unbound drug; however, alterations in protein binding have not been shown to affect AUC. Furthermore, no major gender difference in protein binding has been demonstrated.[45] Nevertheless, it appears that females achieve a higher [caffeine] and also may have a greater duration of exposure to caffeine than males following a given dose. Therefore, it is possible that females may have a greater ergogenic and metabolic response to a given dose of caffeine because these pharmacodynamic responses are dependent on [caffeine].

Unlike the results of Collomp et al.,[42] Schlaeffer et al.[43] and Kaminori et al.,[22] the authors' results are internally consistent and are in agreement with previous pharmacokinetic literature, which has demonstrated no effect of exercise on the metabolism and elimination of drugs similar to caffeine. The Cl_{AUC} and $t_{1/2}$ of these drugs are not affected by exercise because they are not limited by hepatic blood flow, have a large Vd and a low-hepatic extraction ratio.[45,46,47] The internal consistency of the data may be due to the controls because the male and female subjects were matched for level of fitness, activity levels, and caffeine habits, and had a similar percent body fatness. Furthermore, the authors controlled for factors known to alter the intrinsic ability of the liver to metabolize caffeine, such as diet, smoking, drug use, and menstrual cycle phase.

VI. GENDER, EXERCISE, AND CAFFEINE EXCRETION

Caffeine metabolism by CYP1A2 functions to convert caffeine into water-soluble products for elimination. Caffeine metabolites are excreted by the kidney and appear in the urine as quickly as they are formed due to active renal secretion. Only a small percentage (1 to 5 percent) of ingested caffeine is excreted unchanged in urine due to renal tubular reabsorption.[6] Ironically, sport agencies such as the International Olympic Committee (IOC), monitor caffeine intake by urine [caffeine] alone.

Caffeine is considered a controlled substance in sport with the IOC urine [caffeine] limit set at 12 µg/ml. There is limited research evaluating the impact of exercise on the elimination of caffeine. Drug testing is based on one postexercise urine sample. The single standard does not take into consideration gender, exercise intensity or duration, the environmental conditions, or the physiological status of the athlete (e.g., dehydrated vs. euhydrated). The use of a single set standard has been criticized since a 15.9-fold inter- and intraindividual variability in urine [caffeine] has been noted at rest in men and women.[48] A portion of this variability may be due to the fact that the researchers did not evaluate differences in the urine [caffeine] between the male and female subjects.

van der Merwe et al.[49] evaluated the influence of exercise (30 min of running at 75 percent VO_{2max}) and excessive sweating on urinary [caffeine] following a 450 mg dose of caffeine. Exercise caused a significant decrease in urine flow and caffeine excretion. However, the urine [caffeine] were similar with and without exercise (8.28 ± 1.31 µg/ml vs. 8.34 ± 2.27 µg/ml, respectively). The researchers concluded that excessive sweating during long-distance running would not lead to a violation of the maximum permissible urine [caffeine]. The results of this study are difficult to interpret because no attempt was made to quantify the sweat loss during exercise. Furthermore, the large variability in urine [caffeine] may have occurred because each subject ingested a different caffeine dose when based on body weight (5.7 to 7.6 mg/kg).

The effect of exercise may not be the same for men and women. The gender of the nine endurance-trained athletes in the study by van der Merwe et al.[49] was not reported. Duthel et al.[50] reported that caffeine elimination at rest was similar for both sexes, yet moderate exercise (75 min of cycling at 50 percent VO_{2max}) resulted in a fivefold and a twofold decrease in caffeine elimination in women and men, respectively. This was associated with a significantly greater decrease in urinary flow in women. Unfortunately, menstrual status and OCS use was not controlled for in this study and there was no attempt to quantify sweat losses during exercise.

In the previously discussed study, the authors examined the impact of gender and exercise on urine [caffeine]. There was no gender difference in weight loss due to sweating (women = 1.25 ± 0.13 kg vs. men = 1.82 ± 0.29 kg) following 90 minutes of exercise at 65 percent VO_{2max}. Additionally, the authors found no gender differences in urine [caffeine] both at rest (women = 7.66 ± 0.81 µg/ml (range: 3.57 to 10.0 µg/ml) vs. men = 9.18 ± 0.76 µg/ml (range: 5.34 to 10.2 µg/ml) and during exercise (women = 6.10 ± 0.56 µg/ml (range: 4.29 to 8.43 µg/ml) vs. men = 7.12 ± 0.61 µg/ml (range: 4.95 to 9.16 µg/ml)). Furthermore, when a greater heat stress during the exercise was applied to the women (as confirmed by body temperatures and weight loss due to sweating), there was no effect on the postexercise urine [caffeine] (6.18 ± 0.18 µg/ml (range: 2.9 to 10.0 µg/ml). These results indicate no effect of gender or exercise (with and without an additional thermal stress) on the metabolism and excretion of caffeine; however, it also suggests that these factors have no effect on caffeine reabsorption. Interestingly, a 2- to 3-fold variation in urine [caffeine] was noted between subjects in the present study even though the subjects received the same relative caffeine dose based on their body weight. Furthermore, no subjects achieved a urine [caffeine] greater than the IOC limit of 12 µg/ml. The dose of caffeine given to the subjects in the present study was 6 mg/kg, which has been demonstrated to a potent ergogenic aid[12,51,52,53,54] (Figure 13.1).

As previously discussed, limited research suggests both a gender difference and an effect of exercise on the metabolism and elimination of caffeine. However, due to the methodological problems and internal inconsistencies of these data, it is impossible to conclude an effect of these factors on the pharmacokinetics of caffeine. Data demonstrate that eumenorrheic women, tested during the follicular phase of the menstrual cycle, may attain higher [caffeine] than well-matched men, but there is no gender difference or effect of exercise on the metabolism of caffeine and urinary [caffeine]. The authors expect that amenorrheic women would respond similarly to eumenorrheic women in the follicular phase of the menstrual cycle.

VII. GENDER, CAFFEINE, AND TISSUE SENSITIVITY

As demonstrated in Figure 13.1, there is a great deal of evidence that caffeine is an effective ergogenic agent over a wide range of exercise durations. It is not clear how caffeine mediates ergogenic effects (various reviews discuss the possible mechanisms of action;[2,3,4] however, caffeine is known to be an adenosine antagonist and in physiological concentrations many of its actions on tissues are through this mechanism. What is not known is whether these actions result in the enhanced work capacity or whether other mechanisms independent of adenosine receptor antagonism are involved. Adenosine receptors are found in most tissues, particularly in the central nervous system and adipose tissue. In the latter tissue, adenosine acts permissively with insulin to increase glucose uptake and to promote lipogenesis. Caffeine antagonism of the adenosine receptors is a strong lipolytic signal. However, to the authors' knowledge, there has been only one study that has examined adipose tissue for possible gender differences in adenosine receptors. Xu et al.[55] investigated adenosine receptor antagonism in lean and obese Zucker rats. They measured tolerance to a glucose injection (ip) and also examined A1 receptor binding of cerebral cortex and adipose plasma membranes. Although chronic A1 antagonism upregulated receptor number in the adipose tissue, there were no gender differences in either brain or fat tissue.

However, regional differences may exist in human fat cells. Mauriege et al.[56] compared abdominal and femoral adipocytes in lean and obese women. Removing adenosine from the environment did not alter the inhibition of lipolysis by insulin in the femoral adipocytes. However, in the absence of extracellular adenosine, the abdominal adipocytes of lean women had no lipolytic response to insulin, although those from obese women showed a marked inhibition. Unfortunately they did not include males in the study.

Although functionally, adenosine has been shown to have actions on carbohydrate metabolism in skeletal muscle,[57,58,59] attempts to identify receptors in skeletal muscle[60,61] (van Soeren, unpublished) have shown in rat muscle that the A2 subtype exists, particularly in slow twitch muscle. None of these studies has addressed gender differences and it is not known if human muscle also has adenosine receptors.

The only investigation that the authors are aware of that has reported specifically any aspect of gender-specific effects of caffeine on muscle is by Kalow,[63] but it did not address adenosine receptors. Caffeine in pharmacological doses stimulated Ca++ release and produces contractures in skeletal muscle. Patients potentially susceptible to malignant hyperthermia are screened via a test using this property. Muscle biopsies from those who do suffer from this disorder show a high sensitivity to caffeine, i.e. a caffeine-induced contracture occurs with a lower caffeine concentration than in healthy controls. These investigators retrospectively examined the results of approximately 1200 patients (54 percent women) who were found not to have malignant hyperthermia. Muscle from men was shown on average to have a greater sensitivity to caffeine (4.3 compared to 4.8 mM caffeine for men and women respectively) and both father-son and brother-brother comparisons demonstrated a strong heritability relationship although mother-daughter did not and that of father-daughter had a moderate relationship. These findings suggest that men might be more responsive to those aspects of caffeine in which the muscle is stimulated directly.

Mitsumoto et al.[64] separated single, skinned muscle fibers from biopsies of human subjects, identified them as fast- or slow-twitch and determined their sensitivity to caffeine. They found that the slow-twitch fibers responded to a much lower concentration (2.7 vs. 6.9 mM caffeine), which is consistent with the possibility that such fibers have more adenosine receptors. Human muscle is approximately 50:50 fast- and slow-twitch, and if their data is averaged (4.8 mM) it compares very well to the values of 4.3 and 4.8 mM reported by Kalow.[63] In addition, they present a figure of their original data and 5 of 15 subjects were women. The authors have attempted to tabulate their data by gender and estimate the mean values for fast-twitch fibers to be very similar for the men (49 fibers) and women (14 fibers) (6.5 and 6.3 mM, respectively). In contrast, the data for men (18 fibers) and women (16 fibers) for slow-twitch fibers (2.4 and 3.0 mM respectively) indicate a 25 percent difference, which is consistent with that of Kalow.[63] The latter assumed that the mechanism involved was the ryanodine receptor, but it is also possible that adenosine receptors are involved. Unfortunately comparable data are not available for other tissues.

Finally in a preliminary report, Pinto and Tarnopolsky[65] tested 11 men and 12 women (no menstrual cycle control) with a variety of neuromuscular measures including peak twitch torque, maximal voluntary contraction, peak motor unit activation, and tetanic force. A number of these measure are obtained by direct neuromuscular stimulation of the peroneal nerve. Caffeine ingestion (7 mg/kg) resulted in an improvement of only one measure, peak-twitch torque, and the increase was similar in both groups.

VIII. GENDER, CAFFEINE, AND METABOLISM

It is clearly established that one common metabolic effect of caffeine ingestion is stimulation of lipolysis although it is not clear that the active muscle necessarily oxidizes the extra fatty acids.[1,2,3,4] Caffeine ingestion is associated with an increased sympathetic tone and thus the stimulation of lipolysis could occur from a direct caffeine antagonism of adipocyte adenosine receptors or from increased beta-adrenergic stimulation of the adipocytes. It is well-known[66,67] that there are regional differences in the metabolism of adipocytes and also gender differences in both distribution of fat and metabolic sensitivity of male and female adipocytes from the same region. As mentioned previously, only Xu et al.[55] have examined potential gender differences in the distribution of adenosine receptors, but there are gender differences in alpha and beta adrenergic receptor density. Jensen and coworkers[68] demonstrated the importance of this *in vivo* by infusing epinephrine into resting men and women. The men responded to the extra catecholamine by doubling the FFA release from the leg fat. Women had 70 percent more fat mass in their legs then did the men, yet showed no increase in fatty acid release from the legs and had an increased mobilization from the upper body. Just as in the previous section, there is very limited information, but it supports the theory that adipose tissue of women would be less sensitive to caffeine-induced lipolysis.

In a limited study of four men and four women (no controls for menstrual cycle), Cadarette et al.[69] reported that following caffeine ingestion and after prolonged exercise, plasma FFA and glycerol concentrations were higher in the women. Recently, in a preliminary report, Bosman et al.[70] summarized a more detailed investigation. They tested well-trained men (n = 8) and women (n = 8) (in the follicular phase) during 90 minutes of exercise at 65 percent of VO_{2max} followed by exercising to exhaustion at 75 percent of VO_{2max}. Caffeine resulted in no gender differences in RER or circulating glycerol, fatty acids or total triglyceride concentrations during the exercises.

Previous research has noted that men had greater FFA concentrations at rest than women matched for habitual caffeine intake.[71] In the study referred to previously in which the authors compared the caffeine pharmacokinetics of men and women both at rest and during moderate exercise, they also studied their metabolic responses. The men had higher glycerol concentrations than the women, but these were present from the beginning of the protocol and the changes over time were not different for either glycerol or fatty acids. Although the absolute change in glycerol concentrations from precaffeine ingestion levels were not different between the males and females, both in the resting trial and the exercise trial the relative change was significantly greater in the females than the males (Figures 13.2a and 13.2b). Additionally, the relative change in FFA was significantly greater in the females in the exercise trial but not in the resting trial (Figures 13.2c and 13.2d). It generally is accepted that glycerol is a more accurate indicator of lipolysis. Although these results are preliminary, they suggest that female adipocytes are more sensitive to caffeine-stimulated lipolysis both at rest and during exercise.

There have been a number of reports of gender differences in plasma catecholamines. It has been demonstrated that women have lower values of plasma epinephrine at rest[72] or during exercise[73,74] or during a variety of sympathoadrenal stimuli.[72] The data for circulating norepinephrine are less clear; perhaps because it is washed out of various tissues after it has functioned as a sympathetic neurotransmitter. Thus a mixed venous norepinephrine concentration is not a very sensitive measure of activ-

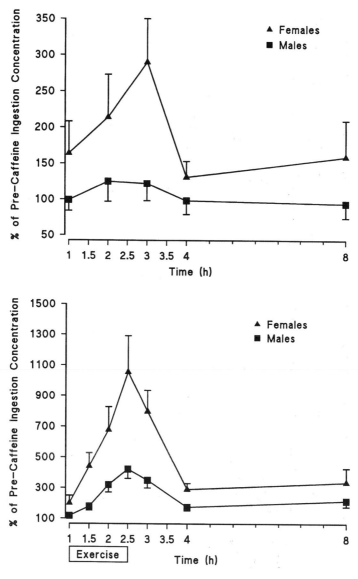

Figure 13.2a and 13.2b The percent change in glycerol concentration relative to the precaf-feine ingestion concentration in the resting trial (a) and the exercise trial (b). Females are represented by the solid triangle and males are represented by the solid square.

ity of the sympathetic nervous system. Muscle is a major contributor to the circu-lating norepinephrine, and differences in muscle mass could lead to lower circulating levels in women even if the activity of the sympathetic nervous system was the same in both sexes. However, there are studies in which women and men are compared for the amount of activity in the muscle sympathetic nerve activity (MSNA) via direct microneurographic recordings in the peroneal nerve. Jones et al.[75] reported

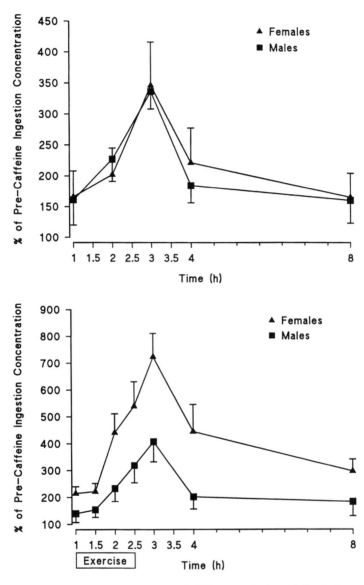

Figure 13.2c and 13.2d The percent change in FFA concentration relative to the precaffeine
ingestion concentration in the resting trial (c) and the exercise trial
(d). Females are represented by the solid triangle and males are
represented by the solid square.

that women at rest consistently had lower MSNA than men. Although Ettinger et
al.[76] did not find a difference at rest, they found that women had less than 25 percent
of the increase in MSNA seen in the men during static forearm contractions. Menstrual cycle status was not controlled for in any of the studies that examined catecholamines, but Ettinger et al.[76] found that postmenopausal women and premeno-

pausal women both showed an age-matched gender difference in MSNA. The lower MSNA activity should be reflected in lower plasma norepinephrine concentrations(Chapter 5).

IX. GENDER, CAFFEINE, AND PERFORMANCE

There is no area of research where there is a clear understanding of possible gender differences. However, the limited data in most aspects reviewed thus far suggest that women are less responsive to caffeine. However, this does not mean necessarily that women will be less responsive to the ergogenic effects of caffeine. As pointed out earlier, the hepatic P450 system in women may be influenced by estrogen such that women experience a greater peak caffeine and a more prolonged exposure to plasma caffeine. In addition, it is far from clear what aspects of caffeine ingestion result in the ergogenic response. It is clear that glycogen sparing is not critical nor is the increase in epinephrine or fatty acids[2]. As a result one cannot predict with confidence whether there should be a gender difference in endurance or performance.

Studies have shown that caffeine can influence both energy intake and expenditure. Tremblay et al.[14] noted that caffeine suppressed energy intake in males but not in females. There have been investigations examining the thermal (VO_2) responses of women and men to caffeine ingestion. Perkins and Williams[10] found that caffeine increased the metabolic rate in men but not in women. The former study demonstrated this at rest and during mild exercise. However, this study failed to consider or document the menstrual status of the women. One should not conclude that women cannot increase their metabolic rate because Bracco et al.[77] clearly illustrated that women do increase their metabolic rates in response to caffeine ingestion. Unfortunately the latter investigation did not compare men and women. Nevertheless, the results once again would suggest that women are less responsive to caffeine.

In contrast, Butts and Crowell[7] (Figure 13.1) had men and women (no menstrual cycle controls were employed) exercise to exhaustion at 75 percent of VO_{2max}. Caffeine did not affect the exercise VO_2 response and neither group had a statistically significant ergogenic response (perhaps because the caffeine was administered in coffee[78]), but following caffeine ingestion the women exercised 8.6 minutes (14.4 percent) longer as compared to 2.1 minutes (3.1 percent) for the men. However, an absolute amount of caffeine was administered to every subject and thus the women received about 20 percent more caffeine per kg body weight and plasma concentrations were not reported. In the study mentioned previously by Cararette et al.[69] the subjects (4 women and 4 men) ran at 80 percent VO_{2max} until exhaustion, but did not report gender-specific results. However, both in this study and that by Butts and Crowell,[7] one female subject had a massive increase in endurance.

In the recent study by Bosman et al.[70] referred to previously in which all the women were tested in the follicular phase, there were no gender differences in exercise VO_2 following caffeine ingestion. Subjects exercised for 90 minutes at 65 percent VO_{2max} and then at 75 percent VO_{2max} to exhaustion. Caffeine did not increase endurance statistically; the data for the men were 16.36 and 18.60 minutes for the placebo and caffeine trials, respectively, and the corresponding data for the women were 7.70 and 10.08 minutes. Thus the men and women improved by 2.34 and 2.38 minutes, respectively, or 13.7 and 31.0 percent of the placebo times. Once again there was a tendency for the women to have a greater relative increase in endurance.

As with the other areas reviewed, there is very little known and rarely have the women and men been well-matched or the reproductive status of the women been considered. However, these few studies would suggest that at rest and in mild exercise, men have a greater metabolic response to caffeine and that possibly women respond more to caffeine during endurance activity. The latter is highly speculative at this time.

X. SUMMARY

In this chapter the authors attempted to review the current information regarding gender differences in the main aspects of caffeine and metabolism: the hepatic metabolism of caffeine, the various metabolic signals mediating the effects of caffeine, and the ergogenic effects of caffeine. Each of these is a complex issue, and there have been so few studies conducted in any one area that it is impossible to reach conclusions. Unfortunately in several instances, investigations of men and women have failed to allow for the potential influence of the hormones associated with the menstrual cycle and/or the use of oral contraceptives. The authors have attempted to summarize the information, to suggest where gender differences could occur, and, most important, to illustrate how caffeine can be a valuable research tool to study possible gender differences.

There have been occasional reports that gender and/or exercise may influence caffeine metabolism, but within each of these studies the data lack internal consistency. When one carefully selects men and women matched for fitness, nutritional factors, adiposity, and caffeine habits, women in the follicular phase of the menstrual cycle have caffeine pharmacokinetics that are very similar to those of men. However, the women have a higher peak plasma caffeine concentration and it remains elevated for a longer period of time. The authors found that neither exercise nor exercise with dehydration influence either these results or the urinary concentration. The possible influence of the hormonal changes in the luteal phase and/or oral contraceptive use remain to be studied.

The known caffeine signals include increased catecholamine activity (both SNS activity and epinephrine secretion) as well as direct actions of caffeine and its metabolites. Possible gender differences in the former have not been studied with respect to caffeine, but generally men have a greater catecholamine response to stressors. Methylxanthines are thought to mediate their affects by antagonizing adenosine receptors. The authors do not know if gender differences exist in humans for adenosine receptors in such critical tissues as the brain, adipocytes, skeletal muscle, and the liver. This is clearly an aspect where caffeine could be employed as a tool to establish if receptor differences exist. Preliminary data suggest that women are more responsive to caffeine in terms of adipocyte lipolysis. The authors speculate that either women have more adenosine receptors on adipocytes or the receptors are more critical in inhibiting lipolysis.

There have been very few studies examining possible gender differences in ergogenic responses. It is impossible to speculate what differences could occur and they may be specific for a given exercise intensity. It is now evident that caffeine can be ergogenic in exercises that result in exhaustion ranging from a few minutes to more than an hour. It is very likely that the limiting factors are different in these various circumstances and thus caffeine must affect different mechanisms. Once again it would appear that caffeine could be a useful probe to study the limiting factors in these conditions.

REFERENCES

1. Conlee, R.K., Amphetamine, Caffeine, and Cocaine, in *Ergogenics — Enhancement of Performance in Exercise and Sport,* Lamb, D.R. and Williams, M.H., Eds., Wm. C. Brown, Ann Arbor, MI, 1991, 285.
2. Graham, T.E., The possible actions of methylxanthines on various tissues, in *The Clinical Pharmacology of Sport and Exercise,* Reilly, T. and Orme, M., Eds., Elsevier Science B. V., Amsterdam, 1997, 257.
3. Graham, T.E., Rush, J.W.E., and van Soeren, M.H., Caffeine and exercise: metabolism and performance, *Can. J. Appl. Physiol.,* 19, 111, 1994.
4. Tarnopolsky, M.A., Caffeine and endurance performance, *Sports Med.,* 18, 109, 1994.
5. Spiller, G.A., Ed., *Caffeine,* CRC Press, Boca Raton, FL, 1998.
6. Arnaud, M.J., Metabolism of caffeine and other components of coffee, in *Caffeine, Coffee, and Health,* Garattini, S., Ed., Raven Press, New York, NY, 1993, 43.
7. Butts, N.K. and Crowell, D., Effect of caffeine ingestion on cardiorespiratory endurance in men and women, *Research Quarterly for Exercise and Sport,* 56, 301, 1985.
8. Chad, K. and Quigley, B., The effects of substrate utilization, manipulated by caffeine, on post-exercise oxygen consumption in untrained female subjects, *Eur. J. Appl. Physiol.,* 59, 48, 1989.
9. Donelly, K. and MacNaughton, L., The effects of two levels of caffeine ingestion on excess postexercise oxygen consumption in untrained women, *Eur. J. Appl. Physiol.,* 65, 459, 1992.
10. Perkins, R. and Williams, M.H., Effect of caffeine upon maximal muscular endurance of females, *Med. Sci. Sports,* 7, 221, 1975.
11. Graham, T.E. and Spriet, L.L., Performance and metabolic responses to a high caffeine dose during prolonged exercise, *J. Appl. Physiol.,* 71, 2292, 1991.
12. Jackman, M., Wendling, P., Friars, D.. and Graham, T.E., Metabolic, catecholamine, and endurance responses to caffeine during intense exercise, *J. Appl. Physiol.,* 81, 1658, 1996.
13. Spriet, L.L., MacLean, D.A., Dyck, D.J., Hultman, E., Cederblad, G.. and Graham, T.E., Caffeine ingestion and muscle metabolism during prolonged exercise in humans, *Am. J. Physiol. (Endocrinol. Metab. 25),* 262, E891, 1992.
14. Tremblay, A., Masson, E., Leduc, S., Houde, A., and Despres, J., Caffeine reduces spontaneous energy intake in men but not in women, *Nutr. Res.,* 8, 553, 1988.
15. Kalow, W. and Tang, B.-K., Use of caffeine metabolite ratios to explore CYP1A2 and xanthine oxidase activities, *Clin. Pharmacol. Ther.,* 50, 519, 1991.

16. Vistisen, K., Poulsen, H.E.. and Loft, S., Foreign compound metabolism capacity in man measured from metabolites of dietary caffeine, *Carcinogenesis*, 13, 1561, 1992.

17. Horn, E.P., Tucker, M.A., Lambert, G., Silverman, D., Zametkin, D., Sinha, R., Hartge, T., Landi, M.T., and Caporaso, N.E., A study of gender-based cytochrome P4501A2 variability: A possible mechanism for the male excess of bladder cancer, *Cancer Epidemiology, Biomarkers & Prevention,* 4, 529, 1995.

18. Relling, M.V., Lin, J.-S., Ayers, G.D., and Evans, W.E., Racial and gender differences in N-acetyltransferase, xanthine oxidase, and CYP1A2 activities, *Clin. Pharmacol. Ther.,* 52, 643, 1992.

19. Bartoli, A., Xiaodong, S., Gatti, G., Cipolla, G., Marchiselli, R., and Perucca, E., The influence of ethnic factors and gender on CYP1A2 mediated drug disposition: A comparative study in caucasian and chinese subjects using phenacetin as a marker substrate, *Ther. Drug Monit.,* 18, 586, 1996.

20. Carillo, J.A. and Benitez, J. CYP1A2 activity, gender and smoking, as variables influencing the toxicity of caffeine, *Br. J. Clin. Pharmacol.,* 41:605–608, 1996.

21. Catteau, A., Bechtel, Y.C., Poisson, N., Bechtel, P.R., and Bonaiti-Pellie, C., A population and family study of CYP1A2 using caffeine urinary metabolites, *Eur. J. Clin. Pharmacol.,* 47, 423, 1995.

22. Kamimori, G.H., Somani, S.M., Knowlton, R.G., and Perkins, R.M., The effects of obesity and exercise on the pharmacokinetics of caffeine in lean and obese volunteers, *Eur. J. Clin. Pharmacol.,* 31, 595, 1987.

23. Caraco, Y., Zylber-Katz, E., Berry, E.M., and Levy, M., Caffeine pharmacokinetics in obesity and following significant weight reduction, *Int. J. Obes. Relat. Metab. Disord.,* 19, 234, 1995.

24. Lane, J.D., Steege, J.F., Rupp, S.L., and Kuhn, C.M., Menstrual cycle effects on caffeine elimination in the human female, *Eur. J. Clin. Pharmacol.,* 43, 543, 1992.

25. Balogh, A., Irmisch, E., Klinger, G., Splinter, F.K., and Hoffman, A., Elimination of caffeine and metamizole in the menstrual cycle of the fertile female, *Zentralbl. Gynakol.,* 109, 1135, 1987 (Abstract).

26. Balogh, A., Irmisch, E., Wolf, P., Letrari, S., Splinter, F.K., Hempel, E., Klinger, G., and Hoffmann, A., Effect of levonorgestrol and ethinyl estradiol and their combination on biotransformation reactions, *Zentralbl. Gynakol.,* 113, 1388, 1991, (Abstract).

27. Rietveld, F.C., Broekman, M.M.M., Houben, J.J.G., Eskes, T.K.A.B., and van Rossum, J.M., Rapid onset of an increase in caffeine residence time in young women due to oral contraceptive steroids, *Eur. J. Clin. Pharmacol.,* 26, 371, 1984.

28. Patwardhan, R.V., Desmond, P.V., Johnson, R.F., and Schenker, S., Impaired elimination of caffeine by oral contraceptive steroids, *J. Lab. Clin. Med.,* 95, 603, 1980.

29. Abernethy, D.R. and Todd, E.L., Impairment of caffeine clearance by chronic use of low-dose oestrogen-containing oral contraceptives, *Eur. J. Clin. Pharmacol.,* 28, 425, 1985.

30. Aldridge, A., Bailey, J., and Neims, A.H., The disposition of caffeine during and after pregnancy, *Seminars in Perinatology,* 5, 310, 1981.

31. Mackinnon, M., Sutherland, E., and Simon, F.R., Effects of ethinyl estradiol on hepatic microsomal proteins and the turnover of cytochrome P-450, *J. Lab. Clin. Med.,* 90, 1096, 1977.

32. Jennings, T.S., Nafziger, A.N., Davidson, L., and Bertino, J.S., Gender differences in hepatic induction and inhibition of theophylline pharmacokinetics and metabolism, *J. Lab. Clin. Med.,* 122, 208, 1993.

33. Scavone, J.M., Greenblatt, D.J., Abernethy, D.R., Luna, B.G., Harmatz, J.S., and Shader, R.I., Influence of oral contraceptive use and cigarette smoking, alone and together, on antipyrine pharmacokinetics, *J. Clin. Pharmacol.,* 37, 437, 1997.

34. Pantuck, E.J., Pantuck, C.B., Garland, W.A., Wattenberg, L.W., Anderson, K.E., Kappas, A., and Conney, A.H., Stimulartory effect of brussels sprouts and cabbage on human drug metabolism, *Clin. Pharmacol. Ther.,* 25, 88, 1979.

35. Kappas, A., Alvares, A.P., Anderson, K.E., Pantuck, E.J., Pantuck, C.B., Chang, R., and Conney, A.H., Effect of charcoal-broiled beef on antipyrine and theophylline metabolism, *Clin. Pharmacol. Ther.,* 23, 445, 1978.

36. Boel, J., Andersen, L.B., Rasmussen, B., Hansen, S.H., and Dossing, M., Hepatic drug metabolism and physical fitness, *Clin. Pharmacol. Ther.,* 36, 121, 1984.

37. Frenkl, R., Gyore, A., and Szeberenyi, Sz., The effect of muscular exercise on the microsomal enzyme system of the rat liver, *Eur. J. Appl. Physiol.,* 44, 135, 1980.

38. Day, W.W. and Weiner, M., Inhibition of hepatic drug metabolism and carbon tetra-chloride toxicity in Fischer-344 rats by exercise, *Biochem. Pharmacol.,* 42, 181, 1991.

39. Michaud, T.J., Bachmann, K.A., Andres, F.F., Flynn, M.G., Sherman, G.P., and Rod-riguez-Zayas, J., Exercise training does not alter cytochrome P-450 content and microsomal metabolism, *Med. Sci. Sports Exerc.,* 26, 978, 1994.

40. Dossing, M., Effect of acute and chronic exercise on hepatic drug metabolism, *Clinical Pharmacokinetics,* 10, 426, 1985.

41. Wilkinson, G.R. and Shand, D.G., A physiological approach to hepatic drug clearance, *Clin. Pharmacol. Ther.,* 18, 377, 1975.

42. Collomp, K., Anselme, F., Audran, M., Gay, J.P., Chanal, J.L. and Prefaut, C., Effects of moderate exercise on the pharmacokinetics of caffeine, *Eur. J. Clin. Pharmacol.,* 40, 279, 1991.

43. Schlaeffer, F., Engelberg, I., Kaplanski, J., and Danon, A., Effect of exercise and environmental heat on theophylline kinetics, *Respiration,* 45, 438, 1984.

44. McArdle, W.D., Katch, F.I., and Katch, V.L., *Exercise Physiology,* Lea & Febiger, Philadelphia, PA, 1991.

45. Gleiter, C.H. and Gundert-Remy, U., Gender differences in pharmacokinetics, *Eur. J. Drug Metab. Pharmacokinet.,* 21, 123, 1996.

46. Ylitalo, P., Effect of exercise on pharmacokinetics, *Annals of Medicine,* 23, 289, 1991.

47. van Baak, M.A., Influence of exercise on the pharmacokinetics of drugs, *Clin. Pharmacol. Ther.,* 19, 32, 1997.

48. Birkett, D.J. and Miners, J.O., Caffeine renal clearance and urine caffeine concentrations during steady state dosing. Implications for monitoring caffeine intake during sports events, *Br. J. Clin. Pharmacol.,* 31, 405, 1991.

49. van der Merwe, P.J., Luus, H.G., and Barnard, J.G., Caffeine in sport. Influence of endurance exercise on the urinary caffeine concentration, *Int. J. Sports Med.,* 13, 74, 1992.

50. Duthel, J.M., Vallon, J.J., Martin, G., Ferret, J.M., Mathieu, R., and Videman, R., Caffeine and sport: role of physical exercise upon elimination, *Med. Sci. Sports Exerc.,* 23, 980, 1991.

51. Graham, T.E. and Spriet, L.L., Metabolic, catecholamine, and exercise performance responses to various doses of caffeine, *J. Appl. Physiol.,* 78, 867, 1995.

52. Mohr, T., van Soeren, M.H., Graham, T.E., and Kjaer, M., Caffeine ingestion and metabolic responses of tetraplegic humans during electrical cycling, *J. Appl. Physiol.,* (in press).

53. van Soeren, M.H. and Graham, T.E., The effect of caffeine ingestion on metabolism, exercise endurance and catecholamine responses following short-term withdrawl, *J. Appl. Physiol.*, (in press).

54. Greer, F., Friars, D., and Graham, T.E., The effect of theophylline on endurance exercise and muscle metabolism, *The Physiologist,* 1996 (Abstract).

55. Xu, B., Berkich, D.A., Crist, G.H., and LaNoue, K.F., A1 adenosine receptor antagonism improves glucose tolerance in Zucker rats, *Am. J. Physiol. (Endocrinol. Metab.)*, (in press).

56. Mauriege, P., Prud'homme, D., Lemieux, S., Tremblay, A., and Despres, J.-P., Regional differences in adipose tissue lipolysis from lean and obese women: existence of postreceptor alterations, *Am. J. Physiol. (Endocrinol. Metab. 33)*, 269, E341, 1995.

57. Fuglevand, A.J., Winter, D.A., Patla, A.E., and Stashuk, D., Detection of motor unit action potentials with surface electrodes: influence of electrode size and spacing, *Biol. Cybern.*, 67, 143, 1992.

58. Vergauwen, L., Hespel, P., and Richter, E.A., Adenosine receptors mediate synergistic stimulation of glucose uptake and transport by insulin and by contractions in rat skeletal muscle, *J. Clin. Invest.*, 93, 974, 1994.

59. Vergauwen, L., Richter, E.A., and Hespel, P., Adenosine exerts a glycogen-sparing action in contracting rat skeletal muscle, *Am. J. Physiol.*, 272, E762, 1997.

60. Challis, R.A.J., Richards, S.J., and Budohoski, L., Characterization of the adenosine receptor modulating insulin action in rat skeletal muscle, *Eur. J. Pharmacol.*, 226, 121, 1992.

61. Sajjadi, F.G. and Firestein, G.S., cDNA cloning and sequence analysis of the human A3 adenosine receptor, *Biochem.*, 1179, 105, 1993.

62. Greer, F., Graham, T.E., and Nagy, L.E., Characterization of adenosine receptors in rat skeletal muscle, *Can. J. Appl. Physiol.*, 22:23P, 1997, (Abstract).

63. Kalow, W., Pharmacogenetic variability in brain and muscle, *J. Pharm. Pharmacol.*, 46, 425, 1994.

64. Mitsumoto, H., DeBoer, G.E., Bunge, G., Andrish, J.T., Tetzlaff, J.E., and Cruse, R.P., Fiber-type specific caffeine sensitivities in normal human skinned muscle fibers, *Anesthesiology*, 72, 50, 1990.

65. Pinto, S. and Tarnopolsky, M.A., Neuromuscular effects of caffeine on males and females, *Can. J. Appl. Physiol.*, 22, 48P, 1997, (Abstract).

66. Bouchard, C., Despres, J.-P., and Mauriege, P., Genetic and nongenetic determinants of regional fat distribution, *Endocrine. Rev.*, 14, 72, 1993.

67. Coppack, S.W., Jensen, M.D., and Miles, J.M., *In vivo* regulation of lipolysis in humans, *J. Lipid Res.*, 35, 177, 1994.

68. Jensen, M.D., Cryer, P.E., Johnson, C.M., and Murray, M.J., Effects of epinephrine on regional free fatty acid and energy metabolism in men and women, *Am. J. Physiol. (Endocrinol. Metab. 33)*, 270, E259, 1996.

69. Cadarette, B.S., Levine, L., Berube, C.L., Posner, B.M., and Evens, W.J., Effects of varied dosages of caffeine on endurance exercise to fatigue, in *Biochemistry of Exercise. International Series of Sport Sciences,* Knuttgen, H.G., Vogel, J.A. and Poortmans, J., Eds., Human Kinetics, Champaign, 1982, 871.

70. Bosman, M.J., Tarnopolsky, M.A., Roy, B.D., and Martin, J.E., Caffeine increases lactate during endurance exercise in males and females, *Can. J. Appl. Physiol.*, 22, 6P, 1997 (Abstract).

71. Cocchi, M., Siniscalchi, C., Rogato, F., and Valeriani, A., Free fatty acid levels in habitual coffee drinkers in relation to quantities consumed, sex and age, *Ann. Nutr. Metab.*, 27, 477, 1983.

72. Kahan, T., Eliasson, K., and Hjemdahl, P., Influence of age, sex and hypertension in studies of circulatory and sympatho-adrenal responses to stress, in *Stress, The Role of Catecholamines and Other Neurotrons*, Usdin, E., Kvetnanasky, R., and Axelrod, J., Eds., Gordon and Breech Sci. Publishers, New York, 1984, 883.

73. Gratas-Delamarche, A., Le Cam, R., Delamarche, P., Monnier, M., and Koubi, H., Lactate and catecholamine responses in male and female sprinters during a Wingate test, *Eur. J. Appl. Physiol.*, 68, 362, 1994.

74. Tarnopolsky, L.J., MacDougall, J.D., Atkinson, S.A., Tarnopolsky, M.A., and Sutton, J.R., Gender differences in substrate for endurance exercise, *J. Appl. Physiol.*, 68, 302, 1990.

75. Jones, P.P., Snitker, S., Skinner, J.S., and Ravussin, E., Gender differences in muscle sympathetic nerve activity: effect of body fat distribution, *Am. J. Physiol. (Endocrinol. Metab. 33)*, 270, E363, 1996.

76. Ettinger, S.M., Silber, D.H., Collins, B.G., Gray, K.S., Sutliff, G., Whisler, S.K., McClain, J.M., Smith, M.B., Yang, Q.X., and Sinoway, L.I., Influences of gender on sympathetic nerve responses to static exercise, *J. Appl. Physiol.*, 80, 245, 1996.

77. Bracco, D., Ferrarra, J.-M., Arnaud, M.J., Jequier, E., and Shutz, Y., Effects of caffeine on energy metabolism, heart rate, and methylxanthine metabolism in lean and obese women, *Am. J. Physiol.*, 269, E671, 1995.

78. Graham, T.E., Hibbert, E., and Sathasivam, P., The metabolic and exercise endurance effects of coffee and caffeine ingestion, *J. Appl. Physiol.*, 1998.

79. Collomp, K., Caillaud, C., Audran, M., Chanal, J.L., and Prefaut, C., Influence de la prise aigue ou chronique de cafeine sur la performance et les catecholamines au cours d'un exercice maximal, *C. R. Soc. Biol.*, 184, 87, 1990.

80. Costill, D.L., Dalsky, G.P., Fink, W.J., and LeBlanc, J., Effects of caffeine ingestion on metabolism and exercise performance, *Med. Sci. Sports*, 10, 155, 1978.

81. Falk, B., Burnstein, R., Rosenblum, J., Shapiro, Y., Zylber-Katz, E., and Bashan, N., Effects of caffeine ingestion on body fluid balance and thermoregulation during exercise, *Can. J. Appl. Physiol. Pharmacol.*, 68, 889, 1990.

82. Pasman, W.J., van Baak, M.A., Jeukendrup, A.E., and de Haan, A., The effect of different dosages of caffeine on endurance performance time, *Int. J. Sports. Med.*, 16, 225, 1995.

83. Sasaki, H., Maeda, H., Usui, S., and Ishiko, T., Effect of sucrose and caffeine ingestion on performance of prolonged strenuous running, *Int. J. Sports Med.*, 8, 261, 1987.

84. Trice, I. and Haymes, E.M., Effects of caffeine ingestion on exercise-induced changes during high-intensity, intermittent exercise, *Int. J. Sport Nutr.*, 5, 37, 1995.

85. Callahan, M.M., Robertson, R.S., Branfman, A.R., McComish, M.F., and Yesair, D.W., Comparison of caffeine metabolism in three nonsmoking populations after oral administration of radiolabeled caffeine, *Drug Metabolism and Disposition*, 11, 211, 1983.

86. Bonati, M., Latini, R., Galletti, F., Young, J.F., Tognoni, G., and Garattini, S. Caffeine dispostion after oral doses, *Clin. Pharmacol. Ther.*, 32:98–106, 1982.

87. Newton, R., Broughton, L.J., Lind, M.J., Morrison, P.J., Rogers, H.J., and Bradbrook, I.D. Plasma and salivary pharmacokinetics of caffeine in man, *Eur. J. Clin. Pharmacol.*, 21:45–52, 1981.

88. Cheng, W.S.C., Murphy, T.L., Smith, M.T., Cooksley, W.G.E., Halliday, J.W., and Powell, L.W. Dose-dependent pharmacokinetics of caffeine in humans: Relevance as a test of quantitative liver function, *Clin. Pharmacol. Ther.*, 47:516–524, 1990.

89. Kaplan, G.B., Greenblatt, D.J., Ehrenberg, B.L., et al., Dose-dependent pharmacokinetics and psychomotor effects of caffeine in humans, *J. Clin. Pharmacol.*, 37:693–703, 1997.

Index

A